EXAMINATION REVIEW
FOR

PRACTICAL NURSES

EXAMINATION REVIEW
FOR
PRACTICAL NURSES

by ARLENE SPEELMAN, R.N., M.S.

Formerly Director, Dixon State School of Practical Nursing, Dixon, Illinois: Director of Nurses, Copley Memorial Hospital, Aurora, Illinois; Sonoma State Hospital, Eldridge, California; State Hospital South, Blackfoot, Idaho. Formerly Psychiatric Nurse Instructor, University of Colorado and Peoria State Hospital, Peoria, Illinois.

G. P. Putnam's Sons   *New York*

Copyright © 1962 by G. P. Putnam's Sons

Library of Congress Catalog Number: 62-17586

Fourth Impression

MANUFACTURED IN THE UNITED STATES OF AMERICA

CONTENTS

PREFACE

One of the objectives of any Practical Nurse School is to prepare its graduates to take and to pass the State Board Licensing Examination. This book has been prepared to give the graduate additional practice with the One Best Answer type of question. Once an individual becomes familiar with the mechanical aspects of this type of testing process, it should then be possible to concentrate more fully on the intent of each question.

The graduate who is preparing for the State Board Examination is urged to think through the questions in this book just as he/she would the questions on the licensing examination. These questions will be stated differently than the ones prepared by your own instructors. The state board questions will be different too. Use the knowledge you already have to reason out the one best answer. It is much more important to be able to combine information from several sources to arrive at a logical answer than to 'parrot' the words of the text or the instructor.

This book will be of greatest value if the user does not circle her choice of answers in the book. Then each time you look at a question you will need to practice all your examination skills. The IBM answer sheets are included to increase your ability to work from an examination paper to an answer sheet without writing in the test booklet.

After a thorough review of these questions you should be convinced that material understood will be there when you need it, while most memorized items remain in their isolated compartments and do not join forces with other items into a meaningful whole.

A good command of the special medical vocabulary is essential to success. If the various terms also give rise to a detailed picture in the 'mind's eye', the graduate will find it easier to reject those answer choices that are impossible and make a better selection of the remaining answers that have some merit. One of the best ways to remember the principles of Inflammation is to re-experience your own reaction to the required Typhoid Fever immunizations. How can you miss the symptoms now?

Study the INTRODUCTION carefully. The questions in this book have been prepared to check the user's test taking skills. The author has deliberately stated questions and answer selections in such a way that the careless, unthinking person will find an incorrect answer attractive. Continued awareness of special test taking skills will make it possible for you to achieve a higher score on the content you know.

The author wishes to express deep appreciation to Mr. George P. Oberst for his faith and encouragement that provided the stimulus for this book.

I am especially indebted to Mr. Milton Sacks who read the manuscript and offered constructive criticism as well as supportive enthusiasm.

The author is most grateful to her mother, Mrs. Sada Frentress, for her assistance in many of the tedious details of preparing the contents of such a manuscript for submission to the publisher.

Mr. Richard H. Miller, Nursing Editor of G. P. Putnam's Sons has been most helpful in introducing a novice to the intricacies of format, proofreading and other responsibilities that must be assumed by an author.

I am sincerely grateful to my many students from whom I have learned so much.

Arlene Speelman

INTRODUCTION

Should the teacher be the only one to understand the tricks of test construction? Too often the student who really knows the subject does poorly on an examination because her test-taking skills are underdeveloped and she has become "confused." At the risk of being criticized for giving away "trade secrets," this section has been written to prepare the graduate to cope with the ONE-BEST-ANSWER type of examination question.

The grade in such examination is usually based on the number of questions answered correctly. A question omitted is just as incorrect in the final count as those for which a poor guess was made. Answer every question. Fewer mechanical errors will be made if each question is answered in order. The answer sheet can be checked lightly near the question numbers to indicate those that need more thought if time permits. Be sure to erase these marks thoroughly before handing in the answer sheet.

One mechanical error which can produce tragic results is selecting the correct answer for Question 6, for example, and then filling in the corresponding space for Question 7. Such a mistake will throw your answers off for the remainder of the test. A second mechanical error with the same results is answering Questions 6 and 7 in the spaces provided for Question 6. You will then be answering Question 8 in the blanks intended for Question 7, etc. The intention to mark space 2 but filling in one of the other four spaces instead, is a third mechanical error. The IBM answer sheet is set up with spaces for five choices. The majority of the test questions will have only four. Be sure to think "space 4" and not "the last space," or you will find yourself filling in space 5. The machine that grades the answer sheets will be set for one of the first four spaces and you will be charged with an error. It is wise to check every tenth question to be sure that mechanical errors have not been made. The grading machine will not be sympathetic to your pleas of, "But I meant . . . ."

Examples of common mechanical errors:

1.

	1	2	3	4	5
3		▮			
4					
5				▮	

Answer space 4 is correct for Question 4. Space 4 has been filled in after Question 5 and all the spaces following Question 4 are left blank. Question 5 will now be recorded in the spaces for Question 6, etc.

2.

	1	2	3	4	5
3	▮		▮		
4					
5					

Selection 1 is chosen for Question 3 and is so marked. Selection 3 is chosen for Question 4 but is marked in the third space after Question 3. The test taker will then answer Question 5 in the spaces provided for Question 4, etc.

Read each question carefully. Each word plays an important part, but one word does not necessarily carry more weight than another. What is the intent of the base statement? Are there words in it that will limit the answer to a specific group based on age, sex, color, religion or disease condition? The selection of a general answer, one that would apply to several groups would not be correct.

EXAMPLE:

The hospital nurse could expect a
newly admitted patient to be _

a. afraid
b. irritable
c. lonesome
d. dressed

    1. all of the above
    2. a only
    3. a and d
    4. all except d

NOTE that there is nothing in the base statement to supply any identifying information
about the patient's age, sex, condition
(medical-surgical-emergency), etc. Such a
question must be answered in terms of ANY
patient or ALL patients and what might be
true about them. It would not be possible to
state that any of these four answer selections
would never be true of a newly admitted
patient. The only choice to be considered,
then, is 1, "all of the above."

Note what the addition of just two words to the base statement can do to your thinking about a correct answer.

EXAMPLE:

The hospital nurse could expect that
any newly admitted infant might be

a. afraid
b. hungry
c. sick
d. irritable

    1. all of the above
    2. a only
    3. a and c
    4. none of the above

WHAT YOU KNOW
    The patient is an infant, newly
    admitted to the hospital.

WHAT YOU DO NOT KNOW
    Sex
    Specific age in months
    Condition or reason for admission.
    The time of day or night.

Your knowledge of the characteristics of an infant will tell you that fear of strange people and strange surroundings can be expected. This makes it possible to consider selection 1.

The base statement gives no clues to the nutritional status of the infant. Perhaps it has just been fed before it came to the hospital. Selection b will not be true of any infant.

Are all infants sick or irritable because they have been admitted to the hospital? Perhaps the child is here for X rays or other diagnostic procedures or correction of a cogenital abnormality such as club foot. In such cases both c and d must be rejected. The correct selection must be No. 2, or "a only."

Some students find it easier to determine the intent of the base statement by changing it to a question. The example just cited could be changed to read, "WHAT can the hospital nurse expect of a newly admitted infant?"

A WHY question will require a cause or a reason for an answer; a WHEN question is asking for a consideration of time; a WHERE question is asking for place; a WHO question is asking for identi- fication of a person or group of persons; a HOW question is asking for procedure or method; and a WHAT question is seeking an explanation, information, or identification of an object, mood or feeling.

There are certain words that can be considered KEY words, others that are precautionary. At- tention to these key words will help to limit the answer selections that can be successfully considered.

EXAMPLE:

The only way to stop the progress of gangrene
is

    1. to apply a tourniquet
    2. to give concentrated doses of penicillin
    3. to isolate the patient
    4. to remove the dead tissues

    The wording of this base statement tells you that there is just one selection that can possibly be correct. The word STOP will also help you to arrive at No. 4 as the correct answer.

EXAMPLE:

The best way to move a postoperative patient
from the Operating Room to his own room is to
place him

    1. on a stretcher from his ward unit
    2. in his own bed
    3. on a stretcher from the Operating Room
    4. on a special transfer cart

    It is not unlikely that any one of these methods would be popular in some hospitals. This is not the kind of question to be answered in terms of practice in your teaching hospital. What method is best for the PATIENT? If the patient is moved from the operating table to his own bed, the surgeon will be available to specify positioning. There is usually more space in the Operating Room than in the patient unit to make this transfer and often there is more help. If the patient is conscious, he will feel more secure in the bed than on a narrow cart. So, although none of the four selections can be considered incorrect, selection 2 fulfills the directions of the base statement for the "best way."

    Other key words are chief, one, greatest, least, few, seldom, often, many, frequent, most, usually. Can you add to this list? These words place limits on the answer selections to be considered correct. In some base statements the key word or words have been underlined. Always pay close attention to underlined words, since the test maker uses this method to tell you to attach special importance to them as a guide for selecting the correct answer.

    Danger words, such as all, always, never, none, and only, and others with similar meanings, appear in the answer selections. In the base statement they would be considered key words. Their presence in the answer selections tends to rule them out as incorrect. How many situations in medicine and nursing qualify as "always" or "never" situations? Usually some exception can be found. Ask yourself if a fact is always true for all patients, for all diseases, for all parts of the country, etc. Seldom can you answer in the affirmative. A word of caution . . . do not automatically rule out answer selections in which these words appear. The phrasing of the base statement may be such that one of these words must appear in the correct answer. Just be sure that you are aware of those words that imply there are no exceptions and proceed cautiously.

    The test taker should also be alert to the grammatical construction of the base statement. If the verb in the base statement is singular, the correct answer must be singular. If the verb in the base statement is plural, the correct answer must also be plural. Read the base statement and an answer selection through to the end. Does it make sense as it is written? If the base statement and the answer selection do not make a complete sentence, the selection is probably not right. The test maker is most likely to write the base statement and the correct answer and then fill in with three or four nearly correct or incorrect selections. The correct answer will undoubtedly complete the base statement in a grammatically correct manner, one or more of the incorrect selections may not.

Another habit of the test maker, based on writing the correct answer first, is to use more words in this selection. Check the longest answer selection carefully. As you go through the questions in this book, look for the number of times the longest answer selection is the right one . . . in spite of the fact that the author has tried to make one incorrect selection just as long as the correct one.

Do not be upset if you find yourself selecting the same answer number for four, five, or six or more consecutive questions. There is no pattern of answers, no attempt to have so many questions with selection No. 1 correct and an equal number with selection No. 2 correct, etc.

The test taker can accept the information in the base statement as correct. Use this information to help you answer other related questions.

Read the base statement and the answer selections as they are written. Do not add words of your own or leave out some that change the meaning. Be very careful not to let your past experiences color the meaning of the base statement or the answer selections. This is especially true in the Growth and Development Section. You have all had childhood experiences, and many of you are or have been responsible for raising a family. Unless you look at each question objectively, you may tend to answer it in terms of the way you behaved or the way you would have liked to be treated. But you must keep in mind that the person who wrote the question did not know about the things you have experienced. Before you select an answer you agree with emotionally or reject one for subjective reasons, consider the theoretical principles you have been taught. When the base statement mentions "the patient" are you guilty of thinking about 80-year-old Mrs. Jones with the broken hip and answering accordingly? Have you failed to appreciate that the base statement included any patient with a broken hip, regardless of sex or age? Although it is a good study habit to recall the symptoms, medications, and treatments of a specific patient who is quite typical of a disease condition, it can interfere with your objective reasoning if you accept this patient image as representative of all patients with this diagnosis.

I have had students complain that the base statement sounded differently when I read it out loud and that the intended meaning and the correct answer selection were clearer. As you read the base statement silently to yourself, concentrate on words that you emphasize. If you were reading aloud these words would stand out. Consider them as special clues.

EXAMPLE:

One might expect an aggressive patient to
enjoy an activity such as

    1. knitting
    2. woodwork
    3. raveling burlap
    4. modeling

Notice as you read this statement aloud that your voice is raised and the volume increased on the words aggressive and activity. The word aggressive distinguishes this patient from other behavior types and the word activity specifies a type of action rather than a mood, a thought, or other idea. The graduate with test-taking skills would not need experience in psychiatric nursing to be able to think this question through to a correct answer.

Some questions will ask you to select an answer that you might give to a patient, a visitor, the doctor, or the head nurse. Often the base statement asks for an answer that will REASSURE or EXPLAIN. Observe carefully the wording of the answer selections. One may be completely correct, but the terminology used would be understood only by the doctor or another nurse. If the answer is to be given to a lay person, find a second answer selection that provides the same information in simpler words. How reassuring can the practical nurse be if she counters the patient's questions with, "You'll have to discuss that with your doctor."? Does such an answer really fulfill the demands of the base statement? Questions of this kind are intended to test the judgment and tact of the graduate as well as her understanding of the limitations of the practical nurse in supplying information. Give these questions careful thought. What reassurance or explanation can you give without making statements that are beyond the responsibility of the practical nurse.

Some questions will ask you to select the one answer selection that is different, the one that does not fit with the other selections. Only careful reading of the base statement will point out what is expected as an answer selection.

EXAMPLE:

Check the one inflammation that is not considered an upper respiratory condition:

    1. sinusitis
    2. tonsillitis
    3. laryngitis
    4. bronchitis

Selections 1, 2, and 3 involve parts of the anatomy described as upper respiratory. The bronchi are part of the lungs and are in the lower respiratory tract. Selection 4 is the only one that meets the demands of the base statement.

Questions listed by letters (a, b, c, d) can be approached in a special way.

EXAMPLE:

To bathe a patient safely in a low bathtub, bend to pick up an article from the floor, or lift a patient, the nurse's knowledge of body mechanics should warn her

    a. to flex knees
    b. to bend at the hips
    c. to keep the back straight
    d. to keep the feet apart, one ahead of
       the other

      1. a, b, and c
      2. b, d, and c
      3. a, c, and d
      4. c, d, and b

Look at "b". How does one bend at the hips? This selection must be incorrect. Now, look at the answer selections 1, 2, and 4. Each includes the letter "b" which we decided must be incorrect. You are left with selection 3 as the only possible correct answer.

So, look for these lettered choices you know are correct and for those you know are incorrect and then determine the combinations possible to arrive at the best answer.

Often the base statement will give you a clue that the expected answer is the one that reads, "None of the above." Such a base statement may begin, "Which treatments, if any, will be best for . . . ?"

When all the answer selections are correct, look for the one answer that includes the other three selections.

EXAMPLE:

The psychiatric treatment of a patient will be influenced by

    1. the physician
    2. the nursing staff
    3. the relatives
    4. all the factors that affect the patient

Selection No. 4 incorporates selections 1, 2, and 3 and also allows for the fact that the patient may not have any relatives.

When the examination is set up after the pattern of the Integrated Nursing Arts Examination in Section 7, it is most important that the explanatory material preceding a group of questions be read carefully, understood, and kept in mind while considering the answer selections. Such information may influence the correct answer selection throughout a series of questions on one situation.

EXAMPLE:

Basic information has previously told the test taker that Mrs. X is in a highly agitated state and has been transferred to the Hydrotherapy Department and placed in a cold wet sheet pack. One of the questions concerning the care of Mrs. X is this:

The nurse will check the pulse at

    1. the radial artery
    2. the brachial artery
    3. the temporal artery
    4. the dorsalis pedis artery

The fact that Mrs. X is in a cold wet sheet pack which envelopes her body, beginning at the neck and incorporating the toes, makes it impossible for the nurse to check the pulse at any but the temporal artery. If the test taker fails to use the information previously given, the answer selected will probably be No. 1, which would be incorrect.

If only one caution could be stressed in taking this kind of examination it would be this . . . . DO NOT CHANGE YOUR ANSWERS ONCE YOU HAVE MADE A SELECTION UNLESS YOU HAVE A DEFINITE, LOGICAL REASON FOR DOING SO. If, on the basis of some other question, you are sure you have made a wrong selection, then make a change. Otherwise, remember that you had a reason for choosing that particular answer, whether that reason is clear to your conscious mind or whether information available at this moment only to your subconscious mind influenced your decision. If your second attempt is still a guess, stay with your first one. In the long run there is a greater chance that your first choice will be right and the second one wrong.

As you review for the State Board Examination, there are several pointers to keep in mind:

1. In a one-day testing situation you cannot possibly be examined on all the course content presented to you in one year.

2. The people who wrote the examination questions are not familiar with your particular practice area: they don't know which of several textbooks you used or the special material provided by your teachers. Don't study by memorizing various aspects of your curriculum. Concentrate instead on basic principles

3. All graduate practical nurses in the 50 states take the same examination. Look for an answer selection that could be considered correct in any part of the country. Recognize the importance of knowing general principles underlying your course content. These principles will not vary from state to state, although the method of applying them may be different from hospital to hospital in the same city.

4. Don't concentrate your study on the rare diseases or those that are confined to special hospitals. The examination questions will be interested in testing your knowledge of disease conditions, medicines, and nursing procedures that are prevalent wherever you might work.

A final word of caution. The skill you may achieve by applying these tips on test taking can be no substitute for sound knowledge. Such skill can, however, give you a better chance to demonstrate what you really know. Practice these principles first on the set of questions that follows, then on the questions in the pages of this book. GOOD LUCK.

THE FOLLOWING ARE PRACTICE QUESTIONS TO TEST YOUR SKILL IN THE TEST-TAKING TECHNIQUES JUST DESCRIBED. IT IS NOT INTENDED THAT THE TEST TAKER KNOW THE CONTENT BEING EXAMINED. IT IS HOPED THAT THE GRADUATE WILL CAREFULLY THINK THROUGH EACH QUESTION, SINCE IN EACH THE CLUES GIVEN IN THE BASE STATEMENT ALLOW FOR ONLY ONE CORRECT ANSWER.

1. One of the first symptoms seen in cancer of the mouth is

1. constant pipe smoking
2. an inadequate intake of vitamins
3. a complete blood count
4. a sore that fails to heal

2. A serious after effect of rheumatic fever is

1. loss of appetite
2. heart damage
3. headache
4. diagnosed by the doctor

3. The only safe way to approach a violent patient is with

1. an empty stomach
2. weapons for your protection
3. plenty of help
4. a strait jacket

4. The best equipment to use to give a patient oxygen is

1. artificial respiration
2. an open window
3. a drug to relax breathing muscles
4. an oxygen mask

5. The age group most likely to be affected by a first attack of rheumatic fever is

1. the 8 to 10 group
2. the female child
3. the underprivileged group
4. the mentally retarded

6. A physical change is made in a glass bottle when you

1. boil it
2. drop it
3. soak it in a disinfectant
4. break it

7. A chemical change would be made in a piece of iron when water is added to make it

1. rust
2. chip
3. break
4. pliable

8. The chemical formula for bichloride of mercury would be

1. $HgCl_2$
2. Hg
3. $HgCl$
4. $HgCl_6$

9. The basic unit of matter is an element. When several basic chemical elements are mixed together, we produce a

1. reaction
2. explosion
3. tension
4. compound

10. When oxygen combines with hemoglobin in the blood stream, the compound is called

1. carbon dioxide
2. metabolism
3. oxidation
4. oxyhemoglobin

11. When a glass of water freezes, it will occupy

1. more space
2. less space
3. the same amount of space
4. only slightly less space

12. Picture ice on the river. With this picture in mind, you could correctly say that

1. ice will not stay unless the weather is below zero
2. ice is heavier than water
3. water is heavier than ice
4. ice forms when oxygen evaporates

13. A saturated solution may be described as

1. a dangerous solution
2. one in which no more of the substance will dissolve
3. one which must be prepared by the pharmacist
4. a pharmacy prescription

14. When a solid substance does not dissolve in the solute, observation will show that

1. a mixture exists
2. the solid particles sink to the bottom
3. the result can correctly be called a suspension
4. the solution is ineffective

15. An occupational therapy project intended to help the patient release emotional tension would be

   1. rug weaving   3. metal pounding
   2. knitting   4. pottery

16. The colors a patient chooses to work with often are an expression of his mood. One would expect a depressed patient to select

   1. pastel shades
   2. reds, oranges, and purples
   3. blues and greens
   4. dark, drab colors

17. A regressed patient often gets satisfaction from working with

   1. yarn
   2. the loom
   3. clay and paints
   4. lumber

18. If a patient makes an article in Occupational Therapy to give to his wife and he knows it is something she does not like, he is taking this opportunity to express his

   1. affection   3. fears
   2. hostility   4. improvement

19. The way a patient works on an occupational therapy project often proves the old saying

   1. "Don't count your chickens before they are hatched"
   2. "A stitch in time saves nine"
   3. "Honey will catch more flies than vinegar"
   4. "Actions speak louder than words"

20. A patient with a great desire to be destructive can benefit from

   1. cutting carpet rags
   2. work with modeling clay
   3. work on a loom
   4. a creative project

21. It is often easier to get a senile patient interested in

   1. a new activity
   2. producing something for the hospital
   3. an activity he has done before
   4. a passive activity

22. Often the best occupational therapy project for the patient who feels guilty about not paying for his hospitalization is to encourage him

   1. to make a gift for his family
   2. to make something for the ward attendant
   3. to make something the hospital can use
   4. to create something for himself

23. The hyperactive patient visits Occupational Therapy for the first time. The most successful project will be one that

   1. can be completed quickly
   2. requires concentrated attention
   3. must be done in a group
   4. requires close supervision by the therapist

24. The patient who is afraid of new situations and experiences will work best on an occupational therapy assignment that requires

   1. considerable supervision
   2. concentration
   3. extensive physical energy
   4. repetition

ANSWER SHEET FOR PRACTICE QUESTIONS
(pp. xiii-xiv)

SCORES

1 ____ 5 ____

2 ____ 6 ____

3 ____ 7 ____

4 ____ 8 ____

NAME ____ (LAST, FIRST, MIDDLE) DATE ____ DATE OF BIRTH ____ AGE ____ SEX ____ (M OR F)

SCHOOL ____ CITY ____ GRADE OR CLASS ____ INSTRUCTOR ____

1 ____ 2 ____ 3 ____ 4 ____ NAME OF TEST ____ PART ____

DIRECTIONS: Read each question and its numbered answers. When you have decided which answer is correct, blacken the corresponding space on this sheet with the special pencil. Make your mark as long as the pair of lines, and move the pencil point up and down firmly to make a heavy black line. If you change your mind, erase your first mark completely. Make no stray marks; they may count against you.

SAMPLE:

1. Chicago is
   1—1 a country
   1—2 a mountain
   1—3 an island
   1—4 a city
   1—5 a state

1 2 3 4 5 (answer 4 marked)

Each question has answer spaces 1 2 3 4 5.

1	31	61	91	121
2	32	62	92	122
3	33	63	93	123
4	34	64	94	124
5	35	65	95	125
6	36	66	96	126
7	37	67	97	127
8	38	68	98	128
9	39	69	99	129
10	40	70	100	130
11	41	71	101	131
12	42	72	102	132
13	43	73	103	133
14	44	74	104	134
15	45	75	105	135

BE SURE YOUR MARKS ARE HEAVY AND BLACK.
ERASE COMPLETELY ANY ANSWER YOU WISH TO CHANGE.

16	46	76	106	136
17	47	77	107	137
18	48	78	108	138
19	49	79	109	139
20	50	80	110	140
21	51	81	111	141
22	52	82	112	142
23	53	83	113	143
24	54	84	114	144
25	55	85	115	145
26	56	86	116	146
27	57	87	117	147
28	58	88	118	148
29	59	89	119	149
30	60	90	120	150

Printed by the International Business Machines Corporation, Dayton, N. J., U. S. A.

IBM FORM I. T. S. 1000 B 108

DISCUSSION OF THE PRACTICE QUESTIONS:

1. WHAT is one of the first <u>symptoms</u> seen in cancer of the mouth?

    Selection 4 is the only selection which qualifies as a symptom. Selection 1 and 2 might be predisposing causes.

2. WHAT is a <u>serious</u> after effect of rheumatic fever?

    Selection 2 is the only one that fulfills the specification of "serious," although Nos. 1 and 3 might be classified as aftereffects.

3. WHAT is the only <u>safe</u> way to approach a disturbed patient?

    SAFE for whom? The patient? The nurse? Since the base statement does not specify which, the answer selection must be one that will be as safe as possible for both the patient and the nurse. This will make selection 3 correct.

4. WHAT is the best <u>equipment</u> to use to give a patient oxygen?

    Selection 4 is the only one mentioning equipment, therefore the only one that fulfills the requirements of the base statement.

5. WHAT <u>age group</u> is most likely to be affected by a first attack of rheumatic fever?

    The words age group limit the correct answer to selection 1, which is the only answer specifying age.

6. HOW is a <u>physical</u> change made in a <u>glass</u> bottle?

    Unless you thought about this one carefully you checked selection 2. But does every glass bottle change physically just because it is dropped? The correct answer is selection 4, which tells us that the glass bottle is now physically changed to a collection of pieces of glass.

7. WHAT <u>chemical</u> change will be made in a piece of iron if water is added to it?

    Selection 1 is the only chemical change listed. Selections 2, 3, and 4 would be physical changes.

8. WHAT is the chemical formula for bichloride of mercury.

    The formula for mercury is Hg. This appears in each of the tour selections. Cl is the formula for chloride, but it appears in three selections. You should know that "bi" means two. Therefore the only possible answer is selection 1.

9. WHAT is produced when several basic elements are mixed together?

    Read the base statement and selection 2: "we produce a explosion." Is this grammatically correct? No. Eliminate this at once as a possible answer. If we mix several things together we produce a new product. Thus selection 4 must be the correct answer.

10. WHAT is the compound called when oxygen combines with hemoglobin in the bloodstream?

    If you did not know the answer to question 9, the base statement of question 10 should have been used to help you. Here we have mixed oxygen and hemoglobin and called it a compound. Selection 4 brings together part of the word oxygen and the entire word hemoglobin. This is the only logical answer you could have selected.

11. HOW much space will a glass of water occupy when it freezes?

    Have you ever filled the ice-cube tray with water to the brim? What did the ice cubes look like after they were completely frozen? Didn't they extend above the level of the ice-cube tray? What happens if a bottle of milk is left outside until it freezes? Can you see that selection 4 must be right for this question?

12. Where is the ice as you see it on the river? It is on top and the water is underneath it. You would be sure of this if you walked on the ice, it broke, and you got wet. Therefore water must be heavier than ice for the ice to stay on top. Selection 3 is correct.

13. HOW can a saturated solution be described?

   Selection 2 is the only one that can be called a description. The other three selections might be true of some solutions, but they do not describe a saturated solution.

14. WHAT do you see when a solid substance does not dissolve in the solute?

   The word "observation" requires an answer that tells what can be seen. Selection 2 is the only one meeting the requirements of the base statement.

15. WHAT occupational therapy project will help a patient release emotional tension?

   Male or female? You don't know, so to be safe select a project that will release tensions and be acceptable to either sex, any age group. Selection 3 best satisfies the base statement.

16. WHAT colors would you expect a depressed patient to select?

   The base statement has already given you some information in the first sentence. Using this information, the graduate will correctly select No. 4.

17. WHAT can the regressed patient do that will provide satisfaction?

   Your understanding of the word "regressed" is essential. This is one of the mental mechanisms. We tend to "go backward" to a period of pleasanter experiences when we cannot cope with current problems. The small child enjoys smearing experiences; so, too, the regressed patient as he or she plays with clay or paints. Selection No. 3 is correct.

18. WHAT emotion is the patient expressing when he makes his wife a gift he knows she does not like?

   When the base statement is turned into a question such as this, it becomes obvious that the correct answer is selection 2.

19. HOW does the way a patient works prove an old saying?

   The base statement implies action on the part of the patient in the words "way a patient works." Selection 4 is the only one involving action.

20. WHAT activity will benefit the patient with a great desire to be destructive?

   Which of the activities listed allows the patient to be destructive without being scolded or censured for the destruction? Selection 1, "Cutting carpet rags" allows the patient to destroy clothing, materials of other sorts and still gain approval for the work.

21. HOW can the senile patient best be interested in some activity?

   What is a common characteristic of the senile group? Resistance to change. Therefore the senile patient will often respond best to an activity he has done previously, one which will not require him to learn new rules, etc. Selection 3 is correct.

22. WHAT is the best type of occupational therapy project for the patient who feels guilty about not being able to pay for his hospitalization?

   If the patient could do something useful to the hospital he might feel he was paying his way in some measure. Selection 3 best fulfills the requirements of the base statement.

23. WHAT type of project will be most successful for the hyperactive patient who is visiting Occupational Therapy for the first time?

   The test taker should have a visual picture of a hyperactive patient. This can be medical, surgical, or pediatric, as well as psychiatric. Such a patient is in continuous motion, jumping from one activity or one idea to another. If he is to make anything successfully in O.T., it must be something that can be completed quickly. Otherwise he will lose interest and be doing something else.

24.   WHAT work assignment is best for the patient who is afraid of new situations and new experiences?

    If the person is afraid of the new, it could be expected that he would be more comfortable doing something that was familiar. The more often a task is performed the more comfortable one feels doing it. Therefore the repetition provided for in selection 4 best meets the requirements of the base statement.

    WORK your way through the questions in this book by analyzing the intent of the base statement and trying to select objectively the answer that best provides the information called for in the base statement. With practice you will find that appraisal of the questions and the answer selections becomes rapid enough to permit you to complete an examination within the specified time.

PERSONAL HYGIENE

(Answer sheet p. 297)

The emphasis in this section is on the health aspects of greatest concern to the individual nurse. Patients can be taught effectively only by the nurse who believes and practices the health habits she is passing on to them. Each nurse should feel a responsibility for concentrating on good health practices until they become a habit.

1. Personal health, as a <u>general term</u>, must include

   1. physical and mental adjustment
   2. the absence of all handicaps
   3. regular physical examinations
   4. a planned program of food, sleep, and activity

2. One of the best ways a practical nurse can <u>teach</u> good hygiene is

   1. to have complete understanding of this course
   2. to set a personal example
   3. to copy the habits of some doctor or nurse she knows
   4. to be active in health groups

3. It should be easier for the practical nurse to follow good health rules and prevent illness when she understands that

   1. good health is necessary to any nurse
   2. illness costs more in time and in misery than prevention
   3. it is so easy to spread disease
   4. her health sets an example for others

4. The best way to deal with a health problem is

   1. to talk about it
   2. to select a doctor who is a specialist and follow his advice
   3. to get the opinions of others who have the same problem
   4. to admit that there is a problem and get the necessary help

5. The practical nurse student who has a goal to work toward will find it easier

   1. to balance work, play, diet, and rest for the best results
   2. to forget health habits in the thrill of studying
   3. to accept all tasks assigned to her
   4. to spend all her time studying

6. The best way to rest the eyes during a long study period is

   1. to change activity frequently
   2. to look off into the distance frequently
   3. to study different subjects
   4. to change from a reading to a writing assignment

7. Eyestrain is increased when the student studies at night with only

   1. the ceiling light on
   2. one assignment to work on
   3. a study lamp on
   4. the light shining over her shoulder

8. Fluorescent lights are hard on the student's eyes if they begin

   1. to flicker   3. to hum
   2. to get dim   4. to cause a glare

9. The study condition most likely to cause eyestrain and headache is the presence of

   1. a draft   3. glare
   2. fatigue   4. indigestion

10. The only person who is qualified to make a diagnosis of a disease that is causing eye symptoms is

   1. an optician   3. an ophthalmologist
   2. an optometrist   4. a pediatrician

11. Poor health will often affect study habits because it interferes with the ability

   1. to read   3. to stay awake
   2. to listen carefully   4. to concentrate

12. In the busy school day the practical nurse student will be wise if she uses her lunch period for

   1. concentrated study
   2. a time of recreation
   3. reading in the library
   4. practicing memory work

13. The time of day the student plans to use for most of her home study should depend on

   1. her home responsibilities
   2. the course she is studying
   3. whether she is an early or a late starter
   4. whether she is reading, memorizing, or writing a report

14. The student who tries to study when she is tired will find that she is

   1. wasting her time
   2. not remembering what she studies
   3. soon asleep
   4. using too much energy for a little accomplishment

15. The ability to study will be lessened if the student brings to her study periods

   1. problems that worry her
   2. food to nibble on
   3. more than one subject to be learned
   4. a large number of tasks

16. A recreational activity that may relax a student can be

   1. something useful
   2. any change from studying
   3. something unnecessary
   4. difficult for the interested student to find

17. When studying becomes difficult because she cannot stay awake and her head aches, the student is advised

   1. to go to bed
   2. to change activities
   3. to wear glasses
   4. to see an eye doctor

18. A bath intended only to cleanse the skin would be taken at a temperature considered to be

   1. cold   3. warm
   2. cool   4. hot

19. Detergent soaps may not be best for people with dry skin because they

   1. have a mineral oil base
   2. do not make a lather
   3. do not remove all the dirt on the surface and in the pores
   4. remove too many of the natural skin oils

20. A bath is important even if the skin does not look dirty because there will always be wastes on the body surface such as

   a. dead skin cells
   b. sweat
   c. sebum
   d. cosmetics

   1. all of the above
   2. a only
   3. b, c, and d
   4. a, b, and c

21. The person who wishes to prevent perspiration odor will select

   1. a stick deodorant
   2. a liquid antiperspirant
   3. one of the deodorants
   4. an astringent powder

22. A substance that closes the sweat glands and prevents perspiration is called

   1. deodorant   3. deodorizer
   2. antiperspirant   4. antiseptic

23. The people with the most problems of body odor are

   1. small children who hate to wash
   2. women of child-bearing age
   3. men who refuse to shave under their arms
   4. older people who become careless about changing their clothes

24. Each member of a family may need a different brand of deodorant because

   1. people react differently to the various ingredients
   2. the deodorant effect depends on the reaction to the perfume
   3. different skin textures need a different combination of ingredients
   4. of their age differences

25. The perspiration odor will be greater in any adult who has

   1. long-sleeved clothing
   2. long hair under the arms
   3. protective dress shields in clothing
   4. too many worries

26. It is not true that hair that has been shaved off will

   1. grow longer and coarser
   2. grow back in fairly soon
   3. be easily removed a second time
   4. grow in the original color

27. The time between shampoos should depend on

   1. the odor of the hair
   2. the physical condition of the individual
   3. the amount of natural hair oil produced
   4. the brand of shampoo used

28. Hair growth may be increased by thorough daily hair brushing that will

   1. increase the supply of nourishment to the roots by improving blood circulation
   2. keep dust particles from settling on the scalp
   3. prevent a collection of dandruff on the scalp
   4. massage the hairs and bring extra food to the tips of the hairs

29. Gray hair appears when

   1. pigment is no longer produced
   2. the pigment changes color
   3. hair dyes change the pigment
   4. responsibility becomes too great for the physical condition of the person

30. If you were at home all day, the recommended way to keep foods from causing dental decay is

   1. frequent inspection for food
   2. to rinse the mouth with an antiseptic solution
   3. to eat some fruit
   4. to brush the teeth after each meal

31. Dental decay can be corrected only by

   1. adequate diet
   2. daily oral hygiene
   3. removing the decay
   4. full mouth X-rays

32. The practical nurse has a professional responsibility to keep her teeth in good repair and her breath "sweet" because

   1. she must work so closely with so many people
   2. she is expected to practice what she teaches
   3. professional people need to stick together
   4. the only way she can remember the best hygiene principles is to practice them

33. A regular daily toothbrushing routine will remove food particles and will thus

   1. prevent all tooth decay
   2. keep the gums healthy
   3. lessen the chance of bad breath
   4. add to one's nutritional state

34. Food particles are best removed from the cracks and crevices of the teeth if the toothbrush is directed

   1. across the surface of the teeth
   2. from the inside toward the outside
   3. back and forth
   4. away from the gums

35. The type of toothbrush recommended as most effective in cleansing the teeth is one that has

   a. bristles of even length
   b. bristles longer at the tip of the brush
   c. firm but not rigid bristles
   d. a low cost

      1. d only
      2. a and c
      3. b and d
      4. all except b

36. To be classified as normal, fatigue must be relieved by

   1. 8 hours of sleep
   2. a couple of hours rest
   3. change of activity
   4. recreation

37. The physically healthy person who is always tired should look for the cause in

   1. an analysis of food intake
   2. the attitudes of others
   3. lack of motivation on the job
   4. unsolved emotional problems

38. If you spend all day Sunday <u>sitting</u> at your desk studying, you will feel "tired all over" because

    1. you are bored
    2. you failed to get fresh air
    3. waste products have accumulated in the blood stream
    4. lack of physical activity has made you sluggish

39. Too many employers and workers fail to appreciate the degree of fatigue that is built up when

    1. environmental conditions are not right
    2. feelings of resentment exist toward the job or the supervisor
    3. coffee breaks are not allowed
    4. the lunch period is too short

40. "On-the-job" relief of fatigue can often be obtained by

    1. a change of activity
    2. sitting quietly at the nurses' station for a few minutes
    3. listening to soothing music
    4. opening the windows wide

41. Sleep is the time for rebuilding and repair of body tissues because

    1. body activities are slowed up
    2. food supplies are not being used as energy
    3. emotional tension does not interfere
    4. the heart beats faster

42. When an individual <u>frequently</u> finds it difficult to sleep, he should suspect the cause is

    1. overfatigue
    2. hard work
    3. boredom
    4. emotional tension

43. An older person often complains of insomnia when the real reason lies in his

    1. eating habits
    2. sleeping habits
    3. decreased need for sleep
    4. emotional frustrations

44. When good posture habits are practiced, the general health will be better because

    1. all the organs have room to work
    2. the appetite is increased
    3. breathing is easier
    4. the person will be more interested in his surroundings

45. Observers would suspect that the student who always sprawls in her chair would also tend to be

    1. the best student
    2. uninterested
    3. careless
    4. very efficient

46. A chair that will give the student the most <u>support</u> is one that

    1. has arms
    2. has a wide seat
    3. allows the student's feet to touch the floor
    4. protects the back from the waist up

47. Poor posture takes less energy because good posture must fight harder against

    1. the wish to be different
    2. the force of gravity
    3. the shape of the chair
    4. the size of the shoe heels

48. At any age the kind of exercise and the amount of exercise taken should be influenced by

    1. the degree of fatigue afterward
    2. a doctor's advice
    3. the current fad
    4. the degree of dignity demanded

49. The shoe salesman tells you that you have flat feet and recommends a shoe with a special arch. You should

    1. respect his superior knowledge
    2. buy arch supports and wear them instead
    3. do nothing unless your feet bother you
    4. exercise your feet faithfully each night.

PERSONAL HYGIENE

50. When you are buying shoes to wear on duty, keep in mind that the most comfortable will be those that

    1. are larger for the left foot than for the right
    2. follow the shape of your foot
    3. fit because the foot has been X-rayed
    4. have a wedgie heel for added support

51. When you must stand quietly in one place for a long time, fatigue will be less if you

    1. wear old shoes for comfort
    2. spread your feet to broaden your base of support
    3. wear sandals to give foot freedom
    4. have a rigid arch support in your shoes

52. The best time to buy shoes to wear on duty and be sure that they will be comfortable for an entire shift is

    1. before your feet have a chance to swell
    2. early in the morning, shortly after the stores open
    3. about noon, when your foot has reached its largest size
    4. at the end of your work day

53. A habit that <u>seriously</u> affects mental health is

    1. viewing problems objectively
    2. expressing emotions
    3. talking about problems
    4. bottling up emotions

54. A mentally healthy person finds it <u>easy</u> to be

    1. happy   3. jealous
    2. angry   4. comfortable

55. A most important reason to work toward improving mental health is to make possible a satisfying adjustment

    1. to the elements of the environment
    2. to all problems
    3. in interpersonal relationships
    4. to people in authority

56. A start toward carrying out the rules of good mental health begins by

    1. inheriting good qualities
    2. living in a satisfactory environment
    3. trying to understand the needs of people
    4. accepting yourself

57. If you have an understanding of your own emotional feelings and needs, you will be better able

    1. to have faith
    2. to understand and tolerate others
    3. to love your neighbors
    4. to be critical

58. One of the most important aids to good mental health in a child is

    1. the inheritance of a strong nervous system
    2. a family of mentally healthy adults
    3. a chance to solve all his problems
    4. a strict disciplinary program

59. One of the characteristics of a mentally healthy person is the ability

    1. to collect all the facts before making a decision
    2. to find expert help with problems
    3. to make a decision, right or wrong
    4. to side-step a problem

60. A mentally healthy person will work toward a goal that is

    1. high
    2. determined by parental guidance
    3. realistic, in terms of abilities
    4. similar to those in his immediate group

61. A person is considered <u>tolerant</u> if he can become acquainted and interested in

    1. political activities
    2. a whole group, even if some are different
    3. all religious faiths
    4. the problems of many people

62. An important emotion that the emotionally healthy person is not afraid to express is

    1. anger   3. hate
    2. attention   4. love

63. From birth to death, one of the important basic needs of human beings is

    1. financial security   3. to be wanted
    2. education   4. to be successful

64. A mentally healthy person is described as one who feels comfortable about himself. This would include

    1. building up self-confidence by showing superiority
    2. accepting his own shortcomings, as well as respecting and recognizing his abilities
    3. being over-critical of his performance to stimulate improvement
    4. an intense display of emotion in most situations

65. A recommended way of relieving the tensions of unconscious personality conflict and thus remain mentally healthy is

    1. to "blow your top" at regular intervals
    2. to attend sports events as a spectator regularly
    3. to take active part in "destructive" sports
    4. to enjoy sports by reading fiction

66. A principle of growth and development that should be practiced by the nurse who wants to stay mentally healthy stresses

    1. sticking to goals reasonable to reach
    2. running away when problems get too great
    3. pushing problems that cause worry into the unconscious
    4. wishful thinking to overcome feelings of inferiority

67. When you are new in a community, it is possible to select an able physician if you

    a. ask people whose opinion you respect
    b. ask the Chamber of Commerce
    c. check with the secretary of the local Medical Society
    d. use the American Medical Directory at the Library

       1. all of the above   3. c and d
       2. c only   4. a, b, and d

68. The best way to tell a qualified physician from a quack is by knowing that

    1. he has no treatments he keeps secret
    2. he has an office and a listed phone number
    3. he does not refuse to make night calls
    4. he has a state license to practice

69. It is dangerous to go to a quack for medical help because he

    1. is in business only for profit
    2. lacks the knowledge and skill to treat the sick
    3. widely advertises his treatments
    4. discourages advice from qualified doctors

70. A specialist is different from a general practitioner because he

    a. does not ask about personal problems
    b. cares only for a special class of diseases
    c. is considered an expert in his chosen field
    d. is not friendly and is always in a hurry

       1. all of the above   3. b only
       2. a and d   4. b and c

71. One real advantage of having a "family doctor" is the fact that he is able

    1. to add information about your job, personal, and financial troubles to the story you tell him
    2. to understand the limits of your ability to pay his fees
    3. to check the whole family in one house call
    4. to make a diagnosis because he knows what is wrong with other members of your family

72. If you receive information by mail telling of the wonderful results of a new medicine to cure deafness, arthritis, cancer, etc., the best thing to do is

    1. throw it in the wastebasket
    2. turn the material over to the postal authorities
    3. give it to a friend who needs it
    4. order a trial supply to find out the ingredients

73. It is wise to find another doctor if you feel you cannot

    1. understand his bedside manner
    2. pay high fees for home visits
    3. have confidence in his decisions
    4. get enough appointments to talk about your troubles

74. If a good general practitioner has been selected, your family can be sure that in time of real trouble he will know when

    1. hospitalization and surgery are needed
    2. laboratory tests should be done
    3. to ask permission for an autopsy
    4. to call in a specialist on the case

75. Alcohol is often wrongly thought of as a stimulant because it

    1. allows the drinker to relax
    2. increases the appetite
    3. allows the primitive impulses to act with less restriction
    4. increases his ability to be sociable and more talkative

76. The person who is on a steady diet of alcohol will be

    1. poorly nourished
    2. overweight
    3. unable to work
    4. tense and irritable

77. The depressant effect of alcohol is best understood when the drinker becomes

    1. irritable and argumentative
    2. happy and noisy
    3. destructive
    4. unconscious

78. To be classed as a social drinker, a person must be able

    1. to take a drink at meal time
    2. to drink or leave it alone
    3. to have a drink to get started in the morning
    4. to serve liquor in his home

79. The individual who is classed as an alcoholic is one who has allowed his habit

    1. to interfere with his home life
    2. to increase
    3. to change his personality
    4. to become too expensive

80. The social drinker has slipped over the line to the alcoholic group when he

    1. behaves foolishly as a result of the alcohol
    2. takes too many of his daily food requirements in the form of alcohol
    3. prefers to drink alone
    4. must have a morning drink to get started

81. The teen-ager would not be so likely to take the first dose of an addicting drug if he were properly informed that later on

    1. the drug would get more expensive
    2. the drug would be harder to get
    3. failure to get the next dose would bring on distressing physical symptoms
    4. he would be fined and imprisoned for the illegal habit

82. The only person who can afford to be a drug addict without in some way injuring society is the one

    1. who peddles the dope
    2. who can easily pay as much as one hundred dollars a day for the drug
    3. who can take it or leave it alone
    4. who can be sure of getting his daily supply

83. A person may be a slave to a habit-forming drug, yet when the drug is taken away he

    1. has no physical withdrawal symptoms
    2. can find a satisfactory substitute
    3. is not upset emotionally
    4. suffers no ill effects

84. The one drug taken most often by addicts and the one with the most dangerous results is

    1. codeine   3. phenobarbital
    2. morphine   4. heroin

85. The cost of drug addiction gets increasingly higher because the addict develops

    1. an idiosyncrasy to the drug
    2. a tolerance to the drug
    3. an allergy to the drug
    4. a taste for a different drug

86. The Federal Government tries to prevent drug addiction as a result of self-medication by

    1. making narcotics impossible to get from a drug store
    2. making it illegal for a lay person to own a hypodermic syringe and needle
    3. requiring a prescription for the original dosage and for any refills
    4. inspecting all ships that arrive from other countries

VOCATIONAL ADJUSTMENTS

(Answer sheet p. 299)

This section contains questions on study techniques, on the requirements, characteristics and adjustments desirable for the practical nurse, on the legal aspects of nursing care, and on information of importance to the new graduate.

1. The recommended way to memorize information is to <u>budget</u>

   1. a daily time for study
   2. short, frequent study periods
   3. study time in the early morning
   4. time for oral review

2. A carefully prepared study plan is a help to the student because it allows her

   1. to do all her work in advance of the "due date"
   2. to get housework and study done in the time available
   3. to take part in recreational activities
   4. to do better work in a shorter time

3. The best way to study for <u>most</u> of your classes is

   1. to outline each lesson in detail
   2. to practice the methods you expect will be used to conduct the class
   3. to prepare and write out answers to essay questions
   4. to anticipate the questions that might be asked on an examination

4. The best <u>approach</u> to a <u>new</u> assignment is

   1. to underline important ideas
   2. to read the summary at the end of the lesson
   3. to skim it
   4. to look up all the new words

5. Except for periods budgeted for memorizing other study periods should be long enough to allow for

   1. self-recitation
   2. a warm-up period
   3. complete review of all classes previously studied
   4. completion of the assignment

6. Last minute cramming to allow the student to pass an examination is <u>dangerous in a nursing program</u> because

   1. the material has to be memorized
   2. the student knows only the words and not the meanings
   3. facts and procedures get mixed up
   4. the material is too quickly forgotten

7. The more you dislike a topic or a course, the more difficult it will be for you

   1. to concentrate long enough to study your assignment
   2. to stay awake
   3. to make adequate notes
   4. to take an examination successfully

8. It has been recommended that the way to develop an interest in a subject you now dislike is

   1. to study until you become an expert
   2. to discuss your dislike with the teacher
   3. to study it only when you feel your best
   4. to learn more about it than you are required to know

9. Many slow readers have difficulty increasing their reading speed because they

   1. move their lips when they read
   2. do not skim the assignment first
   3. have no interest in finding out their mistakes
   4. try to memorize the material

10. Skimming a new assignment will help the student

    1. to pick out the main points of the topic
    2. to prepare for the daily quiz
    3. to get the over-all idea of the subject
    4. to learn the new vocabulary

11. Real study of an assignment will be interfered with if the student

    1. underlines the material in first reading
    2. makes many notes
    3. looks up words that are unfamiliar
    4. studies in a group

12. Before a new assignment is started, it has been recommended that the student quickly review the notes of the last class in the course as an aid to

    1. saving time
    2. passing the course
    3. fitting the new assignment into the total picture
    4. improving the student's ability to make good notes

13. The student who has read the assigned material before class has the advantage of

    1. reading from her notes if called on
    2. being prepared to answer all questions
    3. knowing what information she needs to have explained
    4. feeling well prepared

14. The kitchen or the dining room table is not the best place to set up your study area because

    1. there will be too many distractions
    2. you will be tempted to keep one eye on the television
    3. you will be reminded of too many household tasks still to be done
    4. the area reminds you of food and you cannot settle down to complete concentration

15. Practical nursing is the wrong vocation for the person who

    1. is lazy
    2. does not enjoy people
    3. is dull mentally
    4. does not like to study

16. Self-confidence can best be achieved by first defining

    1. goals that are not too high to reach
    2. all liabilities
    3. the reasons for the need to improve
    4. the word itself

17. The best cure for a feeling of failure is

    1. to talk out the causes of the failure
    2. to find an excuse for it
    3. to do something you can do well
    4. to begin to prepare to succeed the next time

18. To be able to avoid repeating a failure, it is first necessary

    1. to have professional guidance
    2. to locate the cause of the failure
    3. to control your temper
    4. to understand your emotional make-up

19. Discipline is a valuable trait in a practical nurse because she is often called on

    1. to supervise the behavior of patients
    2. to obey orders
    3. to carry out orders at once without explanation
    4. to take over in case of an emergency

20. The belief you have in your ability to succeed defines

    1. self-respect   3. self-discipline
    2. self-control   4. self-acceptance

21. If you feel the pain the patient is suffering so strongly that you cannot make him take deep breaths and cough as ordered, you are being influenced by

    1. empathy   3. transference
    2. sympathy   4. identification

22. If a friend criticized you for spending a year in a practical nurse school when you could get a diploma by correspondence and work as you learned, you would enlighten her by explaining

    1. "I'm too lazy to study by mail"
    2. "A diploma from an approved school of practical nursing is necessary before the licensing examination can be taken"
    3. "It is still necessary to go to the headquarters of the correspondence school to do the practical work"
    4. "A correspondence course can be taken successfully only by a high school graduate who has learned how to study and concentrate"

23. If you find it possible to understand the pain that makes the patient refuse to try to cough, yet you continue to insist that he try, this is an example of

1. empathy
2. sympathy
3. transference
4. identification

24. <u>Whenever</u> two human beings have any contact with each other, there is some exchange of

1. ideas
2. thoughts
3. greetings
4. feeling

25. It is much easier to like the patient who

1. indicates that he likes you
2. looks like your father
3. is neat and tidy
4. respects your authority

26. When you express a dislike for a newly assigned patient because he threw his oral hygiene tray at you, your feeling is the result of

1. empathy
2. sympathy
3. transference
4. identification

27. Prejudices are most likely to be directed toward persons or groups that are

1. too aggressive
2. tricky and sly
3. dirty and indifferent
4. different from your own

28. Prejudices are usually based upon experiences with

1. one person or a small group
2. many members of a different group
3. children at school
4. fellow employees

29. An extremely sick patient will probably not appreciate behavior habits of the nurse such as

a. chewing gum
b. smoking in uniform
c. using vulgar language
d. using a fragrant deodorant

1. all of the above
2. b only
3. a and b
4. a, b, or c

30. The education of a practical nurse is different from nurse aid training because the emphasis is on

1. understanding the patient
2. more complicated nursing procedures
3. the "why" as well as the "how" in patient care
4. the cause and the treatment of many common diseases

31. The student practical nurse who has been in school 6 or 7 weeks should recognize the importance of refusing

1. to feed a bed patient
2. to do anything for the patient without a written doctor's order
3. to feed a patient by putting a tube into the stomach
4. to care for a patient who needs an enema

32. Idle gossip is so damaging to the victim because

1. loss of self-respect is the end result
2. it spreads so fast
3. everyone repeating the gossip adds one more untruth
4. once said, the words cannot be called back

33. A basic goal in practical nurse education is to teach the student to be

1. an expert nurse
2. a safe practitioner of nursing
3. patient and tolerant of all behavior
4. skilled in rehabilitation techniques

34. The practical nurse student uniform should not be worn into the corner tavern because

1. it is not hygienic
2. the uniform will become contaminated
3. the student's behavior is identified with the school
4. the public will be sure the beer will affect the nursing ability

35. The unsuccessful personality in nursing belongs to the one who

1. is temperamental
2. is bashful
3. becomes easily upset by unpleasant sights and smells
4. does not like people

36. The patient may be afraid to ask the nurse for the bedpan if the approach of the nurse has made the patient feel

    1. the nurse is already overworked
    2. an aide should do the "dirty" work
    3. elimination is the patient's problem
    4. unwanted

37. An objective attitude toward the behavior of the patient will allow the nurse to analyze the behavior

    1. by asking the patient his reason
    2. and make accurate reports to the head nurse and doctor
    3. and identify the mental mechanisms in use
    4. without allowing emotions to influence her judgment

38. A warm, kindly feeling toward a patient will be easy if you identify the patient with

    1. some member of your family
    2. a classmate
    3. an instructor
    4. some loved one

39. If the nurse is able to put herself in the place of the patient and accept his behavior because she appreciates how he feels, she is credited with the quality of

    1. objective attitude
    2. empathy
    3. transference
    4. therapy

40. When you begin to prepare Mrs. X for her evening meal, she angrily throws all the care equipment on the floor and then bursts into tears. It would be evidence of your objective attitude if you

    1. scolded the patient crossly for her behavior
    2. cleaned up the mess and got a fresh supply of materials
    3. left this patient alone and did not attempt to give her care
    4. asked other employees what treatments had just been done or who had been visiting the patient

41. Nursing the difficult, demanding patient will be easier for the nurse who accepts such behavior as

    1. release of hostilities toward relatives and the doctor
    2. beyond any control
    3. the reaction to the total situation and not an expression of dislike for one nurse
    4. resentment against the hospital room, the poor food, no visitors, and an irritable physician

42. It is not only courteous, but also time saving if the nurse remembers to answer the telephone

    1. at the first ring
    2. and identify the service, the person answering, and her title
    3. and write out the message given, repeating it to the caller
    4. and explains that she is new on the service and cannot give out information

43. The practical nurse is more likely to be involved in a legal suit as a result of her community actions when she unthinkingly

    1. gives her children aspirin for a cold
    2. offers her services in the first aid tent at the county fair
    3. uses poor nursing techniques
    4. practices medicine without a license

44. After the morning bath, Mrs. X, aged 85, asks you to leave the cotton bath blanket on, next to her, because she is warmer with it on. You recognize that the best total care of this patient will require you

    1. to refuse, since this is a violation of your procedure
    2. to refuse but offer to close the window if she is cold
    3. to leave the bath blanket on and explain to the instructor why you did it
    4. to agree that the room is cold and add an additional wool blanket rather than leave the bath blanket in place

45. Emotional identification with a patient and the patient's illness is called

   1. empathy
   2. transference
   3. sympathy
   4. symbolism

THE NEXT THREE QUESTIONS ARE BASED ON THE FOLLOWING SITUATION:

Your brother brings his small child to you because she is sick. He asks you to use the knowledge and skill learned at the practical nurse school to care for her.

46. As a student practical nurse, you will recognize that it will be most acceptable for you, in this situation,

   1. to do nothing until the doctor sees the patient
   2. to give the child an aspirin to relieve pain and lower fever
   3. to give an enema
   4. to take the temperature, pulse, and respiration

47. You will explain to your brother that you are limited in what you can do because

   1. a diagnosis is important before treatment is started
   2. you have not yet discussed this type of disease in class
   3. you have not yet been given a license to practice
   4. practice of all your procedures requires instructor supervision

48. Your best advice to your brother regarding the care of his child is

   1. to let her rest in bed for a few days and watch her closely
   2. to assume it is a communicable disease and keep the child away from other members of the family
   3. to insist the child be seen by a physician
   4. to advise him to employ a practical nurse who has a state license to care for her

49. The practical nurse will not be criticized for hugging and making a fuss over a patient if

   1. the patient is the same sex as the nurse
   2. the patient is a child
   3. the supervisor is not a rigid personality
   4. the patient has enough intelligence to understand why the nurse behaves in this manner

50. The nurse will not be influenced by personal feelings of dislike for a demanding, irritable patient if she recognizes that

   1. it is best to continue nursing care and ignore the patient
   2. such behavior is a symptom
   3. the patient is looking for the same type of behavior from the nurse
   4. she can ask to care for a different patient tomorrow

51. In a legal suit against the hospital and its nursing personnel the degree of responsibility placed on the actions of each person will be based on

   1. the amount of insurance each person carries
   2. the duties assigned to each group of employees
   3. the level of education and training each has had
   4. the amount of authority each person has

52. The ability to work well with patients of all ages and all personality types requires a deep appreciation of the importance of

   1. respecting individual differences
   2. doing only the jobs you enjoy
   3. getting complete information about the patient
   4. teaching the patient skills he did not have before hospitalization

53. The name and address of the person who can supply the L.P.N. with information concerning licensure in another state can best be obtained by

1. asking the director of the school
2. checking the January or July issue of the American Journal of Nursing
3. writing the governor
4. asking the executive secretary of the Department of Registration and Education

54. The practical nurse who has developed attitudes necessary to good nursing care will be constantly reminded that her most important assignment is

1. acceptance of professional nurse supervision
2. care of the patient
3. to remain cheerful
4. acceptance of any assignment

55. A characteristic of a mature person that will help the practical nurse to work in harmony with the professional nurse is an ability

1. to adjust to the patient
2. to find an easy way to do the job
3. to do only what she is told
4. to accept constructive criticism

56. The L.P.N. who is assigned to work with the professional nurse must expect to prove her abilities. Until the R.N. has been shown the quality of care to expect, the L.P.N. would be wise

1. to check with the professional nurse before doing more than routine patient care
2. to limit her activities to those duties usually assigned to an aide
3. to ask for directions for all procedures
4. to do procedures only as she was taught in practical nurse school

57. The L.P.N. in a soiled, wrinkled uniform impresses others with her

1. industry
2. willingness to pitch in
3. responsibility
4. carelessness

58. To those who work with the L.P.N., the full uniform represents

1. a level of education and performance achieved
2. the limitations of nursing care to be done by the practical nurse
3. a threat because of the pin and the cap
4. the degree of authority

59. A carefully planned, well-written letter of application will give a prospective employer

1. a good initial impression
2. enough information to enable him to hire you
3. no need to check further on your references
4. a complete picture of all your past activities

60. The graduate practical nurse who has absorbed the principles taught her will recognize the courtesy of

1. making an appointment to talk with the employing person
2. typing all letters of application
3. giving at least 2 months' notice of resignation
4. accepting all assigned duties without complaint

61. Before persons are listed as references, the practical nurse should

1. know the person's ability to write a good letter of recommendation
2. be sure that the reference will be satisfactory
3. be sure that they still hold the same position
4. have permission to use the names

62. It is a wise practical nurse who follows up a personal interview with

1. frequent telephone calls to see if the job is filled
2. a thank-you note for the time spent in the interview
3. pressures from important people in the community
4. a letter to the hospital administrator requesting special consideration

63. The length of time you will remain on a job after your resignation is handed in should be based on

    1. the ease with which you can be replaced
    2. the termination of your vacation time
    3. the attitude of your employer
    4. the amount of responsibility your position carries

64. A letter of resignation hastily written in a moment of anger may be responsible for

    1. a request to leave immediately
    2. a poor reference from this job
    3. a loss of terminal vacation
    4. loss of privileges for the remainder of the employment

65. Once a resignation has been handed in, the wise practical nurse will

    1. work hard to get a good reference
    2. continue to fulfill her duties conscientiously
    3. let the new worker carry the responsibility so that she can learn
    4. spend most of her time at the nurses' station talking about her new job

66. The education of a graduate practical nurse makes her legally responsible for her actions. No such nurse can really afford to be without adequate

    1. liability insurance
    2. supervision
    3. witnesses
    4. malpractice insurance

67. Before the L.P.N. accepts a new position, she should carefully consider

    a. what she can give to the job
    b. the quality of maintenance provided
    c. the likes and dislikes of the employer
    d. what the job can do for her

        1. all of the above
        2. a only
        3. a, b, and d
        4. a and d

68. After the practical nurse obtains all the information she possibly can about a position, she should then carefully consider

    1. the salary and personnel policies
    2. whether she is fitted for the job in education and experience
    3. her opportunities for doing more advanced procedures and techniques
    4. the hours of work and the holidays given

69. When she is considering several positions, the courteous practical nurse will

    1. tell each hospital the salary others have offered
    2. refrain from mentioning that she has other interests
    3. notify each hospital when she has accepted a position
    4. not let the other hospitals know when she has decided against them

70. If the graduate practical nurse has set future goals for himself, or herself, it then becomes possible

    1. to study toward this goal
    2. to look for financial assistance to achieve these goals
    3. to look for job opportunities that will add to or improve abilities needed to reach these goals
    4. to demand experiences that lead to promotions in the line of interest

71. When a nurse practice act is permissive, the law is designed to protect

    1. the patient   3. the nurse
    2. the employer   4. the title, L.P.N.

72. If the practical nurse who is licensed under a permissive law moves to a state that has a mandatory license law, she must expect

    1. to take another licensing examination
    2. to be licensed before she can begin work
    3. assignment as a nurse aide until her credentials are cleared
    4. to buy a permit to work.

GROWTH AND DEVELOPMENT

(Answer sheets pp. 301-302)

This section is concerned with the emotional foundations for behavior from birth through the geriatric years. Recognition and acceptance of the role of personality and emotions in behavior demonstrated by the healthy and the sick of all ages will increase the effectiveness with which the nurse will understand people. It is of prime importance that she first begin to understand herself.

1. When you can recall, and talk about childhood experiences long forgotten as you drive through the town where you grew up, you recognize that these memories have been stored in your

   1. conscious mind
   2. id
   3. subconscious mind
   4. ego

2. Most of the unconscious mind contains that part of the personality called

   1. the id
   2. the ego
   3. the superego
   4. the conscience

3. The conscious mind contains the experiences and information that you are aware of, and that you use often, and is the location of that part of the personality called

   1. the id
   2. the ego
   3. the superego
   4. the personality

4. The primitive drives with which we are born, such as the reproductive instinct, are carried in that part of the personality called

   1. the superego
   2. the ego
   3. the id
   4. the behavior

5. The personality with which we are born acts on the guiding principle of

   1. pleasure-pain
   2. independence
   3. conflict
   4. pleasure

6. The chief job of the EGO is to act as

   1. censor for all behavior
   2. moderator between the other parts of the personality
   3. a stimulation for creative activity
   4. ruler of the id

7. The ID is that part of the personality that controls actions

   1. at the age of 2 years
   2. at 6 years of age
   3. as soon as there are some experiences "on file"
   4. at birth

8. The degree of development of the Superego depends on

   1. community laws
   2. parental standards and discipline
   3. the behavior of the gang
   4. the examples set by parents

9. Parental behavior that would tend to develop a strict superego in a child would include

   1. the frequent use of "No" in response to childhood experiences
   2. punishment for breaking family rules
   3. immature decisions
   4. approval one day and disapproval the next day for the same action

10. When the id "wants to" and the superego says, "No, it's bad," most of this battle takes place in

    1. the ego
    2. the spirit
    3. the mind
    4. the unconscious mind

11. Any action in response to a stimulus is correctly called

    1. purposeful
    2. voluntary
    3. personality
    4. behavior

12. Anything that produces a change in an individual, whether it comes from inside or outside the person, is called

    1. movement
    2. feeling
    3. a stimulus
    4. a conflict

13. Behavior of some sort can be expected from stimulations that

 a. come from within (physiological)
 b. come from within (emotional)
 c. result from your attitudes toward other people
 d. result from the attitudes of other people toward you

   1. all of the above
   2. a only
   3. a and c
   4. b and d

14. Whenever a person wants two things at the same time and only one can be obtained, the action that goes on until a decision is made is called

   1. indecision   3. efficiency
   2. vascillating   4. a conflict

15. Although the other fellow may still consider you stupid in spite of your actions, the fact that you beat him with your fists when he called you STUPID will

   1. make him respect you later
   2. reduce your tension
   3. make him afraid to say it again
   4. place you in a superior position

16. While the ego is trying to settle a battle between the ID and the SUPEREGO, the person concerned will have feelings of

   1. pleasure-pain   3. guilt
   2. anxiety   4. memory loss

17. The feeling of uneasiness or fear that is called apprehension is different from this same feeling labeled anxiety because apprehension

   1. is unconscious
   2. concerns something in the external surroundings
   3. concerns relationships with other people
   4. occurs while asleep, as in a nightmare

18. The uneasiness felt when the term anxiety is correctly used is present

   1. during a thunderstorm
   2. at examination time
   3. when the id gets its own way
   4. at the unconscious level

19. The tiny infant knows whether its parents love him and want him because he is capable of

   1. empathy   3. insight
   2. sympathy   4. appreciation

20. When childhood experiences enable the child to build up respect for himself, he will, as an adult, have

   1. an understanding of how he grew up
   2. many rewards
   3. fewer anxieties
   4. increased experiences

21. Whenever a baby's basic needs are not satisfied, the result is a feeling of

   1. fear   3. irritation
   2. tension   4. sadness

22. When a baby's basic needs are not satisfied, he continues to complain, hoping that it will be possible

   1. to regain a comfortable feeling
   2. to upset the whole family
   3. to substitute another need
   4. to forget the need

23. All persons, from birth to death, have a basic need for

   1. superiority   3. health
   2. achievement   4. love or affection

24. If the basic needs are not satisfied in childhood, the adult cannot develop maturity because

   1. mental illness prevents adjustments
   2. he continues to seek satisfactions for the basic needs
   3. he will be irritable and impossible to get along with
   4. he will deny that his need still exists

25. Since sucking is important in the satisfaction of hunger, it is understandable why the first stage of personality development is called

   1. the anal phase   3. the oral phase
   2. the latent phase   4. the gang stage

GROWTH AND DEVELOPMENT

26. The child has many upsetting experiences during the anal phase of personality development, since for the first time in his life he finds it necessary

    1. to do as he is told
    2. to be a "good boy"
    3. to make his own decisions about how much love and affection he can earn
    4. to go against his pleasure principle to get his mother's approval

27. The healthy personality development of a baby during the oral phase is helped when its mother

    1. holds and cuddles him during feeding time
    2. helps him to become emotionally independent
    3. lets him get used to doing things for himself
    4. leaves him quietly alone until the bottle is finished

28. The child's conflict during the Oedipal stage has its roots in its need

    1. to understand the different behavior standards for the sexes
    2. to behave in a grown-up way like the parent of the opposite sex
    3. to take mother's love away from father
    4. to depend upon the parent of the same sex and the desire to have the parent of the opposite sex to itself

29. The superego of a mature adult will act

    1. as the ego decides is best, without a fuss
    2. in a warning, instead of a punishing, capacity
    3. to make him feel anxious and guilty when behavior is bad
    4. as the guiding factor in deciding behavior patterns

30. It is especially important for the mother of little girls to understand and recognize what is happening in the Oedipal phase of personality development to prevent or control her own feelings of

    1. jealousy   3. helplessness
    2. inadequacy   4. discipline

31. The kind of behavior shown to other people depends on the balance of personality kept by

    1. the superego
    2. the ego
    3. the id
    4. the fear of punishment

32. The compromises the ego makes between the desires of the id and those of the superego are known as

    1. mental mechanisms   3. empathy
    2. conflicts   4. transference

33. While the ego is trying to control the urges of the id and the restrictions of the superego, the person concerned is aware only of feelings of

    1. apprehension   3. anxiety
    2. conflict   4. security

34. Any kind of behavior from patients can be more readily accepted by the practical nurse who remembers that

    1. all illness brings out the worst behavior
    2. all behavior has a reason
    3. all disagreeable behavior begins at the unconscious level
    4. the patient is never upset with her

35. That part of the personality responsible for deciding which mental mechanism will best modify the unconscious conflict is

    1. the id   3. the superego
    2. the ego   4. the conscience

36. The moderate use of mental mechanisms makes it possible for humans to get along more smoothly. Without them it would be necessary to solve all problems by a process of

    1. allowing the strongest personality part to rule
    2. compromise
    3. retreat into a mental illness
    4. flight or fight

37. In a battle between the id and the super-ego the successful use of a mental mechanism allows the ego

    1. to remain in complete control
    2. to relieve the tensions produced by the conflict
    3. to use the criticisms being pushed by the superego
    4. to express the primitive needs

38. The knowledge of mental mechanisms and their use should make the nurse more understanding of the behavior of others, since she recognizes that they begin

    1. developing at birth
    2. in traumatic situations
    3. in the subconscious or the unconscious mind
    4. as a protection against the problems of adolescence

39. The only way a person can decrease the number of times he resorts to mental mechanisms is

    1. to have a plan of action that will prevent their use
    2. to change those personality traits that bring out their use
    3. to keep out of situations that call for immediate answers or action
    4. to analyze his behavior and identify the mechanisms used

40. The ego uses rationalization in an attempt to explain behavior

    1. acceptably
    2. so that it seems reasonable
    3. as the fault of someone else
    4. did not exist

41. The student who fails an announced examination on the assignment for the day will be using rationalization if he tells his friends

    1. "There is nothing wrong with my paper. The teacher gives the best grades to her pets"
    2. "I'll learn someday that the teacher means what she says"
    3. "I failed the examination only because the teacher's questions were not clear"
    4. "So what? I can always do the test over"

42. One of the greatest dangers in the over-use of rationalization is the inability to

    1. face reality
    2. keep a circle of friends
    3. use other mechanisms successfully
    4. accept and correct mistakes

43. Rationalization results from unconscious feelings of

    1. guilt or insecurity
    2. hostility
    3. primitive urges
    4. dependence

44. The little girl who dresses up in her mother's high-heeled shoes and uses her rouge and lipstick is using the mechanism of

    1. projection   3. regression
    2. identification   4. sublimation

45. Primitive impulses of love and hate cannot be freely expressed, and the healthy personality will ease tensions by use of the mechanism called

    1. regression   3. sublimation
    2. projection   4. rationalization

46. The small child is helped to develop a healthy personality and acceptable standards of behavior by the use of

    1. rationalization   3. projection
    2. suppression   4. identification

47. The child who is encouraged to make mud pies and to finger paint, and thus gives up messing in his food and his feces, has been helped to use the mechanism of

    1. sublimation   3. conversion
    2. identification   4. compensation

48. The things we "forget" because the ego has pushed them into the unconscious mind illustrates use of the mechanism of

    1. suppression   3. repression
    2. regression   4. projection

49. The person who is always suspicious of the attitudes and actions of other people is probably overworking the mechanism of

    1. rationalization
    2. projection
    3. introjection
    4. conversion

50. When vague, unexplained feelings of anxiety are followed by symptoms of headache, the mechanism used is called

    1. substitution
    2. conversion
    3. compensation
    4. identification

51. A man earns his living at a dull, monotonous office job. His <u>hobby</u> of aeroplane acrobatics illustrates his use of the mechanism called

    1. compensation
    2. conversion
    3. sublimation
    4. regression

52. Jimmy has to stay with his grandmother while his mother goes to the hospital for surgery. <u>Conversion</u> will be suspected if he

    1. packs his toys and runs away
    2. tells his friends his mother will not be back again
    3. tells his friends his mother has gone to get him a pony
    4. suddenly develops a high fever

53. The surgeon who lost one arm in World War II becomes a public health and sanitation expert. This will illustrate use of

    1. sublimation
    2. compensation
    3. conversion
    4. repression

54. When unconscious, otherwise unexpressed feelings of hate are worked out by preparing for a job that requires you to be critical of the work of others, the mechanism at work is

    1. sublimation
    2. conversion
    3. repression
    4. projection

55. The man who seldom stops for a red light or a stop sign unless another car is coming freely expresses his objections to teenage driving on the basis of carelessness. This man is using the mechanism of

    1. identification
    2. reaction formation
    3. projection
    4. displacement

56. Fanatical hand washing in an adult may be an outward expression of guilt feelings concerning childhood masturbation which have been

    1. suppressed
    2. regressed
    3. repressed
    4. projected

57. The adult female who controls her family by frequent crying spells in conflict situations is using

    1. regression
    2. introjection
    3. repression
    4. rationalization

58. The graduate nurse who develops a severe diarrhea on the morning of state board examinations is expressing her unconscious tensions by the use of

    1. compensation
    2. projection
    3. conversion
    4. sublimation

59. When the toilet-trained 4-year-old begins to wet his pants after the birth of a baby brother, he is using the mechanism called

    1. rationalization
    2. conversion
    3. displacement
    4. regression

60. The man who repressed his childhood jealousy and hatred of a younger brother and gave up his own ambitions to earn money to help this brother to reach his goals has used the mechanism of

    1. displacement
    2. overcompensation
    3. sublimation
    4. suppression

61. You would recognize the use of <u>displacement</u> by an employee who

    1. pushed a patient out of his path soon after being scolded by a supervisor for poor ward reports
    2. protested that the man on the other shift changed the original reports
    3. argued that he completed the reports in just the form he had been taught in class
    4. told the supervisor to find someone else to do the "darned reports"

62. When primitive urges of the id cannot be expressed or relieved by the mechanism of sublimation, the ego will try to ease tensions by

1. suppression of the urges
2. represssion of the urges
3. attitudes or behaviors just opposite to the desires not being allowed expression
4. denial by criticizing these desires

63. Suppression is different from repression because the foundation lies in

1. the conscious mind
2. the subconscious mind
3. the unconscious mind
4. the id

64. When you are angry at yourself for not putting the ladder where it belongs and you kick the ladder after you have fallen over it, the mechanism you are using is called

1. identification   3. displacement
2. projection   4. repression

65. When you are angry at your boss for not putting the ladder away and you kick the ladder after you have fallen over it, the mechanism at work is

1. identification   3. displacement
2. projection   4. repression

66. The ability to admit a mistake, followed by a detailed explanation of the things in your environment that prevented you from doing the job correctly, illustrates use of

1. projection   3. displacement
2. compensation   4. rationalization

67. The man who criticizes the faults of other employees and denies that he too is guilty of possessing these faults is unconsciously trying to increase his feelings of worth by

1. introjection   3. rationalization
2. projection   4. compensation

68. Conversion is a mental mechanism that allows its user

1. to find an acceptable excuse for his behavior
2. to blame someone or something for his action
3. to escape all responsibility
4. to get relief from emotional problems through physical symptoms

69. An understanding of the mental mechanism identification should help the practical nurse to appreciate how important her actions are in

1. the hospital situation
2. setting a good health example
3. the community
4. stimulating good medical care

70. An understanding nurse will accept the fact that during a painful or a frightening illness the aspect of the personality that pushes more and more to the front is

1. the id   3. the superego
2. the ego   4. the subconscious

71. A punching bag hung at a commonly used entrance to a home and frequently used by all family members would increase their mental health by allowing them

1. to express resentment and hurt feelings
2. to practice skill in self defense
3. to release emotional tensions through an accepted channel
4. to take out all emotions in the medium of physical activity

72. If the prim and proper preacher drank too many alcoholic drinks, the "shocking" behavior resulting would be caused by

1. the foundation built by his parents
2. an attempt to ease frustrations
3. a repressed desire to behave like other men
4. escape of id impulses

73. The practical nurse should find it easier to understand the patient with many functional illnesses, since she recognizes that physical symptoms are a personality adjustment mechanism known as

    1. compensation
    2. conversion
    3. naturalization
    4. projection

74. The ability to adjust to environment and the people in it is dangerously interfered with if there is excess use of the mental mechanism called

    1. sublimation
    2. identification
    3. projection
    4. compensation

75. Dr. X has just advised the mother of a 6-year-old child that surgery must be done at once to remove the appendix. When the nurse gives the child the pre-operative hypo, the child yells and screams. The mother accuses the nurse of being an unskilled beginner, of enjoying procedures that "torture" a child. This nurse, to be effective, must realize that the mother is using the mental mechanism of

    1. projection
    2. identification
    3. displacement
    4. sour grapes

76. The presence of fears and tensions in the sick patient, as well as in the immediate family of the patient, are best revealed to the understanding nurse by the use of the mental mechanism called

    1. rationalization
    2. repression
    3. overcompensation
    4. conversion

77. Old Mr. Jones cannot understand why he should have to stay in bed until the nurse is available to help him up. Each time he gets up without assistance he insists that the nurse yesterday told him to get up, the noise in the hall frightened him and he got up to investigate, etc. Mr. Jones is using the mental mechanism of

    1. rationalization
    2. compensation
    3. displacement
    4. sublimation

78. The repressed frustrations and tensions of the early childhood period may be able to work out of the unconscious mind in the form of

    1. physical symptoms
    2. emotional distress
    3. unexplained anxiety
    4. loss of memory

79. In a family group in which the emotional health of all the members is a major interest the parents will continuously try

    1. to allow each member of the family to express himself freely at any time
    2. to free the children of responsibility so that they will have time to grow up
    3. to limit the wants of each member so the family interests will get most attention
    4. to balance the needs of each member with those of the whole family

80. A family organization known as paternal is controlled by

    1. mother
    2. mother and father
    3. the oldest male
    4. father

81. Cooperative planning for the spending of money is a characteristic of the modern family organization in which

    1. there are no children
    2. both husband and wife work for wages
    3. father is the recognized head of the family
    4. mother is the recognized head of the family

82. The goal of parents' efforts to raise a child is to make it possible for it

    1. to develop behavior acceptable to society as a replacement for instinct behavior
    2. to become a better citizen than the parents
    3. to increase his inborn intelligence
    4. be more productive than either parent has been

83. A happy, healthy family is developed when every member understands that

    1. strict discipline is needed for later good behavior
    2. each member has individual needs
    3. father's role makes him responsible for all aspects of family life
    4. privileges are granted according to the age of each child

84. A child will have great difficulty developing into a <u>mature</u> adult if he is handicapped by

    1. patterns set by immature parents
    2. a lack of material things
    3. responsibility for some chores at home
    4. a rigid discipline with few limitations

85. One of the most important things young parents should recognize is that

    1. a child is an upsetting factor in any marriage
    2. a child must be allowed to develop at its own pace
    3. a child must be treated as a small adult
    4. the weekly income must be increased once a baby arrives

86. Parents cannot be excused when adolescent behavior is not accepted by society, since the child's attitudes are developed

    1. at the age of 10
    2. by parental restrictions
    3. with early family experiences as their foundation
    4. on the basis of the amount of attention supplied by each parent

87. The purpose of teaching parents about normal child growth and development is to help them

    1. ignore "stages" of behavior
    2. be less tense about a child's behavior
    3. understand the child does not need much attention
    4. set higher standards for each child

88. The behavior of the newborn is directed toward obtaining

    1. food
    2. sleep
    3. comfort
    4. attention

89. Many adult personalities would be different if their parents had recognized that the emotional habits of children develop

    1. by imitation of parents' behavior
    2. after the child gets into school
    3. when he is old enough to play with others his age
    4. before 2 years of age

90. If parents can allow the 2 or 3 year-old child to explore his environment, under supervision, he is encouraged

    1. to learn respect for others' property
    2. to look but not touch
    3. to satisfy his curiosity and thus improve his intelligence
    4. to build confidence in his surroundings

91. When a child's request or behavior is met with an angry "NO," he often <u>misunderstands</u> because it is an angry adult's tendency

    1. to soften the penalty later
    2. to shout too loudly
    3. to omit any explanations
    4. to delay punishment until father comes home

92. The feelings of insecurity that develop in a child whose parents quarrel constantly may be expressed by

    1. physical symptoms
    2. jealousy
    3. soiling himself
    4. vomiting and diarrhea

93. Frequent quarreling between parents in the presence of the small child will make the child feel

    1. insecure
    2. in the way
    3. helpless
    4. unloved

94. When one child is always urged to do as well as an older brother or sister, that child will begin to feel that

1. his parents do not want him
2. he is not appreciated for his own ability
3. he is neglected
4. it is not worth the effort to compete for affection

95. The future personality of a child may be damaged when parents are guilty of

1. telling false stories about where babies come from
2. saying "NO" to anything that is pleasurable to the child
3. allowing today and forbidding the same thing tomorrow
4. using a cross tone of voice to discipline

96. The male child who grows up dominated and directed by his mother will find that his contacts with all females will

1. be childishly pleasant
2. be most important
3. be based on distrust
4. make him feel guilty

97. When paternal discipline dominates, and the father always expects his son to do better than the achievements of which the son feels proud, it can be expected that sooner or later the child will

1. fight back
2. quit trying to please
3. learn to set his own goals
4. depend only on his mother

98. The adults in a child's environment should realize that the progress in emotional control of the very small child will be determined by

1. the time people spend making explanations
2. religious experiences of the whole family
3. the examples to which the child is exposed
4. discipline

99. Scolding or punishing the child when the parent is angry will increase any feelings the child already has that

1. he will be physically harmed
2. he is not loved any more
3. favorite toys will be taken away
4. he will be isolated from the rest of the family

100. When parents understand that each child grows and develops at his own rate, it will be easier for them to love each child

1. in spite of his faults
2. just as he is
3. until good behavior is learned
4. in the right amount

101. Regardless of how many children there are in a family, the parents need to give each child the feeling that he

1. must earn their love
2. is the most important
3. must take his turn sharing the love and attention of the parents
4. has a place that cannot be filled by the others

102. When the older child accidentally wets his pants at play, his usual feeling will be one of

1. indifference   3. jealousy
2. fear   4. emotion

103. The recommended way for parents to help the child who has accidentally soiled himself is

1. to restrict his play
2. to make him clean up his mess
3. to assure him that he is still loved
4. to ignore the situation

104. The aspect of toilet training that normally will be accomplished last is

1. bowel control
2. bladder control
3. bladder control at night
4. dependent on the type of clothes the child wears

105. Parents should not expect any kind of toilet training to be effective until

   1. mother can spend all her time with the child
   2. the child understands the reason for holding urine and feces
   3. the child's nervous system can respond to training
   4. the child can eat a selective diet

106. Since it is a normal desire of small children to smear, it is best for the child and parent

   1. to encourage smearing with substitute play materials
   2. to put diapers on in such a way the child cannot remove feces
   3. to let the child satisfy this urge with his food
   4. to allow smearing but insist that this stage be short

107. One of the few ways a small child can express his feelings of anger and frustration toward parents is by

   1. shyness   3. withholding feces
   2. overeating   4. insomnia

108. Once a child has achieved complete bowel and bladder control, parents should recognize that a return to bed-wetting is

   1. laziness
   2. evidence of emotional conflict
   3. a control weapon against the parent
   4. evidence of a serious bladder disease

109. Teaching a small child bowel control will be difficult if

   a. passing of feces is painful
   b. the child has no acceptable way to release anger
   c. other children do not set a good example
   d. the child is still in diapers

      1. all of the above
      2. a only
      3. a and b
      4. a, b and c

110. It is possible to toilet train a very small child, but such training is based on

   1. above average nerve development
   2. stable kidney function
   3. fear of loss of parental approval
   4. a dislike of being warm and wet

111. A normal emotion expressed by the child who is being toilet trained is

   1. hate   3. pride
   2. anger   4. jealousy

112. Frequent periods of constipation in a small child would make an informed observer (usually not the parent) suspect the reason is

   1. fear of getting dirty
   2. a high-fat formula
   3. irregular toilet habits
   4. some physical deformity

113. A child may hold feces until he becomes constipated if his mother places too much stress on

   1. regularity
   2. cleanliness
   3. obedience
   4. behavior development

114. If fluids are restricted and the small child is awakened several times during the night to go to the toilet in an effort to gain total bladder control, the child will feel he is

   1. important
   2. a nuisance
   3. emotionally unstable
   4. being punished

115. Bedwetting is more likely to be a warning sign of emotional stress if

   1. it occurs after toilet training has been successful
   2. it lasts beyond 2 years of age
   3. the child does not get so much attention as he thinks he should
   4. a new baby has been added to the family group

116. Mother is upset when the small child does not eat everything she places before it. This is based on her feelings

1. of anger because food is wasted
2. of fear of criticism for being a poor mother
3. of alarm that the child might be sick
4. that the child's eating habits will be poor all its life

117. The mother who understands normal child development will not be too disturbed when her 9-month-old

1. begins to lose weight
2. refuses all new foods introduced
3. smears in his feces
4. has a decrease in appetite

118. The adult attitude toward food will depend on childhood

1. experiences with a wide variety of foods
2. remembrances of family eating habits
3. associations with food, pleasant or unpleasant
4. ability to chew and digest foods

119. Children cannot be expected to learn to feed themselves unless parents are willing

1. to buy them child-sized utensils
2. to let them practice doing it
3. to let them imitate other family members
4. to provide them with foods they can eat with their fingers

120. A child can develop an interest in foods only if

1. the rest of the family eats all foods
2. the child is allowed to eat alone
3. mother insists that the child feed himself
4. eating is a time of pleasure

121. The recommended parental attitude toward the healthy child's refusal to eat is one of

1. anger   3. punishment
2. concern   4. indifference

122. Mother should understand that the child will develop food dislikes quickly during

1. adolescence
2. the winter months
3. sickness
4. periods of parental tensions

123. A very poor time to give a child a second chance at a food previously refused is

1. when he is already full
2. at the table with the rest of the family
3. at the morning meal
4. in the presence of company

124. If the small child consistently refuses milk, the wise mother will offer

a. cottage cheese
b. custards
c. ice cream
d. eggnog

1. c only
2. a and c
3. b and d
4. all of the above

125. A mother with her first baby should be reassured that feeding problems are less common if she can accept the fact that

1. baby is the best judge of his needs
2. the "book" is not always right
3. a rigid schedule gives the child security
4. such problems result from her own fears

126. A fear is a normal reaction to a situation that is

1. one of danger
2. filled with frustration
3. poorly handled
4. lacking parental approval

127. The tiny infant is most likely to show a fear reaction in the presence of

1. strange smells
2. sudden, loud noises
3. animals
4. relatives

128. Most of the solid foods the infant rejects, he "spits out" because he is objecting to

1. the taste
2. the feel
3. the absence of the nipple
4. the need to chew

129. The best time to introduce a new food in baby's diet is

1. at bedtime
2. following a meal he particularly likes
3. at the noon meal
4. at the beginning of the meal, while he is hungry

130. Fears that will be the most difficult to overcome are those that develop as a result of

1. feelings of inadequacy
2. new experiences
3. loss-of-support activities
4. the fears of the parents

131. Parents often fail to recognize that the child's fears have been produced as a result of

1. feelings of unimportance
2. parental quarreling
3. being different
4. rigid discipline

132. Fears often accompany the unexpressed emotion of

1. anxiety   3. hate
2. tension   4. apprehension

133. Parental overprotection may be the cause of fear because the child is never encouraged

1. to stay alone
2. to join other children
3. to try anything new
4. to play without mother's approval

134. When the child of 3 to 5 develops fears concerning experiences he has not had, these fears will be the result of

1. hate   3. insecurity
2. jealousy   4. imagination

135. An easy way to prevent a child from becoming afraid in a new experience is

1. to give him a detailed explanation
2. to allow him to watch as a spectator
3. to show him pictures first
4. to have him accompanied by a trusted adult

136. A child will be afraid to express his fears if adults

1. make fun of him
2. refuse to listen
3. discuss fearful experiences
4. prove his fears have no foundation

137. A recommended way to help a child get rid of fears is to encourage him

1. to dream about them
2. to act them out
3. to ignore them
4. to laugh at them

138. Parents who refuse to leave any light on after the child goes to bed because they feel that the child will not sleep, should be helped to understand that

1. fears will cause more sleeplessness than the light
2. a small night light may be enough
3. by the age of five, the fear of the dark will disappear
4. the child is afraid only if he is left alone

139. When a child is not allowed to talk out his fears, parents should expect a frequency of

1. destructive behavior
2. hate reactions
3. nightmares
4. daydreaming

140. Anger in a child can produce serious results when

1. he is disciplined
2. he is not allowed to express it
3. his personality is ruined
4. it seems necessary to isolate him

141. A child becomes fearful when he already has feelings of guilt because he cannot

    1. be like the other children
    2. achieve the high standards set for him
    3. take his emotions out on his toys
    4. find the right words to describe his feelings

142. Instead of building up fears by frequently cautioning the child to BE CAREFUL in carrying out the usual daily routines, a parent can best

    1. have him read about how to do things safely
    2. keep harmful articles out of his reach
    3. show him the safe way to do things
    4. supervise all of his activities closely

143. If punishment follows a tantrum, it will increase the child's feeling of

    1. fear   3. resentment
    2. insecurity   4. jealousy

144. A mother can expect that her child's demonstrations of anger will be increased if she

    1. demands immediate obedience
    2. leaves discipline to father
    3. ignores Junior's bid for attention
    4. gets angry too

145. The 2 year-old becomes increasingly angry when adults are unable

    1. to fix a favorite toy
    2. to understand what he is trying to tell them
    3. to include him in their conversation
    4. to find time to read to him

146. It will not be necessary for a child to have guilt feelings over his anger at his parents if they will assure him that

    1. everyone feels angry sometimes
    2. he will never be punished
    3. they are never angry at him
    4. he will feel different as he gets older

147. Parents would be better able to recognize hidden feelings of anger in a child by more careful observation and understanding of

    1. his play and his treatment of toys
    2. his methods to control his environment
    3. his inability to get along with people
    4. his great need for special attention

148. When the child responds with anger to the necessary requests to carry out daily activities, an effective approach may be

    1. to punish for disobedience
    2. to let him choose between two acceptable activities
    3. to isolate the child
    4. to ignore his bids for special attention

149. Parents should understand that anger is a natural emotion for a child to display when

    1. he is told NO
    2. he is exploring his surroundings
    3. there is evidence of lack of affection
    4. father pays more attention to the new baby

150. Instead of a mother becoming angry when her child shows his anger toward her, she should understand that at this time the child is most in need of

    1. isolation
    2. her love
    3. a disciplinary talk
    4. something to keep busy

151. The older child who has been punished for wetting the bed again after the arrival of a baby brother or sister will be further convinced that

    1. he has lost his mother's love
    2. the new baby is an enemy
    3. habit training is not worth the effort
    4. there is no need to love the new baby

152. When parents will not allow a child to express his anger toward them, the <u>natural outlet</u> is anger

    1. toward the cat
    2. toward his toys
    3. toward his playmates
    4. turned inward on himself

153. Jealousy always has its beginnings in the emotion of

    1. love   3. instability
    2. hate   4. fear

154. It is natural for a small child who is unhappy with jealousy to go back to

    1. daydreaming
    2. destructive behavior
    3. tantrums to gain more attention
    4. habits associated with a happier babyhood

155. If parents suspect that a child is jealous of a new baby, they would be wise

    1. to tell the older child that he is still loved
    2. to observe the older child at play
    3. to allow the older child to care for the baby
    4. to prove their love for the older child by giving him presents

156. Parents should <u>suspect</u> that the older child feels jealous of the new baby when he

    1. is very attentive to the baby
    2. is destructive
    3. avoids the new baby
    4. plays with the baby's toys

157. It would be possible to avoid some feelings of jealousy toward the new baby <u>if</u> parents would

    1. explain where the baby came from
    2. keep the child informed of the progress of the pregnancy
    3. make necessary household changes before the new baby arrives
    4. allow the older child to select the baby's clothing

158. A mother can help her child overcome his feelings of jealousy for the new baby by

    1. insisting father take over the responsibility for the older child
    2. planning time to give special attention to the older child
    3. giving him responsibility in the care of the new baby
    4. putting him in a nursery school

159. Parents should expect that <u>some</u> feelings of jealousy toward the new baby will be

    1. best treated by a psychiatrist
    2. deserving of punishment
    3. evidence of delinquency
    4. normal

160. Some emotions a child can "take out" on his toys include

    a. discipline   c. fear
    b. anger   d. jealousy

        1. all of the above
        2. a and b
        3. b, c, and d
        4. a, b, and c

161. Parents thoughtlessly develop feelings of insecurity in a child by

    1. being too busy with household activities
    2. paying too much attention to father
    3. punishing for unacceptable behavior
    4. telling him a bad boy is not loved

162. Parents often force a child to use his imagination to justify his behavior because

    1. parents set a poor example
    2. he fears punishment for the truth
    3. the truth is so uninteresting
    4. parents put ideas in his head

163. When a child breaks something, it is important that mother look for

    1. a good way to discipline
    2. an unbreakable replacement
    3. a more satisfactory play area
    4. the meaning behind the behavior

164. It is not <u>consistent</u> for parents to demand that a child respect the property of other people and then

    1. not provide him with the things other children have
    2. discuss their child with the parents of neighborhood children
    3. give him everything he demands
    4. have no respect for the child's property

165. If Junior blames the "gremlins" for the crayon drawings on his bedroom wall, mother can best control the situation by

    1. taking away the crayons
    2. scolding him for destroying the appearance of the wall
    3. having his room repapered with washable wallpaper
    4. expressing disapproval and letting him know she is aware that he did it

166. A mother's best response to a wild imaginative tale would be

    1. "You are a naughty boy to tell such a lie"
    2. "Don't let your father hear you tell stories like that"
    3. "That's a good make-believe story. Now tell me what really happened"
    4. "That is a good story. Be sure to tell it to Daddy when he gets home"

167. When siblings, aged 3 and 6, quarrel and fight, a mother should know how important it is

    1. to put them to bed until they can be friends
    2. to let them know she does not love them when they are naughty
    3. to limit all play activities until there is peace
    4. to let both children know she loves them

168. When a mother fails to take time out from her care of the new baby to pay attention to Junior's emotional needs, his natural feeling will be one of

    1. neglect   3. rejection
    2. guilt   4. importance

169. Any type of discipline, for child or adult, can be really effective only if it

    1. is the same each time
    2. is applied each time the action is repeated
    3. comes as a complete surprise so that the naughty child never knows what to expect
    4. takes away something the person prizes highly

170. Parents will find that Junior will not pop in and out of bed or demand extra attention after he has gone to bed <u>if</u>

    1. his mother ignores his behavior
    2. he does not feel that his parents are anxious to get him out of the way
    3. his father takes over the bedtime routine
    4. his mother understands why it is important to take a toy to bed

171. John, age 1 year, begins to handle his genital organs when he is undressed for a bath. Such action

    1. can become a serious habit
    2. will not occur if his genitals are clean
    3. results from diapers that are pinned too tightly
    4. is common at this age

172. When John is old enough to sit on the pottie, his mother finds him playing in his feces. The recommended thing for her to do is

    1. to tell him he is a bad boy
    2. to show how displeased she is by such behavior
    3. to clean him up and give him something else to do
    4. nothing

173. If play activities are expected to keep a child too busy to suck his thumb, they must be planned

    1. to keep both hands active
    2. to provide new experiences to keep him interested
    3. to involve other children
    4. to tire him out

174. A small child is not able to experience two emotions at the same time. When he tells his mother, I HATE YOU, he feels guilty and insecure because

1. he really does not mean it
2. good children do not hate their parents
3. he wants to run away from home
4. he expects to lose love as a result of his behavior

175. The goals parents set for their children are often responsible for many frustrations and inner tensions in the child because

1. the child's interests and capabilities are not considered
2. the parent cannot accept behavior that does not further the goal
3. the parent expects continuing perfection
4. the child will make every effort to achieve

176. Parents should recognize that most small children will return, temporarily, to thumbsucking when they need

1. comforting
2. attention
3. rest
4. excitement

177. If parents reverse their orders or requests because the small child tells them NO, the child will later have difficulty developing

1. at his normal rate
2. an ability to think for himself
3. a realistic idea of himself
4. better ways to control the parents

178. The nurse who cares for the hospitalized child must always recognize that there is some threat to his security because

a. he is separated from his parents
b. strange people are caring for him
c. it is the first time he has been away from home
d. sickness is a new experience

1. all of the above
2. a only
3. a and b
4. b, c, and d

179. A good way to help a child overcome the need to tell highly imaginative stories is

1. to provide him with interesting experiences to talk about
2. to restrict his activities until he can face reality
3. to provide him with playmates who will not accept such stories
4. to punish him each time he is guilty of this behavior

180. The term "emotional trauma" refers to

1. an injury that stops personality growth
2. harmful experiences of an emotional nature
3. emotional experiences that have damaging effects on the personality
4. physical injuries that are emotionally crippling

181. A sick child may develop a distrust of his parents who left him to be cared for by nurses, if the nurses are guilty of

1. telling him lies to get his cooperation
2. bribing him
3. hurting him without giving an explanation
4. making fun of him because he is not a "big boy"

182. The nurse who has empathy with a sick child will be able

1. to understand all his behavior
2. to appreciate the problems his parents create
3. to recognize his dislikes and jealousies
4. to anticipate his fears

183. A mother may be unconsciously resentful of the care the nurse gives her sick child because

1. the nurse has not had enough experience
2. she feels incapable of giving good care herself
3. the uniform makes the nurse look impersonal
4. the child indicates that he likes the nurse

184. The nurse who works well with sick children is one who is able

1. to remember her own childhood feelings
2. to sympathize with the child's loneliness
3. to recognize symptoms of regression
4. to understand behavior problems

185. The nurse could get helpful background information about the sick child if she would listen to

a. the morning report
b. staff conferences
c. the child
d. the parents

    1. d only
    2. all of the above
    3. b and c
    4. c and d

186. When the hospitalized child wets and soils the bed, the practical nurse must recognize and accept it as one way in which he is able to express his objections to

1. being cared for by strangers
2. being left by his parents
3. medicines and treatments
4. hospital foods

187. If the sick child wets the bed because he cannot make the nurse understand that he wants to urinate, his natural reaction to discipline for the bed wetting will be

1. fear   3. jealousy
2. anger   4. depression

188. The child may interpret his hospitalization as

a. abandonment
b. rejection
c. overprotection
d. punishment

    1. all of the above
    2. a, b, or d
    3. all except b
    4. a only

189. Observation of the very small child is most important during sickness because

1. his symptoms are more severe
2. his behavior must indicate his discomfort
3. resistance is low at such an age
4. personality problems are more frequent

190. A room for treatment away from the patient-care area would be especially important on the ward for sick children because

1. the child will be more cooperative
2. treatment can be done more rapidly
3. dangerous instruments can be locked up
4. children misunderstand what they see

191. The sick child who does not want the T.L.C. (tender loving care) offered by the nurse may refuse it because

1. such care makes him more lonesome for his mother
2. the nurse frightens him
3. he feels too old for such attention
4. he is too sick to be bothered with unnecessary attention

192. The nurse can encourage chronic invalidism if in her care of the sick child she

1. treats him like a child
2. does not let him do the things he can do
3. helps him enjoy his treatments
4. is stingy with her sympathy

193. When the nurse tells the mother of a sick child, "You have nothing to worry about, we will take good care of your child," the mother's anxiety may be increased because she is afraid

1. the nurse has not had enough training
2. she is not being told the truth
3. the nurse does not appreciate the seriousness of the child's illness
4. the nurse will take her place in the child's affections

194. The nurse who takes care of the sick child must understand the relationship between

1. doctor and child
2. behavior and age
3. sickness and treatment
4. emotions and sickness

195. The small child will feel less insecurity in the hospital if his parents think to provide him with

1. a favorite toy
2. home-prepared foods
3. daily gifts from members of the family
4. news from home

196. The attitude of the nurse toward the sick child's toy must be

1. considerate
2. one based upon the sanitary condition of the toy
3. one of respect, no matter how worn it is
4. one of interest in what makes it work

197. The nurse could ease some of the mother's feelings of guilt for putting her child in the hospital if she would

1. ask questions that would give the mother a chance to explode
2. let the mother stay with the child all the time
3. explain the need for skilled care which the child could not get at home
4. allow the mother to help with some of the child's care

198. If this period of hospitalization is the first time the school age child has ever been away from home for more than a few hours, the nurse should realize that some of the mother's "difficult" behavior is based on a fear

1. of neglect by the nurses
2. of losing her child's love
3. that the child will be in pain
4. that the child will learn to enjoy being away from home

199. The nurse should not be disturbed by the child's crying when it is time for mother to leave the hospital. She should recognize it as <u>a healthy sign</u> because

1. it is good for a child to miss its mother
2. crying gives a child's lungs needed exercise and stimulates deep breathing
3. the child is actively expressing its feelings of anger rather than repressing them
4. only a child who is improving physically will cry

200. The criticism parents make of the kind of nursing care their sick child receives is probably an expression of their

1. anxiety
2. inexperience
3. ignorance
4. differences of opinion

201. Knowledge of <u>normal</u> growth and development patterns should help the practical nurse assigned to a children's hospital ward as she tries

1. to keep the children progressing as they would at home
2. to prevent regression of behavior
3. to recognize the tricks the sick child uses to get attention
4. to be more understanding of the sick child's behavior

202. The mother of three grade-school children prides herself on spending all her time and energy cooking and caring for her family. An informed practical nurse could advise this mother that

1. she is worthy of special praise
2. her unselfish behavior is unusual
3. she is using all her energies to care for her family and is not caring for her own physical health
4. she is failing to develop interests that will keep her occupied as her family gets older

203. The development of a mature adult personality requires that parents gradually

1. insist that the child take care of all his immediate needs
2. cut all emotional strings and let the child find new interests
3. give the teen-ager more and more responsibility for his behavior
4. plan new experiences for the child

204. The "show off" teen-ager or adult is really expressing his fear of

1. "being lost in the crowd"
2. people
3. authority
4. being an ineffective person

205. The parent who "sowed his wild oats" early may not allow his teen-ager to date, to go to boy-girl parties, etc. Such suspicion of his offspring is based on

1. projection
2. genuine concern for its welfare
3. sound information about children today
4. a need to protect the child from the mistakes of the father

206. The anxieties and guilt feelings present in the adolescent are caused by the demands of

1. the id   3. the superego
2. the ego   4. the Oedipus

207. The adult who finds it necessary to exaggerate the truth has not had adequate parental guidance through the childhood problem of

1. obedience   3. property rights
2. discipline   4. imagination

208. Any person interested in preparing for old age will find it important to plan for

1. something to do
2. someone to take care of him
3. a comfortable home of his own
4. money enough to buy all the foods usually enjoyed

209. A healthy attitude toward the aging process requires an individual to accept

1. responsibility for growing old
2. the gradual but steady changes in body function
3. assistance during times of dependence
4. emotional support from his children

210. An emotionally healthy, happy, adjusted geriatric patient has at one time been

1. a most devoted parent
2. an emotionally well-adjusted child and adult
3. helped to emotional health by psychiatric guidance
4. materially successful

211. Mrs. A, a widow age 75, has been living alone for 10 years. She is now considering buying life care in a home for elderly persons because she feels the need of

1. a greater degree of independence
2. a more flexible schedule than she has at home
3. getting away from family supervision
4. more opportunities for companionship

212. Children and relatives of the aging person should expect to see an increase of, or an appearance of, behavior previously controlled. A common characteristic of the aging is

1. forgetfulness   3. selfishness
2. moodiness   4. boastfulness

213. The aging parent who lives in the home of a son or daughter is too often unintentionally encouraged to be

1. useless   3. alone
2. extravagant   4. independent

214. Aged persons have the same basic needs as the small child. To help satisfy these needs, they should be encouraged

1. to live alone
2. to take part in group activities
3. to eat several meals during the day
4. to keep in touch with relatives

215. In a household of young people the oldster will have frequent feelings of

1. indifference   3. loneliness
2. insecurity   4. rebellion

216. The practical nurse who is skilled at putting elderly patients at ease is one who does not demand that

1. the patient keep to a schedule that is best for his health
2. the habits of a lifetime be given up
3. the patient worry about making decisions
4. the patient be completely independent of the nurse

217. The elderly person is encouraged, even when he is sick, to do as many things as possible for himself in order to keep up his

1. economic security
2. emotional independence
3. regression
4. energy

218. The sympathetic practical nurse who cares for the elderly sick patient may be guilty of encouraging the patient's

1. dependence
2. selfishness
3. depressed moods
4. disorientation

219. An older patient's feelings of importance will be increased by the younger nurse who

1. leaves him alone to do as he wishes
2. permits him to watch television
3. listens to his stories of the "old days"
4. waits on him and leaves few decisions for him to make

NUTRITION AND DIET THERAPY
PART I

(Answer sheets pp. 303-304)

PART I of this section is concerned with basic principles of body needs and body uses of food nutrients, plus the specific food needs of the various age groups. PART II covers the diet adaptations that must be made as part of the treatment program for various disease conditions.

1. Over the last 50 years our national dietary intake has gradually improved because of the increased use of

    1. highly sweet foods
    2. flour and cereal foods
    3. potatoes and other vegetables
    4. milk, fruit, and vegetables

2. Recent studies of the meals served in homes in the United States show that many families are still not getting the necessary amounts of

    1. breads and cereals
    2. meat and potatoes
    3. milk and citrus fruits
    4. meat and vegetables

3. The most important reason why the nutritional intake is inadequate in most homes is

    1. lack of money
    2. not enough information about foods
    3. poor eating habits
    4. poor food preparation

4. Hidden hunger is the result of

    1. a lack of important food substances over a long period of time
    2. an empty feeling in the stomach
    3. going without food for 2 or 3 days
    4. a diet made up of fluids that leave the stomach quickly

5. The first important step in improving food habits is

    1. to follow the example of someone you think knows what makes up a good diet
    2. to learn about the different ways the body uses foods
    3. to be aware of the food you are eating
    4. to notice how you feel after you eat

6. Inadequate breakfasts may result in

    1. too little meat and eggs in the diet
    2. a lowering of morning efficiency
    3. lifelong poor food habits
    4. an attempt to "make up" food needs in the other two meals of the day

7. The food habits of an adult will probably be good if

    1. he has had a college education
    2. they were started in eary childhood
    3. he has a chance to read good books and magazines
    4. the income is enough to buy a variety of foods

8. The essential food nutrients are

    1. proteins, fats, and carbohydrates
    2. needed by every person regardless of age
    3. found only in a few foods
    4. vitamins, minerals, and water

9. A good diet is defined as one that

    1. looks and tastes "good"
    2. includes plenty of at least two of the main nutrient essentials
    3. consists of all foods properly prepared
    4. contains adequate amounts of the essential nutrients

10. Two of the most essential food nutrient groups are

    1. proteins and minerals
    2. meat and potatoes
    3. fruits and butter
    4. green vegetables and breads

11. The form of carbohydrate found in the blood is

    1. dextrin
    2. cellulose
    3. glucose
    4. lactose

12. Every food will supply the body with

    1. important minerals and vitamins
    2. complete proteins
    3. some carbohydrates
    4. some heat and energy

13. A menu of navy beans, bread, butter, and ice cream would be lacking in which of the basic food groups?

    1. milk group
    2. meat group
    3. bread-cereal group
    4. fruit-vegetable group

14. Carbohydrates are needed in the diet primarily

    1. to rebuild worn out tissues in the body
    2. to supply material for building bones
    3. to help regulate body processes
    4. to supply heat and energy

15. Lactose is a form of carbohydrate found in

    1. milk   3. apples
    2. toast   4. sugar

16. The carbohydrate stored in the liver is called

    1. glucose   3. lactose
    2. glycogen   4. sucrose

17. The food listed below that belongs to the carbohydrate group is

    1. fruit   3. meat
    2. milk   4. eggs

18. The carbohydrate glycogen is found in large amounts in

    1. fish
    2. cereals and breads
    3. the liver
    4. vegetables

19. One example of a food containing a complete protein is

    1. gelatine   3. navy beans
    2. wheat   4. veal

20. Carbohydrate foods are needed by the body daily to supply materials for

    1. growth and development
    2. heat and energy
    3. tissue building
    4. regulating body processes

21. The end product of carbohydrate digestion that is ready for use by the body cells is called

    1. dextrose   3. lactose
    2. glucose   4. sucrose

22. Whole-grain cereals are considered good breakfast cereals because they

    1. are more easily digested
    2. contain larger quantities of protein
    3. supply greater amounts of carbohydrates
    4. contain more minerals and vitamins

23. When the term "enrichment" is used on the label of breads and cereals, it means that

    1. such foods are better for you than the unenriched products
    2. these products have about the same food value as whole grain products
    3. more milk has been used in the preparation of these products
    4. iron, thiamine, niacin, and riboflavin have been added to the refined product

24. One reason for cooking cereals is

    1. to kill harmful bacteria
    2. to make them easier to digest
    3. to remove the cellulose
    4. to provide a more nutritious food

25. The primary function of protein is

    1. to provide heat and energy
    2. to serve as padding to protect body organs
    3. to keep the body strong and healthy
    4. to build and repair body tissues

26. Each gram of protein will provide the body with

    1. 9 calories   3. 6 calories
    2. 3 calories   4. 4 calories

27. Foods listed below that are known to be good sources of protein are

    1. peas and green beans
    2. bananas, apricots, and plums
    3. meat and milk
    4. whole-grain products

28. Protein foods have nutrient value because they contain

    1. lengthwise fibers
    2. different kinds of amino acids
    3. connective tissue that holds the fibers together
    4. extractives that give meat its flavor

29. When children have inadequate protein in their diets, the result is

    1. underdevelopment of muscle tissues
    2. too few calories for their energy needs
    3. poorly developed bones
    4. gums that bleed easily

30. Most of our daily protein intake should come from

    1. citrus fruits and green vegetables
    2. foods that have been thoroughly cooked
    3. foods easily digested
    4. sources of complete protein

31. If a healthy adult requires 1 gram of protein per kilogram of body weight, how many grams of protein are required by a man weighing 145 pounds?

    1. 51   3. 75
    2. 66   4. 82

32. Amino acids are important because they are

    1. acids found in tart fruits
    2. end products of fat digestion
    3. protein in meat
    4. building units of which proteins are composed

33. A food that contains considerable protein but not of the kind that promotes growth is

    1. milk   3. navy beans
    2. fish   4. fruit

34. Foods that contain all essential amino acids are said to be

    1. emulsified fats
    2. complete proteins
    3. hydrogenated fats
    4. essential

35. If the adult gets too little protein in his diet, it can result in

    1. anemia
    2. retarded growth
    3. decreased ability to digest foods
    4. an increased need for calcium intake

36. Amino acids are

    1. the acids found in fruits
    2. the end product of fat digestion
    3. the building units of which proteins are composed
    4. the acids produced when food does not digest properly

37. Every individual needs some milk daily because it is the best common source of

    1. protein and iron
    2. vitamin A and vitamin B
    3. calcium and riboflavin
    4. calcium and vitamin C

38. Milk cannot be considered a "perfect" food because it lacks

    1. vitamin A and thiamine
    2. phosphorous and vitamin D
    3. vitamins C and D and iron
    4. carbohydrate and vitamin C

39. An intake of the recommended amounts of milk and milk products will not be constipating if

    1. they are not eaten at the end of the meal
    2. used only in moderate amounts
    3. 4 or more servings are also consumed daily from the fruit-vegetable group
    4. they are cooked into foods instead of being eaten alone

40. Milk is least expensive when it is in the form of

    1. skim milk
    2. evaporated milk
    3. nonfat dry milk
    4. buttermilk

41. When milk is heated in cooking

    1. important nutrients are destroyed
    2. its protein coagulates
    3. the digestibility is impaired
    4. it is usually less acceptable as a food

42. The food value of cultured milk (butter-milk, yogurt, etc.) is

    1. increased because of the special bacteria used in the souring process
    2. less, since the souring destroys some of the vitamins
    3. the same as the food value of the milk from which it is made
    4. an important addition to the diets of many people

43. Cheese is important in our diet because

    1. it is quickly digested
    2. it is an economical source of high-quality protein
    3. it is a good source of energy material
    4. it takes only 1/4 ounce to equal 1 cup of milk

44. It is important to cook cheese

    1. at low temperature
    2. mixed with other foods
    3. primarily for the flavor it adds
    4. in small amounts because of its high fat content

45. Eggs are nutritionally important in the diet because

    1. they are complete protein foods
    2. of the numerous ways they may be served
    3. they are good sources of energy
    4. they contain phosphorus and calcium

46. The fat in eggs is easily digested because it is

    1. an animal fat
    2. homogenized
    3. present only in small amounts
    4. emulsified

47. When cooking eggs in water

    1. soft cook them so that they will be digestible
    2. keep the water from boiling
    3. cover pan and boil rapidly for five minutes
    4. boil 10 minutes so that the yolk and white will be firm

48. A mineral found in important amounts in eggs is

    1. calcium   3. iron
    2. thiamine   4. lactose

49. When subjected to a high temperature, the protein of eggs will

    1. become tough and leathery
    2. coagulate
    3. be indigestible
    4. be hard cooked

50. Meats supply important amounts of

    1. vitamins A and C
    2. water and starches
    3. carbohydrates and fats
    4. protein and iron

51. Meat is important in the diet as a source of

    1. cellulose   3. iodine
    2. vitamin K   4. the B vitamins

52. The connective tissue of meat

    1. contains the minerals of the meat
    2. is made more digestible in the cooking process
    3. is an important source of bulk in the diet
    4. gives the meat its flavor

53. Less tender cuts of meat should be cooked

    1. in a pot on top of the stove
    2. by the moist-heat method
    3. by pan-broiling
    4. by the dry-heat method

54. To cook meat in the oven, the temperature should be between

    1. 300-350   3. 400-450
    2. 250-300   4. 350-400

55. Moist-heat cookery requires that the liquid

    1. completely cover the meat
    2. be kept at a simmering temperature
    3. boil rapidly
    4. just cover the bottom of the pan

56. A round of beef can be made most tender cooking it by

    1. braising   3. frying
    2. roasting   4. broiling

57. A shoulder roast of veal would be most tender if

    1. roasted in an uncovered pan in the oven
    2. cooked under the broiler
    3. pan fried
    4. potroasted on top of the stove

58. The best way to pan-broil ground beef is

    1. to place it in a hot, greased skillet and cook it rapidly
    2. to cook it slowly in an ungreased skillet and pour off the fat as it accumulates
    3. to melt enough fat to cover the bottom of the skillet and fry in this fat
    4. to use the broiling rack in the oven, placed three inches from the heat

59. The extractives in meat

    1. give the characteristic flavor and odor when the meat is cooked
    2. tenderize the connective tissue
    3. shorten the preparation time
    4. add valuable nutrients to meat soups

60. A food high in protein is

    1. corn   3. fish
    2. green beans   4. potatoes

61. In the list below foods that may occasionally be substituted for meat are

    1. bread stuffs and cereals
    2. vegetables
    3. bacon and salt pork
    4. dried beans and nuts

62. Most meat is quickly digested because

    1. it is a high-protein food
    2. of its marbling with fat
    3. it has been thoroughly cooked
    4. the extractives stimulate gastric secretions

63. The dry-heat method is used on meat cuts prepared by

    1. potroasting   3. stewing
    2. broiling   4. braising

64. A meat that would be prepared by the moist-heat method is

    1. T-bone steak   3. stew meat
    2. ground meat   4. rib roast

65. Proper storage for fresh meat includes

    1. wiping with a damp cloth and placing uncovered in the refrigerator
    2. washing and wrapping it closely before placing it in the refrigerator
    3. wrapping it loosely and storing it in the coldest part of the refrigerator
    4. keeping it in a closed container in the coldest part of the refrigerator

66. A meal high in fat has the physiological effect of

    1. increasing the muscular contractions of the stomach
    2. producing nausea
    3. slowing up the emptying time of the stomach
    4. making the meal more appetizing

67. When some fat is present in the diet the body can make better use of

    1. the minerals, iron, and calcium
    2. proteins for building body tissue
    3. the vitamins A, D, and K
    4. the carbohydrates, glucose, and glycogen

68. The most important function of fat in the diet is

    1. to supply more calories for heat and energy
    2. to serve as a padding around the organs
    3. to serve as a reserve fuel supply
    4. to promote better health in body tissues

69. A diet very low in fats is usually not well accepted by patients because

    1. fat foods may be nauseating
    2. it is not appetizing
    3. the patient gets hungry too soon
    4. it cannot be prepared attractively

70. When the term "emulsified" is applied to fat in foods it means that

    1. it is difficult to digest
    2. it has been heated to too high a temperature
    3. it has been changed from a solid to a liquid fat
    4. it is in very finely divided particles

71. The practical nurse should be aware that the food value is exactly the same in

    1. fortified margarine and lard
    2. codliver oil and corn oil
    3. butter and fortified margarine
    4. mayonnaise and French dressing

72. A hydrogenated fat is one that has

    1. had vitamins A and D added
    2. been changed from a liquid to a solid form
    3. been treated to break up the fat particles
    4. not been properly refrigerated

73. Care of fat to keep it from becoming rancid includes

    1. keeping it in a tightly closed can on the back of the range
    2. straining all fat drippings before storing them
    3. not permitting the fat to get so hot that it starts to smoke
    4. keeping the fat in a closed container under refrigeration

74. Mineral oil, as it is used in the diet,

    1. is a satisfactory substitute for other oils in salad dressings
    2. is nutritionally acceptable on a reducing diet
    3. interferes with the absorption of digested food substances into the blood stream
    4. belongs to the group of food stuffs called "fats and oils"

75. An example of a food containing an emulsified fat is

    1. pork   3. beef
    2. eggs   4. bananas

76. The food listed below that contains the largest amount of fat is

    1. roast beef   3. liver
    2. mayonnaise   4. bananas

77. A primary function of minerals in the diet is

    1. to promote healthy mucous membrane linings
    2. to aid in the prevention of infection
    3. to promote a healthy digestive tract
    4. to assist in regulating body processes

78. Good bone and tooth structure depend on an adequate supply of

    1. iron, phosphorus, and vitamin C
    2. calcium, vitamin D, and phosphorus
    3. copper, calcium, and phosphorus
    4. iron, copper, and sodium

79. The production of hemoglobin requires a daily intake of foods containing

1. vitamin D　　3. vitamin C
2. copper　　　4. iron

80. An important use of calcium by the body is

1. the stimulation of gastric juice secretion
2. in the coagulation of blood
3. in the prevention of anemia in young children
4. in building good red blood

81. In addition to milk, calcium can be supplied by eating

1. celery
2. whipping cream
3. dark green leafy vegetables
4. whole-grain breads and cereals

82. Which of the following foods would contribute the most calcium in an average serving?

1. creamed peas　　3. cottage cheese
2. custard　　　　4. carrots

83. Iron is needed by the body

1. to aid in the formation of hemoglobin
2. to promote the development of strong bones and teeth
3. to prevent the development of rickets
4. to maintain the acid-base balance

84. The thyroid gland cannot function normally if the diet lacks adequate

1. vitamin K
2. high-calorie foods
3. hemoglobin-building foods
4. iodine

85. Normal bone development will be interferred with when the diet supplies too little

1. vitamin A　　3. vitamin D
2. iodine　　　4. iron

86. An important food source of iron is

1. milk　　3. beets
2. eggs　　4. apples

87. A food that is a poor source of iron is

1. milk　　　3. liver
2. spinach　　4. navy beans

88. The normal clotting of blood depends on an adequate intake of

1. calcium　　　3. thiamin
2. vitamin C　　4. iron

89. An example of a food that leaves an acid-ash residue after being metabolized is

1. eggs　　　3. butter
2. lemons　　4. asparagus

90. An alkaline-ash-forming food is

1. fruit　　3. sugar
2. eggs　　4. meat

91. An excellent source of vitamin A can be found in food such as

1. oranges　　3. cabbage
2. carrots　　4. beets

92. A food, often included in a tossed vegetable salad, that contains large amounts of vitamin C is

1. green pepper　　3. raw carrots
2. celery　　　　4. lettuce

93. Resistance to infection is lowered in the mucous membrane linings of the body when there is too little

1. vitamin A　　　3. vitamin B-12
2. ascorbic acid　　4. thiamine

94. One of the best sources of ascorbic acid is

1. pineapple　　3. carrots
2. spinach　　　4. oranges

95. Vitamin D must be present in the body before use can be made of the intake of

1. iodine
2. calcium
3. iron
4. copper

96. Milk should be used daily because it supplies necessary

1. lactose, which is easily digested
2. protein, which is a complete protein
3. riboflavin
4. fats in an emulsified form

97. The diet of a healthy person should include eggs because they contain valuable amounts of

1. emulsified fats, which are quickly digested
2. iron needed for the formation of hemoglobin
3. vitamin A
4. phosphorus for building good bones

98. A diet deficient in riboflavin could be expected

1. if most of the calories come from enriched breads and cereals
2. when there is too little fat in the diet
3. in the person who does not use milk
4. to occur more often in children than in adults

99. In the presence of a liver disease, the prevention of the absorption of some nutrients results in

1. a copper deficiency
2. incomplete digestion of protein
3. a vitamin K deficiency
4. gradual starvation

100. A food high in thiamine is

1. eggs
2. milk
3. pork
4. tomatoes

101. Spongy, bleeding gums may occur when the diet supplies an inadequate amount of

1. ascorbic acid
2. calcium
3. vitamin A
4. riboflavin

102. Vitamin B_{12} is probably best supplied by a food such as

1. lean meat
2. cereals
3. eggs
4. liver

103. Night blindness may occur as a result of a deficiency of

1. calcium
2. vitamin A
3. vitamin C
4. vitamin D

104. The strength of the walls of the capillaries is reduced (resulting in small hemorrhages) when the diet contains too little

1. riboflavin
2. ascorbic acid
3. vitamin A
4. vitamin K

105. Riboflavin is found in largest amounts in

1. milk
2. meats
3. vegetables
4. fruit

106. The body uses thiamine

1. to maintain healthy nerves
2. to promote the manufacture of red bone cells in the bone marrow
3. to prevent the development of scurvy
4. to maintain proper functioning of the thyroid gland

107. A food that would not supply much vitamin C is

1. pineapple juice
2. fresh strawberries
3. orange juice
4. raw cabbage

108. A student nurse's decision to eat liver once a week instead of taking self-prescribed vitamin B complex concentrate is based on her understanding that

1. liver is cheaper
2. an oral concentrate is poorly absorbed
3. liver contains other nutrients also
4. liver is good for her

109. A food that is not a good source of vitamin A is

   1. lettuce
   2. eggs
   3. green pepper
   4. carrots

110. When mineral oil is taken every day, the body will lose

   1. too much fluid
   2. the fat-soluble vitamins in food
   3. most of the mineral intake
   4. all of the vitamin B

111. Dried beans are of no value for their vitamin B complex content if

   1. they are boiled for a long time
   2. salt is added early in the cooking period
   3. baked at a high temperature in the oven
   4. the water in which they are soaked is poured off

112. The thiamine and ascorbic-acid content of foods is destroyed if

   1. soda is added to foods during cooking
   2. freshly cooked vegetables stand at room temperature
   3. foods are prepared with vinegar or lemon juice
   4. fruits and vegetables are frozen

113. If the greatest number of vitamins in vegetables is to be saved, we must

   a. use the least possible amount of boiling water
   b. cook just until tender
   c. add salt at the end of the cooking period
   d. use the liquid from the vegetable

      1. a, b , and c
      2. b and d only
      3. a, b, and d
      4. a, c, and d

114. Each gram of fat taken as food yields approximately

   1. 4 calories
   2. 9 calories
   3. 6 calories
   4. 12 calories

115. The term "basal metabolism" refers to

   1. the energy requirements of the body
   2. the total number of calories used when the body is at rest
   3. the fuel needs during muscular action
   4. total caloric needs for the day or the week

116. A calorie is

   1. the amount of heat produced when food is used by the body
   2. a unit of measuring heat produced by the burning of food
   3. the amount of energy found in carbo- hydrate foods
   4. the fuel value of foods

117. The highest calorie count would come from

   1. 1 cup of spinach
   2. 1/4 cup of heavy cream
   3. 1 medium banana
   4. 1 egg

118. The number of calories needed by an individual at rest is

   1. called his lowest caloric rate
   2. about 900
   3. increased with age
   4. known as his basal metabolic rate

119. Foods containing cellulose are valuable in the diet because the cellulose·

   1. contains no calories and is not fattening
   2. absorbs water, thus increasing the bulk in the intestines
   3. can stop hunger pangs
   4. can be eaten in large amounts by any individual

120. The mechanical irritation produced by high cellulose foods can be lessened by

   1. boiling
   2. baking
   3. puréeing
   4. peeling

121. Cellulose is found in abundance in

    1. refined flour and cereals
    2. milk and milk products
    3. fruits and vegetables
    4. meat and poultry products

122. A food containing considerable cellulose is

    1. navy beans
    2. enriched white bread
    3. shredded wheat biscuit
    4. round steak

123. Water is valuable to the body because it helps

    1. to prepare foods for more rapid digestion
    2. to regulate body temperature
    3. to decrease peristaltic movement of the digestive tract
    4. to lubricate the digestive tract

124. The body needs for fluids are greatly influenced by

    1. the sex of the person
    2. the adequacy of protein
    3. the activity of the person
    4. the total food intake

125. Much of the water we drink is absorbed into the body from

    1. the stomach
    2. the kidney
    3. the intestines
    4. the small veins in the body

126. Water taken into an empty stomach in the morning

    1. helps to satisfy hunger and prevents overeating
    2. remains in the stomach for an hour or more
    3. stimulates peristalsis and evacuation
    4. tends to improve the appetite

127. An average serving of a vegetable is

    1. 1 cup   3. 1 large cup
    2. 1/3 cup   4. 1/2 cup

128. The body is said to be in "water balance" when

    1. thirst has been satisfied
    2. intake equals output
    3. 6 to 8 glasses a day have been consumed
    4. the amount of urine excreted exceeds the amount of water used

129. When there is an inadequate amount of water in the body tissues

    1. one does not perspire so much
    2. the skin becomes scaly
    3. the condition is called dehydration
    4. the amount of minerals in the diet should be decreased

130. As soon as fresh vegetables are received, they should be

    1. stored in an open container in the refrigerator
    2. washed, covered, and kept cold
    3. kept in a cool place
    4. washed just before they are used

131. Selections from the vegetable-fruit group of the basic four in an adequate diet would number

    1. 2 servings a day
    2. 4 or more servings a day
    3. 1 serving a day
    4. 6 or more servings a day

132. Cooked vegetables will keep their vitamin and mineral content if they are

    1. kept under refrigeration at all times
    2. cooked in small amounts of water until tender
    3. placed in cold water to restore their crispness
    4. cooked rapidly in enough boiling water to cover

133. In selecting a green or yellow vegetable for the day's menu, you would not pick

    1. pumpkin   3. beet greens
    2. head lettuce   4. broccoli

134. When fresh fruits and vegetables are used in a salad which is kept at room temperature for several hours, the resulting nutritive change is

1. a change in color
2. loss of crisp texture
3. a wilted, unappetizing appearance
4. loss of much of the vitamin C content

135. To consider pork safe to eat, it should be cooked

1. at a temperature of 400°F, allowing 15 minutes cooking time per pound
2. until the center of the meat shows no pinkish color
3. at temperatures much lower than that required for beef
4. for a long time at a low temperature

136. Adequate refrigeration of cooked protein foods requires

a. cooling as rapidly as possible
b. storing at a temperature around 50°
c. placing in shallow containers
d. refrigerating as soon as cooled

1. b and d
2. all of the above
3. b, c, and d
4. a, c, and d

137. Washing fruits and vegetables before eating them raw is considered a safe food practice because

1. dangerous sprays or fertilizers are removed
2. farm workers with disease may have harvested the foods
3. such goods are exposed to the germs of many people in the stores
4. all parasites would be removed

138. The chief reason that bacteria and parasites gain entrance to the body through food is

1. insufficient cooking of meat
2. storing of utensils where rodents can reach them
3. insanitary food-handling practices
4. failure to use safety procedures in dressing rabbits

139. The food and drug law considers a food "misbranded" if

1. it contains any substance harmful to the human body
2. a substance has been added, such as a coloring, to hide poor quality
3. a statement of weight, measure or content is not printed on the label
4. packing is done under insanitary conditions

140. Outbreaks of food poisoning most often can be traced to

a. staphylococci bacteria
b. parasites
c. Salmonella organisms
d. chemical poisons

1. a only
2. all of the above
3. a, b, and d
4. a and c

141. The most serious physical disturbance caused by a parasite in food results from ingestion of

1. pinworm
2. trichinae
3. tapeworm
4. ameoba

142. Sickness caused by contaminated food could be prevented by constant attention to the recommended food-handling practice of

1. keeping foods containing protein under continuous refrigeration until ready to use
2. canning nonacid vegetables by the water-bath method
3. washing all raw meat thoroughly before cooking
4. covering an infection on the hand before touching food

143. The practical nurse should know that foods containing the staphylococcus organisms can be heated and that the organism will be

1. killed, making the food safe to eat
2. unaffected
3. removed from all protein foods
4. destroyed but the toxins are unaffected

144. Botulinus poisoning is most commonly the result of

1. eating meats that have not been thoroughly cooked
2. preparation that calls for excessive handling of food
3. eating improperly home-canned nonacid foods
4. holding protein foods at room temperature for a long period

145. Salmonella organisms reach the gastro-intestinal system when

1. cooking equipment is insanitary
2. hands are not washed at frequent intervals
3. fresh fruits and vegetables are not thoroughly washed
4. prepared meat and dairy products are stored at room temperature

146. Chemical poisoning from foods can occur from the use of

1. the green part of sprouting potatoes
2. cooking highly acid fruits in aluminum utensils
3. sulfur dioxide in the drying process for dried fruits
4. sodium benzoate used as a preservative in jams and jellies

147. A food fallacy is described as

1. the scientific beliefs about foods
2. the information passed on by super-stitious people
3. a popular belief about a certain food
4. a misconception about food

148. An individual will not be fooled by food fads and fallacies if his prepara-tion includes

1. a distrust of all agents who have something to sell
2. a fund of information supplied by friends
3. knowledge of the nutritive value of foods
4. an ability to check the truth of ad-vertised items

149. A food fad is a belief about food that is

1. highly publicized in magazines and newspapers
2. advertised on television
3. not established by scientific research
4. handed down from generation to generation

150. The statement "a slice of toast has fewer calories than a slice of bread" is an example of

1. the truth
2. a food fallacy
3. a food fad
4. information that is usable in diet planning

151. The greatest danger of a dietary plan based on food fads and fallacies occurs when

1. competent medical attention is de-layed
2. the foods are expensive
3. nutritional foods are then refused
4. the products are not readily available

152. Foods purchased at so-called "health stores"

1. often are more nutritious than foods purchased elsewhere
2. taste and look better than similar foods from the grocery
3. may be injurious to health
4. usually cost more than similar foods at the grocery

153. Check the one statement below that is a food fallacy:

1. Milk curdles when it reaches the stomach
2. Whole-wheat bread is much less fattening than white bread
3. A tablespoon of butter has the same food value as a tablespoon of margarine
4. Foods cooked in aluminum are just as wholesome as foods cooked in stainless steel

154. Which of the following statements is true?

1. an acid condition of the body is increased by acid fruits
2. milk and cheese are not constipating
3. pasteurizing milk destroys its nutritive value
4. milk is fattening

155. The use of certain laxatives advertised as reducing remedies can result in

1. considerable weight loss
2. irritation of the bowel
3. loss of nutrients in foods eaten
4. excessive excretion of body fluids

156. A food fad adopted by many individuals is

1. the use of nonfat dry milk to increase the protein intake
2. the sweetening of foods on reducing diets with noncalorie sweeteners
3. the use of stone-ground whole-wheat flour in place of regular whole-wheat flour.
4. the drinking of fruit juices for breakfast

157. The practice of taking vitamin concentrates without a physician's advice is not encouraged because

1. most vitamin concentrates are quite expensive
2. a varied diet will supply both vitamins and other essentials
3. it is possible to take too much with adverse affects
4. you are using products that you know nothing about

158. Before adequate plans for family meals can be made, it will be necessary to consider first

1. the amount of money available for each type of food
2. the season of the year
3. the likes and dislikes of all family members
4. the nutritional needs of each member

159. A key nutrient group around which most meals should be planned is

1. breads and cereals
2. protein foods
3. vitamins and minerals
4. fruits and vegetables

160. Indicate which of these food lists will provide the daily calcium requirement for an adult:

1. 1 serving of cereal, 1 glass of milk, and 1 egg
2. 1 serving of meat, 1 serving of a green, leafy vegetable, 2 slices of bread
3. 1 serving of cream soup, 1 serving of fruit, and 1 serving of fish
4. 1 glass of milk, 1 egg, 1 ounce of American cheese

161. The housewife can expect that planning menus several days in advance will

1. increase the difficulty in making the best use of leftovers
2. require too much of her time
3. not be a practical procedure for most housewives
4. save time in shopping for food

162. Foods that are most acceptable as snacks are

1. sandwiches, milk, or cookies
2. candy, pop, or ice cream
3. foods that are low in nutrients
4. foods that contribute more than just calories

163. What is lacking in a menu of baked fish, mashed potato, cabbage salad, bread and ice cream?

1. a source of vitamin C
2. sufficient protein
3. calcium
4. variety in color

164. Which one of the following foods would be considered a "light" dessert?

1. cream pie   3. custard
2. gelatin dessert   4. angel food cake

165. A good food-shopping habit that should result in more economical purchasing is the practice of

1. doing most of your shopping where the clerks know you
2. purchasing by name brand only
3. preparing and using a shopping list
4. shopping several times a week

166. The nutritive value, the color, and the flavor of cooked vegetables will be retained if they are prepared

1. in an open kettle, in boiling, salted water, until they are very tender
2. in a large amount of rapidly boiling, unsalted water, until done
3. in cold water and cooked just until tender
4. in a covered container, in a small amount of boiling, salted water, just until tender

167. Select the one breakfast in the following list that includes the greatest variety of essential nutrients:

1. orange juice, muffins, bacon, butter, jelly, coffee
2. pineapple juice, sweet rolls, butter, coffee
3. cereal, buttered toast, sausage, milk
4. grapefruit, scrambled eggs, toast, butter, milk

168. If a breakfast is planned to include sliced oranges, bacon, eggs, muffins, butter, and coffee, which food should be prepared first?

1. coffee
2. bacon
3. muffins
4. sliced oranges

169. Select from the following list the one meal that could be considered an adequate lunch:

1. hamburger on bun, potato chips, milk
2. macaroni and cheese, pickles, ice cream, coffee
3. egg salad sandwich, carrot sticks, peaches, milk
4. head lettuce salad, muffins, butter, baked apple, milk

170. The plans for the evening meal should give special attention

1. to making it as attractive as possible
2. to including a green or yellow vegetable to secure the day's needs of vitamin A
3. to preparation of foods all of the family members especially like
4. to including essential foods not eaten at previous meals of the day

171. Which one of the following foods is considered highly seasoned?

1. macaroni and cheese
2. breaded tomatoes
3. meat stew with vegetables
4. spaghetti with meat sauce

172. Select from the list below the food that would best classify as a low calorie dessert:

1. bread pudding with orange sauce
2. fruit in gelatin
3. ice cream
4. custard

173. Good nutrition during the preschool years is threatened by the practice of

1. allowing the child some freedom to choose from foods on the table
2. including sweet foods as part of his meals
3. frequent nibbling and piecing
4. allowing unlimited time to eat

174. The preschool child prefers his food served

1. in small amounts and mixed together
2. with considerable seasonings
3. either very warm or very cold
4. in separate small portions

175. The preschool child prefers a texture experience in his food such as that described by

1. the softness of cooked vegetables
2. the firmness of cheese dishes
3. the thickness of cereals and puddings
4. the moistness of meats and eggs

176. On the basis of normal weight increase, the nutritional requirements of the preschool child are

1. increased over those of the infant because he is growing rapidly
2. less than the nutritional requirements of the infant
3. less than the needs of an adult
4. about the same as the needs of an infant

177. The preschool child will learn to form acceptable food habits if

1. he has some freedom to choose between equally essential foods
2. he is urged to eat all of the food served to him
3. he is fed at the family table all of the time
4. he is helped whenever he has difficulty in handling his food

178. The preschool child will more readily accept his meals if

1. the portion sizes are small
2. foods are highly seasoned
3. soups, cereals, and puddings are thick
4. all foods are soft or liquid in consistency

179. The family menu includes broiled steak and mixed raw vegetable salad. From this menu, a 4-year-old child could be served

1. the same foods
2. a soft-cooked egg and creamed peas
3. a broiled beef patty and carrot curls
4. a cream soup and toast strips

180. The nutritional requirements of the preschool child are

1. greater because growth rate has increased
2. not much different from any other age level
3. less, on the basis of weight, than in infancy
4. difficult to achieve because the appetite tends to be less

181. The preschool child should be given food between meals if

1. he appears to be hungry
2. he has played hard and is tired
3. it will make him more contented
4. the foods used are simple and nutritious

182. Desserts that supply a larger amount of the key nutrients are

1. sponge cake
2. cookies
3. milk and egg dishes
4. fruit

183. A child should not be forced to eat food he does not want because

1. it will make him more stubborn
2. this can create a lifetime dislike for these foods
3. he has likes and dislikes just the same as adults
4. it will cause him to dislike the person feeding him

184. Milk is likely to be better accepted by the child of preschool age if

1. it is given to him between meals
2. he can help himself from a small pitcher
3. he is urged to drink it at the beginning of the meal
4. it is always very cold

185. The preschool child can handle food more conveniently

1. if firm foods are in "bite-size" portions
2. with a large curve-handled spoon
3. served on a small flat plate
4. if it has the consistency of thin soup

186. The school-age child frequently eats inadequate amounts of

1. green and yellow vegetables
2. meats, fish, and poultry
3. cereals and breadstuffs
4. butter, sweets

187. The protein source that would be best for a school-age child is

    1. spaghetti with meat sauce
    2. chil con carne
    3. hamburger patty
    4. barbecued beef

188. A frequent cause of inadequate nutrition in the 6-to-12-year-old group is

    1. the very low vitamin A intake
    2. the failure to eat breakfast
    3. the very high total calorie intake
    4. the amount of protein eaten between meals

189. Acceptable after-school snacks are

    1. jelly sandwiches
    2. simple cookies
    3. fruit
    4. milk and egg desserts

190. The foods needed by the 6-to-12-year-old child

    1. are found in the basic four groups
    2. consist primarily of milk, fruit, vegetables
    3. should be prepared in a different way than for the preschool child
    4. are different from foods for adults

191. After-school snacks for the school child should

    1. be discouraged
    2. not be necessary if the child is served three adequate meals a day
    3. include essential foods
    4. be considered an example of poor food habits

192. Many parents are not aware that the young school child's breakfast appetite is upset when

    1. excitement, anxiety, and hurry are associated with going to school
    2. he feels strange
    3. he must get out on the playground with the other children
    4. the day holds many adjustments for him

193. One advantage of providing the noon meal at school where there is understanding supervision is

    1. the shorter time allowed for lunch
    2. longer out-of-doors play at noon
    3. the opportunity for the child to learn to like a greater variety of foods
    4. the relief the mother gets because she does not have to worry about preparing a noon meal

194. If the school child's lunch usually consists of a hamburger, pop, and a candy bar, his nutritional deficiency at the end of the day is in foods such as

    1. potatoes, fruit, and caloric foods
    2. green or yellow vegetables and enough milk
    3. meat, potato, and vegetables
    4. vitamin C, enough milk, and enough calories

195. The dietary requirements of the teen-ager are primarily affected by

    1. his increased rate of growth
    2. his desire for approval from his family or friends
    3. his social interests
    4. resistance to parental supervision

196. The average teen-age boy usually needs

    1. as much food as a moderately active adult
    2. a little less protein than his father
    3. less energy foods than his father
    4. more nutritious food than the average girl

197. The inadequate diet so characteristic of the teen-age girl can be responsible for

    1. endangering health and stunting growth
    2. underweight or overweight
    3. unnecessary difficulties at childbirth
    4. greater incidence of infections

198. A desirable daily milk intake during adolescence is

    1. 1 pint   3. 1 quart
    2. 1 1/2 pints   4. 1 1/2 quarts

NUTRITION AND DIET THERAPY

199. Inflammation of the gums, often found in teen-agers, is usually the result of

   1. insufficient amounts of vitamin-B complex
   2. chewing too many hard foods
   3. inadequate intake of vitamin C
   4. too little roughage in the diet

200. The inadequate diet of the teen-ager, continued through the teen-age period, plays an important part in

   1. producing complexion problems
   2. limiting athletic successes
   3. decreased popularity
   4. preventing optimum physical and mental development

201. Recognition of the desire of the teen-ager for approval in appearance and achievement can be used

   1. to motivate him to develop good food habits
   2. to help him to see the result of poor food habits
   3. to keep him from being interested in "fad" foods
   4. to limit his lunch intake to hamburgers and a coke

202. Emphasis on optimum nutrition standards throughout life increases the chance of

   1. being healthier
   2. finding life more satisfactory
   3. extending the years of productive life
   4. working more successfully

203. A bodily change that often affects the nutritional state of aging persons is

   1. the decrease in activity
   2. a feeling of rejection and loneliness
   3. inadequate money for food needs
   4. a decrease in efficiency of the digestive system

204. To meet the food needs of the adolescent, servings from the meat group should be in the amount of

   1. 1 egg and 1 meat
   2. 3 or more
   3. 2 or more
   4. 1 more than needed by adults

205. Fewer calories are needed in the later years because

   1. the aged tend to have less appetite
   2. work will be reduced for the body processes
   3. there is a gradual decrease in the rate of body metabolism
   4. there is a decrease in the needs for body repair

206. Feelings, common in the aging process, that may affect the nutritional status are

   1. a sense of rejection and loneliness
   2. weakness and insecurity
   3. disgust at the inability to chew foods thoroughly
   4. discomfort from poor digestion

207. Many elderly persons are in a poor nutritional state because

   1. they often refuse to eat citrus fruits
   2. of a dislike for many essential foods
   3. of a special liking for breads, pastries, and cereals
   4. yellow and green vegetables are commonly avoided.

208. Regardless of money available to buy food, many elderly people are poorly nourished because

   1. there may be no one to prepare the meals for them
   2. they either have no teeth or have poorly fitted dentures
   3. foods are not so well digested, absorbed, and put into use
   4. the weekly income is not enough to permit the purchase of essential foods

209. The basic nutritional needs of the healthy older person will

1. require less protein than during the middle years
2. be about the same as those of a younger person
3. be greater than during the teen-age years
4. require smaller amounts of vitamins and minerals than for a younger person

210. It might be easier to get middle-aged people to eat better balanced meals if more publicity were given to the fact that poor nutrition brings about

1. an early death
2. signs of aging earlier
3. decreased mental stimulation
4. many of the diseases caused by overweight

211. The nurse who works closely with elderly patients should recognize that the resistance to new foods, or to the familiar foods prepared in a different way, is one evidence of

1. feelings of insecurity
2. selfishness
3. decreased judgment
4. their reluctance to get old

212. The increased use of salt and sugar as an individual grows older is because

1. of a special liking for very sweet and salty foods
2. of the development of poor food habits
3. such seasonings are familiar ones and are not expensive
4. of a decreased sense of taste and smell

213. It is very difficult to change the eating habits of many elderly persons because

1. they lack interest in improving their health
2. poor teeth interfere with enjoyment of food
3. limited activity reduces the appetite
4. they are too dependent upon others

214. It is recommended that the appetite of the elderly person be stimulated by

1. giving him only small amounts of food at a time
2. using hot clear soups and broths frequently
3. telling him what foods you have and asking him which ones he wants
4. giving only light snacks between meals

215. Which of the following food lists should be emphasized in planning a diet for an older person?

1. whole-grain breads and cereals, meat, potatoes, other vegetables
2. bread, jelly, fruits, butter, milk, and eggs
3. fresh fruits, vegetables, milk, eggs and lean meat
4. bland soft-cooked foods

216. An adequate diet plan for an elderly person must include

1. only those foods particularly liked
2. fewer protein foods than for a younger person
3. liberal use of carbohydrate foods, since they are easily digested
4. as much or more mineral- and vitamin-rich food than would be required in earlier years

217. The nurse might help an aged patient to keep up an interest in food by

1. urging him to eat everything on his plate or tray
2. offering him sweets between meals occasionally
3. including at least one food on his tray that he especially likes
4. telling him how his body needs that food to keep him well

218. When the elderly person has difficulty chewing foods, the nurse might suggest that he

1. eliminate meat and raw vegetables
2. substitute another food
3. use only liquid foods
4. soft cook, chop, or grind essential foods

(Answer sheets pp. 305–306)

1. Every therapeutic diet, given for <u>more than</u> a short time, should aim at

   1. ease of digestion
   2. nutritional adequacy
   3. proper elimination
   4. increase in weight

2. Diet therapy may be defined as

   1. the use of diet to correct existing nutritional deficiencies
   2. the modification of the normal diet to meet the requirements under special conditions
   3. the use of special dietetic foods prepared in a different way
   4. use of a diet free of harsh fibers and of highly seasoned foods

3. A soft diet is a modification of the normal diet emphasizing

   1. extra amounts of milk
   2. sufficient calories for the patient's energy needs
   3. adequate amounts of emulsified fats
   4. simple, easily digested foods

4. Raw-vegetable salads may be included on

   1. a light diet
   2. a soft diet
   3. a regular house diet
   4. a full fluid diet

5. One example of the modification of a normal diet is

   1. the planning necessary to make it nutritionally adequate
   2. the increase or decrease in the amount of bulk or cellulose
   3. the proper preparation of food and attractive service
   4. the consideration of the pathological aspects that affect the diet

6. It is possible to prepare a full fluid diet that

   1. is nutritionally adequate
   2. will include soft mashed potatoes
   3. will be acceptable to all patients
   4. can be used for most patients the day of surgery

7. A diet modification of first importance for pre- and postoperative patients is

   1. an increase in fluid intake
   2. the restriction of all foods for at least 24 hours
   3. an emphasis on protein foods
   4. aimed at improving the nutritional condition of the patient

8. You can increase the nutritive value of the full fluid diet without increasing quantity by adding

   1. milk, pureed vegetables, or strained cereals
   2. fruit and vegetable juices
   3. plain gelatin desserts and custards
   4. glucose, butter, or dry milk powder

9. A high caloric diet is a modification of the normal diet in terms of its

   1. carbohydrates and fats
   2. energy content
   3. fats and proteins
   4. proteins

10. The primary purpose of the clear fluid diet is

    1. to relieve the hunger pangs of the patient
    2. to aid in replacing fluids lost
    3. to provide the patient with a mild stimulant
    4. to make the patient feel cared for

11. The postsurgical diet needs to be high in

    1. easily digested foods
    2. calories and carbohydrates
    3. complete proteins and emulsified fats
    4. proteins, minerals, vitamins

12. The type of diet frequently used immediately following surgery is

   1. a soft diet
   2. a light diet
   3. a full fluid diet
   4. a clear fluid diet

13. The _mechanically_ soft diet is used for patients who

   1. are critically ill
   2. are in the early stages of convalescence
   3. have trouble in chewing their food
   4. have difficulty in cutting their food

14. Current health and mortality statistics tend to prove that the weight desirable at the age of 25 to 30 should be

   1. gradually increased in the later years
   2. less than the recommended weight for age 60
   3. maintained throughout life
   4. considered unsafe at the age of 75

15. The chief reason why people consume more calories than they need is because

   1. their daily activities keep them hungry
   2. they skip breakfast
   3. their recreational and social activities include high-calorie foods
   4. the heaviest meal is eaten in the evening

16. Obesity is more likely to occur during middle age because

   1. leisure time increases the amount of food eaten
   2. metabolism is greatly lowered by glandular imbalances
   3. people participate in more social functions where food is served
   4. food intake remains the same as activity decreases

17. A safe variation from your normal weight is

   1. 10 pounds above or below
   2. 15 pounds above or below
   3. 5%, above or below
   4. within 10% above or below

18. When all members of a family are overweight, it is usually because

   1. the food habits of family members tend to be similar
   2. the causes of overweight have been inherited
   3. the body build of family members is alike
   4. all members of the family like starchy foods

19. The only way to take off unwanted pounds is

   1. to start each day with little or no breakfast
   2. to reduce the calorie intake to less than the energy output
   3. to eliminate all sweet foods
   4. to find a reducing diet you think you can follow

20. Obesity can be a problem at any age level because

   1. breakfast is commonly omitted
   2. food compensates for lack of love and affection
   3. additional calories are consumed with the "coffee-break"
   4. mealtime desserts are usually high in calories

21. Parents often encourage the habit of overeating during childhood by

   1. encouraging excessive appetites to keep up the growth pattern
   2. allowing food between meals
   3. using extra sweets as a reward for being good
   4. allowing the child to get too hungry before a meal is served

22. An effective reducing program emphasizes that the weight loss should be

    1. more rapid during the first few weeks
    2. rapid, to encourage the person to "stay with" the diet
    3. limited to 25 pounds or less per year
    4. limited to 2 pounds per week

23. Prescribed drugs do not solve the problem of weight control because

    1. the diet is not changed
    2. the weight loss will be slow
    3. the psychological effect creates a problem
    4. the weight gain is rapid when the medicine is discontinued

24. An important objective necessary to an effective weight control program is

    1. the correction of faulty eating habits
    2. the steady weight loss of 4 to 5 pounds a week
    3. the elimination of between meal eating
    4. the recognition of the importance of regularly scheduled meals

25. It would be difficult to maintain a good nutritional state on a weight-reduction diet that

    1. concentrated only on the basic four foods
    2. did not include milk or milk products
    3. limited starchy foods to two servings a day
    4. allowed no sweet foods

26. Fad diets are not recommended as a sensible way to reduce and stay reduced because

    1. the foods are usually expensive
    2. the weight loss is often slow
    3. permanent improvement in eating habits will not take place
    4. the person is too often hungry

27. On a long-term reducing plan the most effective loss of excess fat takes place when

    1. foods containing fats are eliminated from the diet
    2. there is a regular schedule of 3 meals daily
    3. there is restriction of fluids along with reduced calories
    4. the diet is composed primarily of protein foods

28. An attempt is made to prevent hunger between meals by providing

    1. low-calorie snacks
    2. large amounts of bulky foods at mealtime
    3. increased liquids between meals
    4. a generous serving of a protein food at each meal

29. The underwight person will gain weight with appropriate between-meal snacks, provided they

    1. are foods that he likes
    2. do not interfere with his appetite for his regular meal
    3. contain large numbers of calories
    4. are made up of easily digested foods

30. A high-iron diet will make use of increased servings of

    1. milk
    2. fruit
    3. green leafy vegetables
    4. bread

31. Foods that interfere with iron absorption are

    1. citrus fruits
    2. starchy vegetables
    3. whole-grain cereals
    4. pastries

32. The dietary program in pernicious anemia must be planned to include foods that are

1. high in protein, vitamins, and minerals
2. high in calories and carbohydrates
3. low in calories to control weight
4. high in emulsified fats

33. A food supplying a better-than-average amount of iron and protein is

1. pork
2. beef
3. spaghetti
4. liver

34. An anemia diet calls for the frequent use of high-iron-content foods such as

1. citrus fruits, yellow vegetables, milk
2. fruits, vegetables, and cereals
3. green leafy vegetables, dried fruits, whole grains
4. cheese, butter, fish

35. If the patient with anemia has the usual accompanying mouth symptoms, the nurse would expect him to find it difficult to eat all but one of the following:

1. acid foods
2. hot foods
3. chewy foods
4. bland foods

36. The dietary treatment of anemia may require

1. an abundance of fluids to promote digestion and absorption
2. high carbohydrate foods
3. a restriction of fats because they slow up iron absorption
4. liberal amounts of milk, cheese, and butter

37. Hemoglobin can be replaced only if the diet is adequate in

1. carbohydrates
2. calories to take care of the energy needs
3. high-quality proteins
4. emulsified fats

38. A patient with an iron-deficient anemia should have a diet that includes a plentiful supply of

a. eggs
b. milk
c. meat
d. green leafy vegetables

1. all of the above
2. a, b, and c
3. b, c, and d
4. a, c, and d

39. The food most effective in the regeneration of hemoglobin is

1. dried prunes
2. liver
3. egg yolk
4. lean meats

40. The anemia patient with a decrease in the number of red blood cells would suffer nutritional problems as a result of

1. interference with the normal absorption of digested foods
2. insufficient storage of glycogen
3. insufficient protein available
4. decreased oxidation of food materials

41. Too much fat in the diet of the anemia patient may affect nutrition by

1. decreasing the appetite
2. slowing up the absorption of iron from the digestive tract
3. making the caloric intake too high
4. increasing the needed calories without adding too much bulk

42. Nutritional anemia may develop if the preschool child's diet consists chiefly of

1. milk
2. green and yellow vegetables
3. meat and eggs
4. fruits and vegetables

43. Anemia in the late stages of pregnancy is the result of

1. hemorrhage
2. too little vitamin C in the diet
3. increased nutritional requirements
4. absence of the intrinsic factor

44. A diet high in calories is desirable in anemia to prevent the body's need

1. to break down fatty tissue
2. to use proteins for energy
3. to accumulate waste
4. to protect itself through thirst

45. The dietary plan for the cardiac patient stresses the importance of modifying

1. the size and the frequency of meals
2. the intestinal irritation by eating soft-cooked fruits and vegetables
3. emotional tensions
4. the acid-base products of metabolism

46. Additional strain on the heart will be avoided if food is

1. given in small amounts at frequent intervals
2. preferably in cooked form
3. well liked by the patient
4. neither too hot nor too cold

47. The diet for the cardiac patient should contain a total caloric count that will

1. be low enough to keep the weight considerably below normal
2. be sufficient to include foods that are well liked
3. be obtained from equal amounts of fats, proteins, and carbohydrates
4. maintain the body weight at slightly below normal level

48. Repair of heart damage will require a protein intake of

1. 1 1/2 grams per kilogram of body weight
2. 1 gram per kilogram of body weight
3. 2/3 gram per kilogram of body weight
4. 2 grams per kilogram of body weight

49. In the list of fatty food substances below, the one that would have the least tendency to slow up the emptying time of the stomach is

1. corn oil   3. butter
2. margarine   4. lard

50. When food remains too long in the stomach of the cardiac patient, a diet change of importance would be

1. the substitution of liquid for solid food
2. the addition of stimulating foods to speed up stomach movements
3. the restriction of the amount and kind of fats
4. a decrease in the number of meals eaten during the day

51. A dietary observation that the cardiac patient must be encouraged to report would be on

1. the foods he especially likes
2. the foods that cause him distress
3. the change in flavor when herbs are used on his vegetables
4. the appearance of the foods on his tray

52. Cardiac decompensation requires a diet that consists of

1. increased fluid intake
2. unrestricted fats
3. normal amounts of tea and coffee
4. easily digested, soft, bland foods

53. A high-fiber food, usually used to help prevent constipation, that would not be served to a cardiac is

1. asparagus tips   3. applesauce
2. broccoli   4. cooked carrots

54. On a low cholesterol diet, which one of the following foods would be omitted?

1. skim milk   3. peanut butter
2. eggs   4. peas

55. The newer trend in diets for the patient with edema

1. restricts sodium and fluid
2. restricts sodium and fluid intake is normal
3. restricts fluid and sodium as desired
4. eliminates potassium and phosphorous

56. A low cholesterol diet will include foods that are chiefly

1. animal proteins and carbohydrates
2. low in sodium
3. low in fats
4. from plant sources

57. A food group high in cholesterol is

1. fruit   3. animal foods
2. vegetables   4. cereals

58. If the cardiac patient is obese, the physician will want him to reduce because

1. an overweight person becomes tired more quickly
2. there is more chance of an obese person having an accident
3. the patient probably will be more comfortable
4. an excess of fat in the tissues means more work for the heart

59. A condition of edema will be controlled by a diet that

1. decreases the amount of animal fats eaten
2. limits intake of high-protein foods
3. restricts the sodium intake
4. reduces the total fluid intake

60. A food that could be digested and assimilated with the least amount of energy by the patient with cardiac decompensation is

1. sliced bananas   3. fruit cocktail
2. applesauce   4. baked pears

61. A type of food that will provide the necessary cellulose in the diet and yet require the least effort to digest and assimilate is

1. raw vegetable salads
2. bran cereals
3. soft-cooked fruits
4. fresh fruit

62. The person who is on a <u>sodium-restricted</u> diet must learn to avoid

a. using salt on foods at the table
b. adding any salt to the food as it is being prepared
c. fresh vegetables or prepared foods with a high sodium content
d. all foods with sodium in them

1. d only
2. a and b
3. all of the above
4. a, b, and c

63. A diet planned to include 500 milligrams of sodium a day is classified as

1. a mildly restrictive diet
2. a severely restrictive diet
3. a moderately restrictive diet
4. a high sodium diet

64. If prepared foods, or partly prepared foods, are to be used in a sodium-restricted diet, it will be necessary for the practical nurse

1. to reheat foods to eliminate the sodium
2. to read the label
3. to taste them before placing them on the tray
4. to add a little sugar to minimize the lack of salt

65. One flavoring that should not be used in a sodium-restricted diet is

1. green pepper   3. garlic
2. parsley flakes   4. prepared mustard

66. One vegetable that would not be included in a sodium-restricted diet is

1. green beans   3. squash
2. spinach   4. lettuce

67. Which one of the following foods would be safe to use in a sodium-restricted diet?

1. "quick" oatmeal
2. commercial canned peas
3. puffed wheat
4. muffin mix

68. A low-sodium diet cannot be accomplished if the meals include

    1. fresh fruit
    2. commercially canned vegetables
    3. meat, eggs
    4. unsalted yeast breadstuffs

69. The patient will accept a sodium-restricted diet if

    1. it is made up of easily prepared foods
    2. he understands how to make food tasty without salt
    3. the nurse insists that he learn to like it because it is best for him
    4. he makes use of salt substitutes

70. The practical nurse will advise the patient who asks about using salt substitutes

    1. to sprinkle them over the cooked food
    2. to mix them into the food as it cooks
    3. to secure the doctor's approval of the kind to be used
    4. to use them only in very small amounts

71. A severely restricted sodium intake would allow sodium in the amount of

    1. 1 gram
    2. 1 teaspoon of salt
    3. 1000 milligrams
    4. 200 to 500 milligrams

72. Unsalted vegetables may sometimes be improved in taste by

    1. using a larger amount of water in cooking
    2. serving them in an attractive dish
    3. adding small amounts of sugar
    4. serving them cooked instead of raw

73. Food groups that are generally low in natural sodium are

    1. milk, eggs, cheese
    2. meat, poultry, fish
    3. leafy greens, milk, organ meat
    4. fruits, vegetables, cereals

74. In any type of kidney disease it is important that most of the protein come from sources

    1. that are readily digested
    2. that carry a high iron content
    3. that are fairly low in calories
    4. of complete protein

75. The diet in acute nephritis during the first few days of the illness will

    1. include large amounts of fluid to flush out the kidneys
    2. be omitted if there is nausea and vomiting
    3. omit all protein foods that increase the work of the kidney
    4. consist of high CHO and moderately low-fat foods

76. A low-protein diet tends to be lacking in adequate amounts of

    1. vitamin A and D
    2. the B complex vitamins
    3. fat and vitamin C
    4. iron and niacin

77. In acute nephritis small amounts of crushed ice or fruit juices may be given

    1. when the patient is suffering from attacks of kidney stones
    2. to help increase the fluid intake
    3. during the early stage
    4. if nausea and vomiting are present

78. A moderately low protein diet is sometimes prescribed in acute nephritis because

    1. foods high in protein contain too much sodium
    2. a minimum intake makes less work for the kidneys
    3. proteins tend to stimulate the secretions of the digestive tract
    4. it will help to restrict the total fat intake

79. After nausea and vomiting have stopped, the first food allowed the patient with acute nephritis is usually

    1. milk   3. soft-cooked eggs
    2. cooked cereals 4. pureed fruit

80. A food suitable to use in a diet for acute nephritis to increase calories without increasing protein is

   1. cereal
   2. jelly
   3. egg yolk
   4. peanut butter

81. When anorexia is present in chronic nephritis, the diet plan may need

   1. to restrict fats
   2. to increase calorie content
   3. to provide 6 small meals
   4. to reduce the amount of fluid

82. In chronic nephritis, if protein loss in the urine is high, the diet must be planned

   1. to stress increased fluid intake
   2. to provide a rest for the kidneys
   3. to supply an increased amount of protein
   4. to reduce the protein supply until the kidneys can handle it better

83. In nephrosis a high-protein diet based on the patient's ideal weight will call for

   1. 2 or more grams of protein per kilogram of body weight
   2. 1 to 1 1/2 grams of protein per kilogram of body weight
   3. 4 grams of protein per kilogram of body weight
   4. 1 1/2 to 2 grams of protein per kilogram of body weight

84. A diet planned to prevent the recurrence of kidney stones must be based on

   1. information about the type of stones formed
   2. acid-ash-forming foods
   3. foods high in fats, sugar, and starches
   4. foods considered neutral

85. In the presence of kidney stones a diet primarily of meat, eggs, and bread-stuffs would be used

   1. if the urine is acid
   2. when the stones are of alkaline composition
   3. when the urinary calculi are acid
   4. to help dissolve the stones present

86. If a diet consists chiefly of fruit, vegetables, and milk, it will probably be inadequate in

   1. ascorbic acid and vitamin A
   2. minerals and vitamins
   3. calories and calcium
   4. iron and protein

87. Glucose found in the blood comes from the metabolism of

   1. dietary sugars
   2. carbohydrates in the foods eaten
   3. starchy foods
   4. CHO, protein, and fat

88. The doctor's dietary prescription for diabetes should be written in terms of

   1. the amount and kind of insulin to be given
   2. grams of protein, fat, and CHO to be allowed
   3. food exchanges to be allowed in each meal
   4. total calories for the day

89. Whenever the diabetic person takes in more food materials than he can metabolize, he is in danger of

   1. acidosis
   2. insulin shock
   3. glycosuria
   4. polydipsia

90. The kind of insulin the patient is receiving will determine the diet plan for

1. the approximate percent of CHO served at each meal
2. dividing the total intake over 5 meals
3. selection of the right kind of CHO
4. determining the exchange lists to use

91. When the amount of insulin produced by the pancreas is not enough to metabolize all the food substances eaten, the nutrient that is not properly metabolized is

1. the amino acids
2. the proteins
3. the glycerol
4. the glucose

92. In the treatment of diabetes the doctor's diet prescription will limit the amounts of

1. carbohydrates and fats
2. sugars and starches
3. proteins, fats, and carbohydrates
4. carbohydrates

93. It is important for the diabetic to appreciate the need for eating foods high in vitamins and minerals

1. to take care of the increased need for these nutrients in blood regeneration
2. to maintain an adequate reserve in the liver
3. to prevent hemorrhages in the capillaries
4. to keep up resistance to infections

94. In diabetes the total caloric intake is usually planned to enable the patient to maintain

1. ideal weight for height and age
2. weight somewhat above normal to provide a reserve fuel supply
3. a slow, steady loss in weight to lessen the work of the pancreas
4. carbohydrate foods at a level at which the insulin can take care of it

95. The diabetic patient under treatment should try to eat all of the foods planned for each meal in order

1. to supply the necessary amount of calories for energy needs
2. to maintain the glycogen reserve in the liver
3. to avoid an insulin reaction
4. to prevent protein depletion and anemia

96. If the family of a diabetic patient is bringing food into the hospital because it is advertised as being "low in starch and high in protein," the first thing the nurse must do is

1. notify the dietitian
2. tell the family they must not bring food to the patient
3. remove the food from the patient's room
4. tell the patient he should not eat them

97. A popular product that may be given to the diabetic child without making dietary changes is

1. diabetic ice cream
2. diabetic canned fruits
3. carbonated beverage sweetened with a noncaloric sweetener
4. a diabetic chewing gum

98. If a diabetic patient dislikes a CHO food on his tray, the nurse may

1. call the doctor about it
2. tell the patient he has to eat it
3. substitute another food containing about the same amount of carbohydrate
4. give the patient an orange to eat

99. Since the diabetic patient is susceptible to infections, he needs

1. an adequate protein intake
2. increased amounts of vitamins A and C
3. a reduction in his weight
4. large amounts of fluids

100. When the patient is getting N.P.H. insulin, dietary plans must include

1. dividing the carbohydrate equally among three meals
2. a bedtime feeding
3. 4 or 6 daily meals instead of 3
4. giving the largest amount of the carbohydrate allowance at the meal that follows the administration of insulin

101. When the Orthodox Jewish patient has diabetes, his religious dietary restrictions make it necessary for the nurse to plan his meals so that

1. highly seasoned foods are seldom used
2. milk and meat are not served at the same meal
3. dried fruits are used instead of fresh fruits
4. rye bread is given instead of white bread

102. The diabetic who has to eat his lunch away from home should usually

1. avoid all high carbohydrate foods
2. eat only fresh fruit and fresh vegetable plates
3. find a restaurant that serves dietetic foods
4. avoid "mixtures" or combination dishes

103. If the diabetic patient refuses to eat his half cup of oatmeal, the nurse can make a substitution of

1. 1 1/2 slices of bread
2. 3/4 cup of Wheaties
3. 2 baking powder biscuits
4. 3/4 cup of cooked rice

104. Which one of the following foods should not be given to a patient on a convalescent ulcer diet?

1. creamed chicken on toast
2. Italian spaghetti with meat sauce
3. cream of asparagus soup
4. beef loaf with cream sauce

105. The patient with a gastric or duodenal ulcer will need to have a normal diet modified because

1. the entire digestive system needs rest
2. an adequate diet is needed in a form that will permit the ulcer to heal
3. constipation must be prevented by generous servings of high-fiber foods
4. the acid-base balance in the body must be maintained

106. A food with a stimulating effect on the flow of gastric juice that must be omitted from the diet of an ulcer patient is

1. milk   3. beef broth
2. fruit juice   4. eggs

107. Foods that decrease gastric motility are

1. rough, fibrous foods
2. high in CHO
3. of liquid consistency
4. high in fat content

108. A vegetable that should not be used on the convalescent ulcer diet is

1. buttered potatoes
2. creamed eggs on toast
3. creamed cauliflower
4. pureed spinach with egg slices

109. If diet is to be used as an important part of the treatment of a gastric ulcer, it will be necessary

1. for the patient to like all of the foods given him
2. for some protein food to be in the stomach all of the time
3. to include foods high in vitamin C to promote healing
4. to season the foods to please the patient

110. A food that tends to slow down the movement of the stomach and to decrease the flow of the gastric juice is

1. Cream of Wheat
2. thin cream
3. lean tender meat
4. pureed fruit

111. The dietary program for an ulcer patient in the convalescent stage consists of

 1. 3 well-planned meals with emphasis on protein foods
 2. foods that make up an adequate bland diet
 3. a bland diet distributed over 6 small meals
 4. small amounts of milk and cream every hour during the period the patient is awake

112. The patient on a Sippy diet program will receive

 1. small amounts of milk and cream every hour
 2. foods to neutralize the HCL of the stomach
 3. a high CHO diet to rest the digestive tract
 4. foods in a form that the patient can tolerate

113. A food that would irritate the ulcerated tissue is

 1. ground meat
 2. mashed potato
 3. pureed pears
 4. oatmeal

114. An acute diarrhea will require a diet modification that will

 1. emphasize a high-protein diet
 2. give a low residue diet
 3. provide extra amounts of soft cooked fruits and vegetables
 4. provide rest for the entire intestinal tract

115. On the first day of an acute diarrhea dietary treatment will consist of

 1. allowing the patient to select the foods he will eat
 2. withholding all food and oral fluids
 3. providing foods that are quickly digested
 4. coaxing the patient to take any food

116. In order to prevent or overcome one of the dangerous results of acute diarrhea, the diet

 1. should be soft
 2. must include chiefly milk drinks
 3. must include high-fiber foods to supply bulk
 4. should be high in fluids

117. The patient with colitis should receive a diet that is

 1. high in protein and fat
 2. low in fat and carbohydrate
 3. nonirritating and high in nutrient essentials
 4. high in calories and carbohydrates

118. A modified normal diet will help a patient with spastic constipation because it will

 1. provide an abundance of high-carbohydrate foods
 2. increase the muscular contraction of the intestine
 3. decrease the fiber content of the foods used in the diet
 4. remove dietary sources of irritation to the intestinal walls

119. A food properly served in a low-residue diet is

 1. cream soup
 2. shredded wheat biscuit
 3. baked apple
 4. buttered carrots

120. A dietary suggestion to correct or prevent atonic constipation is

 1. regular elimination after breakfast
 2. the daily use of a small amount of mineral oil at bedtime
 3. to drink 1 or 2 glasses of water 30 minutes before breakfast
 4. to puree most fruits and vegetables

121. The food that contains the most residue is

 1. cheese   3. meat
 2. apple   4. white rice

122. Dietary treatment of <u>atonic</u> constipation includes a modified normal diet of foods that will

1. prevent irritation of the walls of the intestines
2. stimulate peristalsis by an increased fiber content
3. promote the healing of inflamed intestinal walls
4. provide the patient with high-protein foods

123. An important goal to achieve in the dietary treatment of liver disease is

1. the intake of sufficient calories to result in weight gain
2. the repair of damaged liver tissue
3. the increased intake of alkaline-ash-forming foods
4. gradual improvement of the liver's tolerance for fat foods

124. The prescribed diet for a patient with liver disease would <u>not</u> include

1. large amounts of fat
2. small frequent feedings
3. salt on his food
4. large amounts of protein

125. One of the biggest problems the patient with liver disease presents in relation to his diet is

1. the inability to make foods palatable without salt
2. the inadequacy of the vitamin and mineral content of the allowed foods
3. his refusal to increase his liquid intake
4. his reluctance to eat

126. Better patient acceptance of the prescribed diet in liver disease is obtained when

1. foods are well seasoned and highly flavored
2. it is given in small frequent feedings
3. raw fruits and vegetables are omitted
4. only pureed foods are used

127. Diets generally used for liver diseases are

1. low in protein and fat
2. low in carbohydrate and sodium
3. high in protein and carbohydrate
4. high in fat and cellulose

128. You could double the protein content in 1 quart of milk with very little increase in volume by

1. combining it with 2 tablespoons of baby cereal
2. substituting 1/4 cup of cream for part of the milk
3. adding 2 tablespoons of lactose to the milk
4. adding 1 cup of nonfat dry milk

129. The diet in gallbladder disease must be planned to include

1. plenty of roughage to prevent constipation
2. sufficient calories to prevent weight loss
3. only small amounts of emulsified fats
4. a high fluid intake to prevent dehydration

130. A food to avoid in planning the diet for gallbladder disease is

1. cottage cheese   3. buttermilk
2. creamed eggs   4. green beans

131. A food that probably would be gas-forming for the patient with gallbladder disease is

1. spinach   3. prunes
2. applesauce   4. cucumbers

132. Once the gallbladder has been removed surgically, the patient can expect his diet to provide for

1. gradual return to a full preoperative menu
2. adjustment of the fat intake according to his tolerance
3. only those foods low in fat
4. high-CHO, high-protein foods only

133. To increase calories in an 8 ounce glass of orange juice, add

    1. 1 beaten egg
    2. 1 tablespoon of gelatine
    3. 1 tablespoon of syrup
    4. 1/4 cup of cream

134. An _acute_ fever of _short_ duration requires a dietary intake that includes

    1. plenty of protein
    2. frequent small meals
    3. emulsified fats
    4. fluids in large amounts

135. When the pneumonia patient runs a temperature of 105°F, the increased rate of metabolism requires a diet that

    1. forces fruit juices
    2. is high-caloric, high-CHO
    3. is high-protein, high-fat
    4. keeps some food in the stomach at all times

136. An adequate diet plan for a patient with a fever must consider the physiological changes in the body during the fever. The total caloric needs will be

    1. affected by the destruction of the body proteins
    2. upset when the glycogen supply in the liver is exhausted
    3. increased because metabolism is speeded up
    4. decreased because of fluid accumulation in the tissues

137. One of the symptons of tuberculosis is a low-grade fever present every day. The main objectives of the dietary program for such a patient are

    1. to keep the patient contented during convalescence
    2. to restore wasted tissue and prevent further wasting
    3. to supply a reserve of energy in the form of adipose tissue
    4. to neutralize the toxic effects of the disease

138. The patient is in the acute stage of a disease and his temperature is elevated. Such a patient's diet should be planned

    1. to increase proteins to replace those used to support the fever
    2. to include easily digested fats and carbohydrates
    3. to double the caloric intake
    4. to permit maximum rest of the digestive system

139. In those diseases in which a common symptom is an elevated temperature lasting for _several weeks,_ the diet would need to supply extra amounts of

    1. easily digested carbohydrate
    2. protein foods
    3. pureed fruits and vegetables
    4. high-caloric and high-protein foods

140. The healing and repair of tissues destroyed by tuberculosis will require a diet that includes an abundance of foods high in

    1. proteins, vitamins, and minerals
    2. both cooked and raw fruits and vegetables
    3. iron, phosphorous, and vitamin D
    4. easily digested carbohydrates and fats

141. A food that must be avoided in the diet plan for the typhoid fever patient is

    1. chopped celery creamed with a high protein milk
    2. eggnog made with half and half cream
    3. tea with sugar and glucose added
    4. strained oatmeal gruel with cream and sugar

142. This patient has been ill with a disease in which there have been frequent periods of elevated temperature. During convalescence this patient will require a diet high in

    1. nourishment
    2. easily digested CHO
    3. bland foods
    4. calories with added vitamin supplements

143. The 10-year-old with chronic rheumatic fever will need a diet that places stress on an abundance of foods

1. with high fluid content to replace the fluids being lost
2. that normally require extra sugar and cream
3. such as fruits, vegetables, and protein foods
4. the child especially likes

144. When a disease is characterized by chills alternating with fever, the nurse must recognize the need to increase the intake of

1. all the important vitamins and minerals
2. copper and phosphorous
3. liquids to balance the fluids lost through diaphoresis
4. fresh fruits and vegetables to maintain the acid-base balance

145. A FORCE FLUID order written for a patient with a disease characterized by prolonged elevation of temperature would mean an intake of

1. 1000 to 1500 c.c.
2. 2000 to 2500 c.c.
3. 2500 to 3000 c.c.
4. 3000 to 5000 c.c.

146. The biggest dietary problem that occurs when a patient has a high temperature is

1. his preference for liquid foods
2. his reluctance to take any nourishment
3. the loss of fluid through perspiration
4. rapid absorption of foods ingested

147. The present trend in the dietary program for arthritic patients places the emphasis on

1. an abundance of essential vitamins and minerals
2. avoiding fruits, which tend to produce acidosis
3. the use of protein and carbohydrate foods at separate meals
4. low-fat diets because of the interference with digestion

148. The anemic arthritic patient will probably be placed on a diet that emphasizes

1. an abundance of fluids
2. a high-protein, high-iron diet
3. a restriction of high-fat foods
4. an abundance of high-CHO foods

149. The dietary plan for the patient with arthritis is chiefly aimed at

1. making eating as easy as possible
2. preventing overweight
3. providing food the patient especially likes
4. correcting any existing nutritional deficiencies

150. The patient with osteoarthritis has the most difficulty in the weight-bearing joints. The best diet for such a patient will provide for

1. an adequate supply of energy-building foods
2. maintaining weight slightly below optimum
3. a high-vitamin, high-caloric intake
4. a minimum of gas-forming foods

151. The patient with multiple fractures who must remain in bed in a large body cast for several months will need a diet plan that will include

1. stimulants to offset his periods of depression
2. high-caloric foods to give him enough energy for crutch walking
3. sufficient roughage to prevent constipation
4. low-residue foods because it is hard for him to use a bedpan

152. To prevent an excess of calcium from being removed from bone to help develop new bone, the diet of a fracture patient should include generous amounts of

1. lean meat
2. green and yellow vegetables
3. citrus fruits and tomatoes
4. milk products

153. Present-day dietary treatment of gout is based on the theory that the patient benefits from

    1. a weight gain
    2. some restriction of food sources of uric acid
    3. the maintenance of a low intake of CHO and fats
    4. a restriction of calcium to prevent deposits in the joints

154. A food that should not be used in the diet of an obese patient with gout is

    1. skim milk
    2. fresh fruit in gelatin
    3. small baked potato
    4. fried egg

155. A low purine content will be found in a <u>food group</u> such as

    1. vegetables   3. dry beans
    2. meat   4. organ meat

156. The most suitable menu for a person on a low purine diet is

    1. cream of tomato soup, steak, mustard pickles, asparagus, bread, butter, chocolate cake, coffee
    2. liver, mashed potato, carrots, bread, butter, baked apple, milk
    3. scrambled eggs, baked potato, peas, tomato salad, bread, butter, fruit cup, milk
    4. consomme, creamed sweet breads, tomato slices, whole-wheat bread, butter, raspberries, milk

157. The arthritic patient who has great difficulty feeding himself can often be encouraged by providing foods that he

    1. can manage without spilling
    2. can eat without utensils
    3. can eat without chewing
    4. particularly enjoys

158. Ketosis will result when the diet is

    1. high in CHO and protein
    2. low in glucose and high in fat
    3. high in calories and CHO
    4. low in fat

159. Foods that should be avoided by the patient with gout because of their high purine content are

    1. glandular meats
    2. milk, eggs, and nuts
    3. breads and cereals
    4. beef and veal

160. The chief sources of protein for the patient with gout are

    1. beef and veal
    2. milk and eggs
    3. whole grains and nuts
    4. liver, kidney, brains

161. If the patient with a nervous-system disease has poor muscle coordination, he can be encouraged to feed himself by

    1. offering only brightly colored foods
    2. putting his plate conveniently in front of him
    3. offering foods that can be easily swallowed
    4. using foods that will stick to the spoon

162. To obtain the desired effects of the ketogenic diet, it will be necessary to alter the normal nutritive pattern by

    1. increasing fat and reducing CHO
    2. reducing protein but increasing calories
    3. increasing the vitamins and controlling the minerals
    4. increasing CHO and restricting sodium

163. The foods used in a ketogenic diet in the treatment of epilepsy are intended

    1. to reduce weight gradually
    2. to produce acidosis
    3. to prevent anemia
    4. to provide foods the patient will eat

164. In partial paralysis following a stroke, a food easily swallowed would be

    1. mashed potato   3. vegetable salad
    2. applesauce   4. roast beef

165. One nutritional problem in the use of the ketogenic diet is that

 1. it is difficult to prepare
 2. the protein content is inadequate
 3. the vitamin and mineral content is too low
 4. total calories are too low for the patient's activity needs

166. In multiple sclerosis in which there is tremor of the arm muscles the practical nurse assigned to the diet kitchen will

 1. plan to feed the patient since use of the arm increases the tremor
 2. provide foods in the form that will stick to the spoon
 3. support the arm as the patient feeds himself
 4. provide foods that are soft and easily chewed

167. The food substance most likely to be deficient in the diet of a pregnant woman is

 1. vitamin A
 2. vitamin C
 3. B complex vitamins
 4. protein

168. Studies of thousands of pregnant women seem to prove that there are fewer complications, such as anemia and toxemia, when

 1. the meat intake is moderate in amount
 2. vitamin and mineral concentrates are used
 3. the diet remains adequate throughout pregnancy
 4. the fat intake is reduced

169. An adequate diet throughout the prenatal period is important to the postnatal period. If the mother has had no major dietary deficiencies during the period of pregnancy, after birth of the baby she can expect

 1. to regain her strength more quickly
 2. to be free of all complications
 3. to have an adequate supply of milk
 4. to regain her figure quickly

170. The skeletal development of the unborn baby may be seriously affected if the prenatal diet does not contain adequate amounts of

 a. vitamin A
 b. calcium
 c. phosphorous
 d. vitamin D

 1. all of the above
 2. b only
 3. b and d
 4. b, c, and d

171. To avoid excessive weight gain, the expectant mother ought to concentrate on foods supplying necessary nutrients. A fat with the most nutritive value is

 1. Crisco   3. butter
 2. bacon   4. olive oil

172. The expectant mother is gaining weight too rapidly. The first thing she can do to control this increase is to eliminate from her diet all

 1. bread and cereals
 2. potato and corn
 3. butter and margarine
 4. fried foods and pastries

173. The physician has ordered a pregnant woman to reduce her calorie intake. To assist her in cutting calories without decreasing the amounts of needed nutrients, he will probably

 1. give her a rigid 1000-calorie menu
 2. insist that she omit all starches and fats from her intake
 3. advise her to limit fluid intake to 800 c.c. daily
 4. stress selection of items that come from the essential food groups

174. If an expectant mother is allergic to eggs, she could substitute for her "egg a day"

 1. a serving of cheese
 2. an extra serving of meat
 3. an extra glass of milk
 4. a serving of cereal

175. Which food listed below frequently causes the pregnant woman discomfort?

   1. sweet potato   3. lettuce
   2. green beans   4. raw peaches

176. If skim milk is substituted for whole milk to reduce calories, the diet should include more

   1. butter or margarine
   2. meats, poultry, fish
   3. fruits and vegetables
   4. green and yellow vegetables

177. High-protein foods recommended daily for the pregnant woman include

   1. 1 quart of milk, 1 egg, 4-to-5 ounces of meat
   2. 2 or more servings from the meat group, 1 pint of milk
   3. 1 quart of milk, 1 to 2 servings of meat
   4. 1 1/2 quart of milk, 1 egg, 3 ounces meat

178. The pregnant woman can expect to stimulate peristalsis with a diet that includes 4 or 5 daily servings of

   a. raw fruits
   b. raw vegetables
   c. cooked fruits
   d. cooked vegetables

     1. a and b
     2. all of the above, in combination
     3. c or d
     4. a and d

179. The daily milk intake during pregnancy should be 1 quart. This amount can be expected to supply

   a. the extra protein needs of pregnancy
   b. liberal amounts of easily digested lactose
   c. calcium
   d. riboflavin

     1. all of the above
     2. a only
     3. a and c
     4. all except b

180. The dietary relief of the nausea of early pregnancy includes

   a. liquids only
   b. a dry carbohydrate diet
   c. foods to reduce specific cravings
   d. 6 small meals

     1. all of the above
     2. d only
     3. a, c, and d
     4. b and d

181. Which of the food groups listed below will provide the most adequate daily intake of vitamin C for the expectant mother?

   1. 4 ounces of orange juice and a raw vegetable salad
   2. 6 ounces of grape juice
   3. 1 tomato and a raw vegetable salad
   4. 1 orange, 4 ounces of tomato juice, a raw vegetable salad

182. The food listed below that will supply the most milk in one serving is

   1. gravy   3. creamed asparagus
   2. custard   4. mashed potato

183. Which of the food groups listed below if eaten daily will provide sufficient iron to prevent anemia in both the mother and infant?

   1. 1 serving of citrus fruit, 2 servings of vegetables, 3 servings of breadstuffs
   2. potatoes, milk, fruits, and vegetables
   3. 1 green leafy vegetable, 1 egg, 4-to-5 ounces of meat
   4. 2 tablespoons of butter, 1 quart of milk, 3 servings enriched bread

184. In most instances the caloric intake of the expectant mother needs to be

   1. higher than for the nonpregnant woman because she is eating for two
   2. lower than for normal needs to prevent excessive weight gain
   3. approximately the same as for the non-pregnant woman
   4. gradually increased as the fetus develops and activity decreases

185. Check the one food below that adds little to the nutritional needs of the pregnant woman except calories:

1. rice
2. baked potato
3. oatmeal
4. enriched bread

186. The nursing mother requires 1 1/2 quarts of milk daily. Which combination of foods or food groups listed below will total the needed amount of milk?

a. 8 ounces of a milk beverage at each meal and at bedtime
b. 1/2 cup of cottage cheese
c. 1 ounce of cheddar cheese, 1 cup of milk soup, and 1/2 cup of milk dessert
d. 1/2 cup of custard

    1. all of the above
    2. a and b
    3. a and c
    4. a, b, and d

187. Compare breast milk with cow's milk. Check the following statements that are true:

a. breast milk has more carbohydrate
b. cow's milk contains almost twice as much protein
c. the amount of fat is about the same in each
d. the protein curds are larger in breast milk

    1. all of the above
    2. a, b, and c
    3. a, c, and d
    4. b, c, and d

188. An infant has nutritional requirements, compared with the needs at other age levels, that are

1. so high that vitamin supplements must be added to the diet
2. the highest of any growth period
3. lower than during school years
4. in line with the needs of most adolescents

189. Sugar is added to the infant's formula for the purpose of

1. improving the taste of the formula
2. increasing the caloric content
3. providing extra body-building materials
4. maintaining a normal consistency in the stools

190. The chief nutritive difference in commercially prepared infant formulas, as compared to the formulas prepared at home, is

1. the use of dextro-maltose or lactose for CHO content
2. the addition of lactic acid
3. the use of dry milk powders
4. the addition of minerals and vitamins

191. A definite reassurance to a mother that her infant is progressing favorably is the knowledge that

1. his weight compares with the weight of most children the same age
2. his weight agrees with that stated on the height-weight chart
3. his monthly weight is reported to the doctor
4. gains in height and weight are steady

192. Some source of ascorbic acid should be added to the infant's diet because

1. the supply in the liver is quickly exhausted
2. the vitamin C content of milk is too low to be of any value
3. the vitamin needs of a formula-fed baby are higher
4. food alone cannot supply the vitamin needs of a 6-month-old baby.

193. Fish-liver oils supply the infant's nutritional need for

1. ascorbic acid
2. vitamin B complex
3. iron
4. vitamin D

194. The infant on a formula has its energy needs adequately supplied by

1. use of 1 quart of milk
2. the addition of 3 ounces of orange juice daily
3. the protein content of the milk
4. the lactose and fat in the milk plus the added CHO

195. The iron that the infant needs in its first few months of existence is supplied by the

1. addition of sugar to the milk formula
2. fish-liver oil supplements
3. the reserve stored in its own liver
4. iron content of 1 quart of milk daily

196. It has been observed that foods, other than the formula, given to an infant earlier than age 2 1/2 to 3 months will

1. stimulate more rapid growth
2. result in excess weight gain
3. be almost completely eliminated in the feces
4. prevent anemia

197. Terminal sterilization of formulas is recommended because

1. milk curds are softened by heat
2. the method is safe and quick
3. harmful bacteria are destroyed
4. less vitamin C is destroyed

198. An infant with a respiratory infection should have a diet that

1. is increased in vitamin C and fish-liver oils
2. includes only liquids
3. consists of a diluted skim-milk formula
4. forces sugar water

199. When an infant has diarrhea, his diet should

1. include double the normal amount of water
2. be changed to boiled skim milk only
3. be withheld for 12 to 24 hours
4. consist of scraped apple

200. The most important reason for using terminal sterilization in preparing the infant's formula is the recognition that

1. the method is quicker and just as safe as older methods
2. the chance for contamination of the formula is decreased
3. the milk will not need to be boiled
4. the bottles will not need to be sterilized

201. A normal 4-month infant can be assured of an adequate protein intake if

1. he gets 1 quart of milk a day
2. egg yolk is added to the diet at 6 months of age
3. strained meats are included early in the first year
4. he receives prepared infant cereals twice daily

NURSING ARTS
PART I

(Answer sheets pp. 307-308)

The questions in this section test your basic knowledge of the principles of nursing procedures. The specific equipment and the step-by-step order for each procedure will vary from hospital to hospital, but the skills stressed to make them safe for the patient will be consistent from teaching program to teaching program. This section gives you an excellent opportunity to practice the objectivity discussed in the INTRODUCTION.

1. The nurse will find her bed-making efficiency is increased when she remembers

   1. to strip the bed completely
   2. to get the patient up in the chair
   3. to turn the mattress
   4. to collect all the necessary linen

2. Following the discharge of a patient, the nurse would expect to make up the bed according to the procedure for

   1. the open bed
   2. the closed bed
   3. the occupied bed
   4. the Gatch bed

3. Mrs. X is in a cast that covers her body from the axillary region to the groin. After a bed bath, the nurse would proceed to make

   1. an anesthetic bed
   2. an open bed
   3. a closed bed
   4. an occupied bed

4. The nurse is making the bed while the patient sits up in a chair. To save the physical energy of the nurse, the bed-making procedure specifies

   1. the use of a mattress protector
   2. the use of a draw sheet
   3. that assistance is needed to turn the mattress before the linens are placed on the bed
   4. that the linens be placed on one side of the bed before the nurse goes to the opposite side

5. If a rubber sheet and draw sheet are used, they should be placed on the bed so that their top edges come

   1. to the patient's armpits
   2. 10 inches from the head of the bed
   3. in the exact middle of the bed
   4. to the waistline of the patient

6. If the following types of mattresses were available, which would be best for the patient with a tendency toward pressure sores?

   1. orthopedic
   2. innerspring
   3. horsehair
   4. sponge rubber

7. A new patient is in the admitting office and has been assigned to Room 206. The nurse could expect to prepare this unit for occupancy by

   1. removing the chenille bedspread
   2. opening the bed
   3. opening the windows
   4. removing the extra pillow

8. The procedure for placing the top sheet and the bedspread is intended

   1. to protect the blanket
   2. to add to the professional appearance of the bed
   3. to keep the patient's shoulders covered
   4. to keep the bedspread from soiling

9. An innerspring mattress can safely be turned

   1. daily
   2. when the patient goes home
   3. from head to foot and side to side without bending
   4. by folding from the head to the foot

10. A freshly made bed is quickly upset if

   1. the covers are tucked in tightly at the foot
   2. the doctor visits
   3. the patient asks to use the bedpan
   4. wrinkes are left in the draw sheet

11. If, day after day, the nurse tucks the top bedding tightly over the feet, the result will be

    1. wrist drop
    2. foot drop
    3. poor posture
    4. backache

12. A well-made bed can best be judged by by the

    1. over-all appearance
    2. tightness of the linens
    3. smooth corners
    4. comfort of the patient

13. A closed bed must be opened carefully to avoid

    1. exposing the patient
    2. loosening the top linen
    3. pulling the bottom linen loose
    4. wrinkling the draw sheet

14. The nurse is taught to remove the bed linens one piece at a time. This is important to prevent

    1. loss of personal or hospital property
    2. a laundry miscount
    3. any error in exchange of clean for dirty linen
    4. exposure of the patient

15. On any hospital service the unit should be carefully cleaned after a patient goes home. The psychological value of this cleaning lies in

    1. the satisfaction of the person who cleans the unit
    2. the mental comfort of the next patient to use the unit
    3. the satisfaction one has earned his salary
    4. the need of all of us to do some housekeeping

16. Damp dusting is recommended for hospital furniture and the floor because it will

    1. kill more germs
    2. keep the germs in one unit
    3. preserve the paint
    4. prevent the spread of germs through the air

17. There is one place in a unit that is often missed in the terminal cleaning process, and one that is sure to be used by the next occupant. This place is

    1. the medicine cabinet
    2. the bedside stand
    3. the drawer in the over-the-bed table
    4. the bottom dresser drawer

18. The important principle to practice in cleaning a patient unit after the discharge of a patient is

    1. to start with the bed first so that another patient can use it
    2. send all of the items in the room to the laundry and request clean ones
    3. expect housekeeping employees to clean the unit
    4. start with the cleanest areas and progress to those most contaminated

19. Soiled equipment in a bedside stand, such as the wash basin, bedpan, urinal, and emesis basin can best be cleaned for use by a new patient by

    1. washing and sterilizing
    2. disinfecting
    3. washing and autoclaving
    4. washing with soapy water, rinsing, and drying

20. The person who cleans a patient unit and prepares it for use by another patient should be aware that one of her important responsibilities is

    1. to admit the next patient to that unit
    2. to check and report any equipment out of order
    3. to clean only the items to be used by the next patient
    4. to leave all the windows open to air the unit

21. A chart is considered legal evidence in court. To be of legal value, the signature of the R.N. or the L.P.N. must always be

    1. printed
    2. charted in blue ink
    3. written after each entry on the chart
    4. written

22. The practical nurse violates the charting principles she has been taught and fails in her legal responsibility when she

   1. charts only routine care
   2. fails to chart symptoms in a descriptive manner
   3. records medications and treatments before they are given
   4. permits the patient to refuse a medication

23. The practical nurse has recorded the temperature of an irrigating solution as 150°F instead of 105°F. To indicate this mistake, it will be necessary for her

   1. to recopy the entire chart
   2. to eradicate the mistake and correct it with red ink
   3. to draw a line through the mistake and write under it "ERROR"
   4. to recopy one page

24. Miss X has recorded information about Miss Brown on the chart of Mr. Jones. Since several nurses have recorded observations on Mr. Jones on this same page the nurse must recopy the entire page. Legally, the incorrect page must be

   1. filed in the Record Room
   2. destroyed
   3. filed at the back of the chart
   4. sent to the office of the medical assistant

25. An example of descriptive charting would be

   1. "Mrs X is uncooperative"
   2. "Mrs X refuses food"
   3. "Mrs X is making faces at other patients"
   4. "Mrs X clamps her teeth together when food is offered"

26. When a patient has a high temperature, oral hygiene should be carried out

   1. 3 times a day
   2. at least every 2 hours
   3. before and after meals
   4. as the patient desires

27. The headings on the chart sheets require certain information about the patient. The responsibility for filling in these chart headings belongs to

   1. the head nurse
   2. the night nurse
   3. the person who adds a new sheet
   4. the person who completes the sheet

28. The patient's name is James Stuart. So that there will be no confusion about which is the first name and which is the last name, the nurse should

   1. print the name clearly on all pages of the chart
   2. underline the last name
   3. write the last name first
   4. write the first name, middle initial, then the last name

29. Check the notation on the patient's chart that is <u>incorrect</u>:

   1. "The right ankle appears swollen and pressure with the finger tips produces pitting"
   2. Tosses about, changes position every few minutes. In constant motion"
   3. "General diet. Ate well"
   4. "A complete bed bath will be given as soon as the doctor removes the stitches and changes the dressing"

30. If the nurse is teaching the patient how to brush his teeth, she would explain that the movement of the brush should be

   1. circular
   2. up and down on the outside of the teeth, then on the inside
   3. downward on the upper teeth and upward on the lower teeth
   4. back and forth, sideways from the center of the mouth toward the back

31. Oral hygiene is important before the patient has an operation to prevent

   1. any after effects of the anesthetic
   2. vomiting postoperatively
   3. infection of the salivary glands after the operation
   4. loss of appetite postoperatively

32. When the patient is very sick, oral hygiene should be done

    a. when the patient wakes up in the morning
    b. every hour
    c. before and after meals
    d. at bedtime

      1. all of the above
      2. d only
      3. a, c, and d
      4. a, b, and c

33. The mouth and teeth of the unconscious patient can best be cleaned with

    1. glycerine and lemon juice
    2. gauze sponges
    3. dental floss
    4. a mouthwash gargle

34. A good argument the nurse can use to stress the importance of regular dental prophylaxis is the fact that

    1. people with bad breath are not popular
    2. a sweet breath is evidence of courtesy
    3. general body health can be kept at its best only when the teeth are in good condition
    4. prevention of decay is much cheaper than repair or dentures

35. An effective lubricant to apply to the gums, tongue, cheeks, and lips following removal of sordes is

    1. lemon and alcohol
    2. Listerine and water
    3. lemon and glycerine
    4. cold cream and vinegar

36. The method of cleaning dentures must take into consideration that the material used to make the plates may readily

    1. change shape if hot water is used
    2. be affected by the kind of toothpaste used
    3. slip out of one's hands
    4. deteriorate

37. Dentures must be protected from breaking during the cleaning process by

    1. using ice water
    2. rinsing in salt water
    3. plugging the drain
    4. keeping the running water under low pressure

38. Oral hygiene for the patient with dentures must include

    a. complete brushing of cheeks, tongue, and roof of the mouth
    b. brushing the dentures
    c. rinsing the mouth with mouthwash
    d. soaking the teeth in a pleasant-tasting solution

      1. all of the above
      2. a and b
      3. b, c, and d
      4. b and c

39. It would be an indication of empathy on the part of the nurse if the convalescent patient with dentures is

    1. supervised during the cleaning
    2. left alone while he brushes them
    3. instructed in their correct care
    4. permitted to keep the dentures in his mouth all the time

40. Matted or tangled hair can best be combed if the nurse uses

    1. a small amount of alcohol or vaseline
    2. a vinegar rinse
    3. a coarse-toothed comb
    4. a wire brush

41. Long hair is difficult to care for when the patient is acutely ill. However, the practical nurse must remember that legally

    1. a daily combing is necessary
    2. it can safely be left in braids for days
    3. written permission is needed to cut it short
    4. this is one area of care the patient can do for herself

42. Combing tangled hair will be less painful for the patient if the nurse

   1. brushes the hair
   2. combs from the ends of the hair toward the scalp
   3. cuts out tangles that pull
   4. shampoos the hair before brushing it

43. Combing and brushing the hair are usually the last things done in the complete bath procedure. Clean linens should be protected by

   1. directing the patient to hold her head over the side of the bed
   2. newspapers
   3. covering the pillow with a face towel
   4. removing the pillows

44. Care of the hair must protect the patient from a scalp infection. The nurse should never be guilty of

   1. using the patient's personal equipment
   2. using one set of equipment for several patients without sterilizing them between uses
   3. using a strong disinfectant solution on the comb and brush
   4. roughness in caring for matted, tangled hair

45. The natural oils on the hair shaft interfere with the sudsing of a shampoo. This makes it necessary

   1. to rinse the hair with a grease-cutting solution before applying the shampoo
   2. to use water at a temperature of 120°F or higher
   3. to use a dry shampoo first
   4. to use two or more applications of shampoo

46. The nits of pediculi look like dandruff. One differentiating characteristic of nits is their ability

   1. to move up and down the hair shaft
   2. to dissolve in soap and water
   3. to produce a skin rash
   4. to stick tightly to the hair shaft

47. The nurse should be alert to the presence of head lice (Pediculi capitis) in

   a. eyebrows and eyelashes
   b. beard
   c. moustache
   d. chest hairs

      1. a only
      2. a, b, and c
      3. b or d
      4. all of the above

48. After appropriate treatment, the nits and the pediculi are removed from the hair by fine combing. The best way to destroy the nits and the pediculi is

   1. to collect the combings on newspaper and burn them
   2. to continue the treatment daily for several weeks
   3. to soak the head in vinegar
   4. to shampoo with a surgical-soap solution

49. For the patient who is confined to bed over a period of several weeks, the bed bath is a valuable way

   1. to stimulate circulation
   2. to entertain the patient
   3. to promote sleep
   4. to occupy the patient's time

50. Before the practical nurse starts a bed bath she is advised to visit the patient's room. Such a visit will allow her

   a. to offer the patient the bedpan or urinal
   b. to determine what linens are needed
   c. to judge how long the bath procedure will take

      1. all of the above
      2. a only
      3. b only
      4. a and b

51. Soap that is incompletely rinsed off the skin surface will cause

   1. itching
   2. a rash
   3. macules
   4. decubitus areas

52. The nurse must give a complete bed bath to a very sick patient. The bath for such a patient would be considered a form of

1. active exercise
2. passive exercise
3. hydrotherapy
4. occupational therapy

53. The bed patient who is unable to help himself finds that a good bed bath stimulates

a. circulation
b. digestion
c. respiration
d. elimination

    1. all of the above
    2. a only
    3. b or d
    4. a, c, and d

54. The bath procedure instructs the nurse to place the patient's foot in the bath basin. To do this safely the patient must be able

1. to sit on the edge of the bed
2. to get into the bathtub
3. to flex his leg at the knee
4. to use a foot tub

55. A tub bath for cleansing purposes should be limited to

1. 5 minutes   3. 20 minutes
2. 10 minutes   4. 30 minutes

56. The practical nurse must never give a patient a tub bath unless

1. the patient has had bathroom privileges
2. the doctor has written an order for it
3. the pulse is within normal limits
4. the patient will allow her to remain in the bathroom

57. The patient has had breakfast at 8:00 A.M. The nurse should not plan to give this patient a tub bath before

1. 8:10 A.M.   3. 8:30 A.M.
2. 8:20 A.M.   4. 9:00 A.M.

58. The patient in the bathtub begins a grand mal convulsion. The FIRST thing the nurse will do is

1. call for help
2. pull the plug to let the water run out
3. get the patient out of the tub and on to the floor
4. hold the patient's head out of the water

59. This is the first time Mrs X has had a tub bath since her hospitalization. The nurse should appreciate how important it is for the doctor to know

1. the temperature of the water
2. how long the patient remained in the tub
3. the patient's ability to care for herself
4. the pulse rate, before and after the bath

60. Mr. A is completely helpless. The doctor has ordered daily tub baths to enable the nurse to carry out passive exercises under the water. Such a patient should be

a. placed in the tub before it is filled with water
b. removed from the tub after the water has been drained
c. encouraged to help himself as much as possible
d. stimulated by a water temperature of 86°F

    1. a only
    2. all except d
    3. a and b
    4. all of the above

61. If hangnails are pulled off instead of cut off there is greater danger of

1. trauma   3. pain
2. infection   4. swelling

62. A.M. care is given for the purpose of

1. making the patient appear well when the doctor visits
2. providing hygienic care that will freshen the patient
3. satisfying the hospital policy
4. giving the nurse a chance to observe the patient's condition

63. The patient's nails are best cared for immediately following the bath procedure because

1. the nurse will be more likely to remember it then
2. it more nearly follows the patient's usual hygienic habits
3. dirt and the cuticle are loosened by soap and water
4. the nurse has more time then

64. The nurse should plan to start her A.M.-care assignment with the patient who

1. has bathroom privileges
2. is most demanding
3. has a special diet and his breakfast will be served first
4. has had the most uncomfortable night

65. It is hoped that the nurse's plan of A.M. care will recognize the importance of

1. washing all patients
2. leaving the sleeping patient until the last
3. omitting such care if the patient is acutely ill
4. leaving some patients until breakfast is served

66. The nurse should consider that the A.M. care procedure gives her an opportunity to

1. make the patient help himself
2. prepare the patient to face the new day
3. plan her nursing care on the basis of patient needs
4. guide the patient's mental outlook

67. Oral hygiene is an important part of A.M. care because it often helps the sick patient

1. enjoy his breakfast
2. face the day with a better attitude
3. feel more normal
4. prevent dental decay

68. An accurate oral temperature taken in the early A.M. must be done

1. just before breakfast is served
2. after the oral hygiene procedure
3. before 6:00 A.M.
4. before oral hygiene is done

69. If the evening-care (P.M.-care) procedure is to accomplish its purpose, it is best done

1. before supper
2. before visiting hours
3. after visiting hours
4. when the patient feels sleepy

70. The nurse should use all her nursing skills to enable the very sick patient to sleep well because sleep

1. helps the time pass more rapidly
2. gives body tissues a chance to repair themselves
3. decreases the amount of medicine needed
4. uses less energy

71. Thorough evening care will be of little value if

1. there is more than one patient in a room
2. the doctor does a painful dressing later
3. the patient turns on his radio to go to sleep
4. there are too many nurses on night duty

72. Mrs Y was admitted at 6:00 P.M. The nurse can use the evening care procedure to reassure this patient that

1. the doctor has left orders for sleeping pills
2. other patients will not disturb her
3. there is nothing to fear from the ward noises
4. a nurse will be within call all night

73. A backrub should take the nurse a minimum of

1. 3 to 5 minutes   3. 15 minutes
2. 5 to 10 minutes   4. 20 to 30 minutes

74. Mr. Jones is scheduled for exploratory surgery in the morning. The sensitive nurse will recognize that the time spent in the evening-care procedure can be used to encourage

1. passive exercise
2. the patient to talk
3. bed exercises
4. occupational therapy

75. When a patient lies in bed constantly, day after day, extra massage is welcome

1. on the buttocks muscles
2. over the hip bones
3. over the shoulder blades
4. on the lower back and the neck

76. If the backrub procedure is to require the least amount of energy for the nurse, the patient should be

1. in the center of the bed
2. on her stomach
3. close to the edge of the bed, near the nurse
4. relaxed during the rub

77. A backrub is sure to be uncomfortable for the patient if

1. the nurse's hands are cold
2. the nurse runs her hands lightly over the back
3. the nurse chatters throughout the procedure
4. it takes too long

78. A backrub is used to stimulate circulation. The greatest pressure is applied by the hands

1. on the downward stroke
2. on the upward stroke
3. at the base of the neck
4. in the small of the back

79. A fully developed pressure sore can be recognized by the presence of

1. the bluish color
2. an area of infection and pus
3. the foul odor
4. an area of dead tissue

80. The supervisor is watching the practical nurse during the backrub procedure in an effort to evaluate the interest of the nurse in the patients. The supervisor will be sure to observe

1. the kind of lotion used
2. the position of the patient
3. the length of the nurse's fingernails
4. the conversation of the nurse

81. The massage of reddened pressure areas should be done gently, starting from

1. the outer surface and working toward the center
2. the center and working toward the outer surface
3. the periphery
4. the distal location

82. Lack of nutrition to the tissues is the usual cause of a pressure sore. This is most often the result of

1. prolonged pressure on the part
2. an inadequate diet
3. dehydration
4. a decreased number of blood vessels in the part

83. The nurse would suspect the beginnings of a pressure sore if such objective signs were present as

1. pain, swelling, and cyanosis
2. redness and ulceration
3. redness, heat, and a mottled appearance
4. pain and loss of function

84. The infant, Baby X, has a reddened area on the right ear when you go off duty Friday evening. If this has broken down into a pressure sore by the time you return to duty Monday morning, you would suspect

1. he had not been bathed
2. he had not eaten well
3. his position had not been changed often enough
4. his relatives had cared for him during visiting hours

85. Good nursing care could prevent causes of pressure sores such as

   a. poor circulation
   b. moisture
   c. wrinkles
   d. prolonged weight of the body on one part

      1. none of the above
      2. all of the above
      3. d only
      4. b, c, and d

86. The paralyzed patient must be <u>very carefully</u> watched for evidences of pressure sores because

   1. he cannot feel the effects of pressure
   2. the patient does not complain
   3. nourishment is decreased to the danger areas
   4. the temperature may be high

87. The internal body temperature stays fairly constant as long as the body can

   1. stay alive
   2. keep comfortable
   3. balance the daily heat production with the daily heat loss
   4. keep the brain functioning to bring out homeostatic processes

88. Body heat is lost through

   a. the skin
   b. the bowels
   c. the urine
   d. perspiration

      1. a and d only
      2. a, c, and d
      3. d only
      4. all of the above

89. In cold weather the brain stimulates the skeletal muscles to produce more heat by causing us

   1. to shiver
   2. to feel cold
   3. to feel hungry
   4. to put on more clothing

90. Foods high in fats and carbohydrates provide more fuel to the cells because they are

   1. higher in calories than other foods
   2. more easily digested and absorbed
   3. burned better than any other foods
   4. high in oils which burn easily

91. One way the brain controls the increase or decrease of heat lost is by the regulation of

   1. the kind of food eaten
   2. the room temperature
   3. the emotional stimuli
   4. the production of perspiration

92. A greater amount of body heat will be lost into the environment when the surface blood vessels

   1. contract
   2. dilate
   3. increase the production of sweat
   4. help the skeletal muscles relax

93. Before a thermometer is used, the nurse is instructed to be sure the mercury level is

   1. 94°F   3. 96°F
   2. 95°F   4. 98.6°F

94. When a high temperature quickly drops to normal or below, the process is described as

   1. lysis   3. fever
   2. regular   4. crisis

95. The mercury end of a rectal thermometer is inserted into the rectum for a length of

   1. 1 inch   3. 2 inches
   2. 1 1/2 inches   4. 3 inches

96. The rectal thermometer must be <u>held</u> in place for a period of

   1. 1 minute   3. 3 minutes
   2. 2 minutes   4. 4 minutes

97. If the groin had to be used to check a patient's temperature, the thermometer would be surrounded by body tissue if the patient

   1. held the thermometer in place
   2. remained flat on his back
   3. flexed his knee sharply
   4. had the head of the bed elevated

98. Temperature will not be taken by rectum if the patient has just had

   1. a bowel movement
   2. rectal surgery
   3. a painful dressing
   4. visitors

99. The method of removing saliva or feces from a thermometer begins with

   1. wiping off the thermometer, starting from the center of the thermometer and working toward the bulb end
   2. a hot-water rinse
   3. cleansing with an alcohol cotton ball
   4. wiping off the thermometer, starting from the bulb end and working toward the finger tips

100. A reasonably correct temperature cannot be obtained in the axilla if

   1. the thermometer is left in place too long
   2. a rectal thermometer is used
   3. the patient has just had a drink of water
   4. the armpit is rubbed dry before the thermometer is put in place

101. Temperature, pulse, and respiration are usually checked together because in combination they give the doctor valuable information

   1. about the fighting forces of the body
   2. about the hypothalamus
   3. on the functioning of the body
   4. for a prognosis

102. A temperature reading of 98.6°F is considered normal when it is obtained by

   1. a skin thermometer
   2. the axillary route
   3. the rectal route
   4. the oral route

103. The nurse must recognize that in evaluating a temperature reading the method of taking the temperature must be considered, since

   a. the only accurate method is an oral temperature
   b. a rectal temperature is one degree higher than oral
   c. adjustments must be made in the reading
   d. an axillary temperature is one degree lower than oral

   1. all of the above
   2. a only
   3. b and d
   4. b and c

104. If the patient has both arms in a cast from shoulder to fingers, the nurse would expect to count the pulse at

   1. the radial artery
   2. the temporal artery
   3. the femoral artery
   4. the sciatic artery

105. An artery that can be used to count the pulse must be located

   1. close to the heart
   2. close to the skin surface, over a bone
   3. near an important organ
   4. in the upper part of the body

106. The most important precaution to take if an accurate count of respirations is to be obtained is

   1. to count them without the patient's knowledge
   2. to wait until the patient is relaxed
   3. to use a watch with a second hand
   4. to take the temperature first

107. If a young man's pulse is 64 just before visiting hours and 72 after his sweetheart has left, the nurse would <u>suspect</u> the increase was the result of

1. relaxation from a pleasant visit
2. excitement
3. a quarrel
4. emotional strain of entertaining visitors

108. It is unwise to take the patient's blood pressure right after the meal because

1. the patient may become upset and have indigestion
2. food intake causes a rise in blood pressure
3. it interferes with the digestion of protein
4. the blood will be helping the digestion of food and not be in the arm

109. An accurate blood pressure reading requires the patient to be positioned

1. flat on his back
2. with the arm well supported
3. with the feet higher than the heart
4. before and after the initial reading

110. Blood pressure is normally increased

1. during illness
2. when the patient is tired
3. during an emotional upset
4. before the morning bath

111. The contraction of the heart muscle produces

1. the highest blood pressure reading
2. hypertension
3. the lowest blood pressure reading
4. changes in heart sounds

112. The blood pressure cuff will be wrapped around the upper arm and the stethescope will be placed over

1. the radial artery
2. the dorsalis pedis artery
3. the femoral artery
4. the brachial artery

113. A blood pressure reading listed below that would be considered normal for a man aged 20 would be

1. 140/72   3. 120/64
2. 120/80   4. 130/72

114. The resting phase of the heart-beat cycle is called

1. systole
2. diastole
3. sphygmomanometer
4. pulse pressure

115. The nurse could expect a blood pressure to be higher if

a. the lumen of the blood vessels was small
b. the walls of the blood vessels were rigid
c. blood is thinner than normal
d. the patient is a man

1. c only
2. a and b
3. b and d
4. all of the above

116. <u>If</u> a blood-pressure reading is to give <u>valuable</u> information, it will be necessary for the doctor and the nurse

1. to know the age, previous illness, medication being taken
2. to know the patient's attitude toward the procedure
3. to get the same reading
4. to know the normal blood-pressure reading of the patient

117. When a hot application is applied to the skin, the nurse would expect

a. surface blood vessels to dilate
b. sweat glands to decrease production
c. the skin to become pink
d. the muscles to relax

1. c only
2. a, b, and c
3. all of the above
4. a, c, and d

118. Patients vary in the degree of heat they can tolerate. One thing that will determine the degree of heat the patient can take in a local hot application is

    1. the texture of his skin
    2. his condition
    3. color of his skin
    4. his sex

119. The patient is a conscious adult. Water placed in a hot water bag for such a patient should not exceed

    1. 95°F   3. 125°F
    2. 110°F   4. 135°F

120. An ice bag might be ordered if an acute inflammation of the appendix were suspected because the cold would

    1. decrease the blood supply to the part and slow up pus formation
    2. relieve the pain by contracting the appendix
    3. prevent the spread of the infection
    4. deaden the pain until surgery can be done

121. An ice bag would be applied to an area that had just received a severe blow in an effort

    1. to relieve pain
    2. to reduce swelling
    3. to decrease hemorrhage into the tissue
    4. to lower local elevation of temperature

122. The amount of help the nurse must provide to get food ready for the patient to eat will depend on his

    a. physical strength
    b. previous eating habits
    c. need for attention
    d. muscle coordination

        1. a only
        2. b and c
        3. a and d
        4. all of the above

123. If the patient complains of the weight of the ice bag applied to his chest

    1. remove it at once
    2. suspend it from a bed cradle
    3. use only small amounts of ice in the bag
    4. fanfold the bedding back to lessen weight

124. A common fault of the nurse who is feeding a patient is

    1. to use too large a spoon
    2. to insist that all food on the tray be eaten
    3. to feed according to her own eating pattern
    4. to make it very evident that she has more important things to do

125. Before the tray is brought to the bed patient, the nurse must give the patient an opportunity

    1. to rest
    2. to wash his hands
    3. to get rid of his visitors
    4. to move to the most comfortable position

126. If the nurse uses good body mechanics to carry the tray, she will

    1. support it with her shoulder
    2. use both hands
    3. carry the tray at arms' length in front of her
    4. carry the tray at waist level with her elbows close to her sides

127. The ambulatory patient will have the best appetite if the hospital facilities make it possible for him

    1. to sit up in the chair to eat
    2. to eat with other patients who are pleasant
    3. to eat at the same time he would eat at home
    4. to be introduced to foods he has not eaten before

128. If a rubber ring is used to relieve pressure over the coccyx, it is necessary

    1. to inflate the ring to full capacity for firm support
    2. to place the ring so that the air valve lies between the patient's legs
    3. to pad it with cotton to prevent pressure on the buttocks
    4. to use a straw to inflate the ring sanitarily

129. Most bed patients spend some time lying on their sides. Comfort in this position will be increased by

    1. turning the bed toward the window
    2. elevating the back rest
    3. extending the legs at the hip joints
    4. placing a pillow lengthwise between the legs

130. To keep the feet and legs in good physiological position while the patient is lying on his back, it will be necessary

    1. to place a footboard at the bottom of the mattress
    2. to use foam-rubber doughnuts under the heels
    3. to use sandbags to prevent movement
    4. to miter the sheet and spread firmly for support

131. A good way to keep the weight of the top bedding off the feet and legs is to use

    1. pleats in the bedspread
    2. warm bed socks
    3. a bed cradle
    4. percale or nylon bedding

132. To prevent pressure on the breasts of the female patient while she is lying on her stomach, it will be necessary

    1. to place a pillow under the abdomen
    2. to elevate the head of the bed
    3. to place two pillows under the patient's head
    4. to supply a well-fitted brassiere

133. If the patient is lying on his stomach, pressure on the toes can be prevented by

    1. raising the foot of the bed
    2. a footboard
    3. placing a pillow under the lower legs
    4. cotton doughnuts

134. Deformities that result from the arms and legs rolling outward can be prevented by the correct use of

    1. a footboard
    2. sandbags
    3. a rubber ring
    4. a foam rubber mattress

135. If pillows are to be used effectively as comfort devices, it is necessary that

    1. they be made of foam rubber
    2. they be made of horsehair
    3. a plastic protective cover be used
    4. a variety of sizes be available

136. The first time the patient is permitted to dangle his legs, the nurse should tell him to expect that

    1. he will feel faint
    2. his feet and legs will tingle
    3. he will become breathless
    4. nausea and dizziness will occur

137. When two nurses are needed to get the helpless patient into a chair, both must remember that it is important

    1. to work in unison
    2. to move the patient smoothly
    3. to talk to keep the patient from being fearful
    4. to dress the patient warmly

138. When the patient is getting out of bed with the assistance of the nurse, he should be instructed to place his hands

    1. on the nurse's shoulders
    2. around the nurse's neck
    3. so that the palms are resting on the edge of the bed
    4. so that he is supported by crossing his arms over his chest

139. To prepare a wheelchair so that it will be safe to move the patient into it, the nurse should

    1. make the chair comfortable
    2. be sure that the chair is in good repair
    3. be sure that the wheels are locked
    4. lower the leg rests

140. The best support for the patient who is just out of bed and walking in the corridor will be

    1. hard-soled bedroom slippers
    2. soft, pliable shoes
    3. toeless clogs
    4. his own street shoes

141. The usual reason for the doctor's restraint order is

    1. to keep the patient quiet
    2. to protect the patient
    3. to keep stitches from breaking
    4. to relieve the nurse of extra work

142. Limitation of motion in a part may be necessary

    1. to permit healing of the part
    2. to the over-all treatment
    3. to prevent or control deformity
    4. to facilitate muscle re-education

143. The elderly patient is confused and disoriented. It is often wise to limit his motion by use of

    1. a strait jacket
    2. a cold, wet sheet pack
    3. bedside rails
    4. arm and leg leather restraints

144. A procedure stressed in the personal hygiene of a well person but so often neglected by the nurse in the care of the bedfast patient is

    1. good room ventilation after a bowel movement
    2. a plentiful supply of toilet tissue
    3. handwashing following elimination
    4. provision for privacy

145. If the patient must be prevented from tearing dressings from his eyes, it would be necessary to restrict movement of

    1. his fingers   3. his shoulders
    2. his elbows   4. his head

146. If there is much friction between the restraint and the patient's skin surface, one could expect

    1. the patient to struggle for freedom
    2. redness, heat, and swelling
    3. a jaundiced condition
    4. the part to become cyanotic

147. To keep the restless patient from injuring himself by falling out of bed, a wise doctor may order restraints placed

    1. on all four extremities
    2. on both arms
    3. on both legs
    4. on one arm and the opposite leg

148. To put the helpless patient on the bedpan, the following steps may be necessary:

    a. lift the hips
    b. place the pan against the buttocks
    c. roll the patient to one side
    d. roll the patient on the pan

THE CORRECT ORDER OF THESE STEPS IS

    1. a, b, and d
    2. b and d
    3. c, b, and d
    4. a and b

149. Before a nurse gives a medication, she should know

    a. why the medication is being given
    b. the safe dosage
    c. how long the patient will be on the medication
    d. the expected results

    1. none of the above
    2. a and b only
    3. all but c
    4. all of the above

150. The nurse should be especially careful to take away the bedpan or urinal promptly when it is almost

1. visiting or meal time
2. time for shift change
3. bedtime
4. bath time

151. The nurse should expect the male patient who asks for the bedpan to want also

1. both the head and foot of the bed elevated
2. the urinal
3. to be left alone in the room
4. a laxative

152. A practical nurse who understands how the patient reacts to her behavior and attitudes will realize that constipation may be caused by

1. fear of an enema
2. the need of a laxative
3. her failure to respond quickly to the signal light
4. her expression of disgust at having to empty the bedpan

153. A medication classed as an analgesic and ordered for its palliative effects will be given for the purpose of

1. curing the disease
2. getting the disease under control
3. preventing the disease
4. easing the discomfort

154. The organ through which a medicine is eliminated from the body receives the most concentrated dose of the drug. With this knowledge, the nurse should expect that

1. frequent specimens from this part will be collected
2. symptoms of overdose or cumulation will appear in this part first
3. she will need to check the rate of elimination of the drug
4. an order for "force fluids" will be needed

155. A drug that is given for its local effect can be expected to treat

1. the entire body
2. the circulatory system only
3. one specific part of the body
4. the skin surface only

156. Any very potent medicine will be given to a child in a dose that is

1. smaller than that for an adult
2. the same as that for an adult
3. larger than required for an adult
4. combined with milder medications

157. When the organ through which a drug is eliminated is diseased and working less efficiently, the nurse would expect the ordered dose to be

1. smaller than the usual dose
2. larger than the usual dose
3. in liquid form
4. given by hypodermic

158. The nurse could expect that a drug such as morphine would be given in a larger-than-usual dose when the patient

1. has respiratory complications
2. is in very great pain
3. has edema
4. is not cooperative

159. A drug that is slowly eliminated from the body can produce very serious symptoms when its effects are

1. rapid
2. retarded
3. cumulative
4. habit forming

160. The most rapid effects of a medication will be obtained by giving it

1. orally
2. hypodermically
3. intramuscularly
4. intravenously

161. The greatest harm to the body cells results when the patient's reaction to the drug is one of

1. habituation
2. addiction
3. immunity
4. resistance

162. If oral medications are to be absorbed rapidly for a quick effect, they should be given

1. mixed with food
2. in capsule form
3. when the stomach is empty
4. only after the stomach juices have started to flow

163. When the amount of drug present in the blood stream must be kept at a constant level, the doctor will order a large initial dose, followed regularly by

1. a therapeutic dose
2. a cumulative dose
3. a maintenance dose
4. a tolerance dose

164. When a medicine is given by inhalation for the relief of systemic symptoms, the nurse would expect the effects to be

1. too great
2. difficult to determine
3. very valuable
4. dangerous

165. Under what circumstances would a student practical nurse refuse to give a medication:

1. if the patient is disoriented
2. if the patient is uncooperative
3. if the instructor is not present
4. if there is no written order

166. When a bad-tasting medicine must be given, the nurse is usually allowed to lessen the unpleasantness by

1. diluting the medicine with water
2. giving the patient ice chips before the medicine
3. putting the medicine in fruit juice
4. putting it in a capsule

167. If a drug is absorbed into the circulatory system, yet it has an effect on only one part of the body, its action is described as

1. selective   3. untoward
2. antagonistic   4. stimulating

168. When cough medicines are given to soothe irritated tissues of the throat, the action is described as

1. selective   3. systemic
2. local   4. depressive

169. The diabetic person whose body does not produce enough insulin will be taking insulin by hypodermic. Such treatment is described as

1. anti-infective
2. hormone therapy
3. essential
4. replacement therapy

170. The patient who develops a skin rash from taking aspirin will be reported as having

1. a reaction
2. a tolerance to the drug
3. side effects
4. an idiosyncracy to the drug

171. Tablets that are absorbed into the blood stream through the large blood vessels under the tongue are labeled

1. oral   3. parenteral
2. hypodermic   4. sublingual

172. If the medication normally has a precipitate, the label should read

1. FOR LOCAL ADMINISTRATION ONLY
2. POISON
3. SHAKE WELL
4. FOR EXTERNAL USE ONLY

173. If the practical nurse is to give medicines safely, one of the first principles of administration that she must put into practice is

1. her knowledge of the average dosages of all common medicines
2. her knowledge of the route of administration for each kind of medicine
3. to inquire if there is any doubt about the drug or the dose
4. the strictest sterile technique in their preparation

174. The administration of narcotics under the control of the Harrison Narcotic Law, even if the drug is given orally, requires the nurse

    1. to account for it on an appropriate sign-out form
    2. to give it only for a limited time
    3. to give it only when the order reads P.R.N.
    4. to have her mathematics checked by the supervisor

175. Safe preparation of medicines requires a well-organized medicine cabinet. Such organization will include

    1. a double lock
    2. a separation of medicines for internal use
    3. location next to the nurses' desk
    4. adequate storage space and running water

176. The recommended way to pour liquid medications into a medicine glass is

    1. to hold the glass at eye level and keep the thumbnail on the level to pour
    2. to leave the glass on the counter and look into the glass until the correct level is reached
    3. to hold the glass up to the light
    4. to hold the medicine glass a distance from the bottle

177. Medicines can be most accurately recorded on the chart when the nurse

    1. charts each medication as soon as it is given
    2. checks the doctor's order sheet before each medicine is charted
    3. charts from penciled notes she has in her pocket
    4. charts from the medicine tickets

178. The syringe usually referred to as a "hypodermic" will hold fluid up to

    1. 15 minims   3. 32 minims
    2. 20 minims   4. 45 minims

179. Since the nurse who gives the medication must be sure the patient has taken it, she should appreciate her instructions

    1. always to look in the patient's mouth
    2. to dissolve all pills and capsules so that they cannot be hoarded
    3. to find some way to give the medication by injection if she does not trust the patient
    4. never to leave medicine on the bedside stand for the patient to take ad. lib.

180. Daily care of the medicine cupboard will be much easier for the person assigned this task if each co-worker

    1. wipes off the bottles before returning them to the shelf
    2. washes the medicine glasses
    3. takes his turn at dusting the shelves
    4. keeps the labels upright while pouring

181. To be sure that medicine is still to be given and to check the ordered dose, it is important for the student practical nurse

    1. to read the label
    2. to be able to identify her patient
    3. to compare the medicine ticket with the doctor's order
    4. to ask the instructor to check each medication

182. A medication will be given by hypodermic when it is known the drug will be

    1. irritating to the stomach
    2. changed by the gastric juices
    3. nourishing to the tissues
    4. delayed in its action

183. To get 1 c.c. of medication out of a 1-c.c. ampoule, it will be necessary for the nurse

    1. to use a 5-c.c. syringe
    2. to draw air into the syringe equal to the amount of fluid in the ampoule
    3. to tip the ampoule gradually to get all the medicine drawn into the syringe
    4. to use a needle with a large lumen

184. The usual location for the injection of a hypodermic medication is

   1. into the outer surface of the upper arm
   2. into the gluteal muscle of the buttock
   3. determined by the purpose of the drug
   4. dependent on the amount of fatty tissue present on the extremities

185. The skin area must be cleansed before the hypodermic is given. Cleansing with an alcohol sponge is done by

   1. massaging the entire area thoroughly
   2. starting at the outer limits of the injection site and moving to the center
   3. a spray of alcohol under pressure
   4. starting at the injection site and moving outward

186. To give a hypodermic injection correctly, the needle should be inserted at an angle of

   1. 25°   3. 60°
   2. 45°   4. 90°

187. The preparation of a medication in tablet form for hypodermic injection requires the tablet to be

   1. dissolved in distilled water
   2. crushed before fluid is added
   3. dissolved in sterile water
   4. dissolved in normal saline solution

188. The most effective way to obtain relaxation of the gluteal muscles is to place the patient

   1. on his side, with both legs extended
   2. in a modified Sims position
   3. in the dorsal recumbent position
   4. in the prone position

189. The angle of insertion of the needle for administration of medicine into muscle tissue is

   1. a 30° angle   3. a 80° angle
   2. a 45° angle   4. a 90° angle

190. An intramuscular injection is most often given in the area described as

   1. the deltoid muscle, at a 30° angle
   2. near the inner angle of the upper outer quadrant of the gluteal muscle
   3. near the inner angle of the lower inner quadrant of the gluteal muscle
   4. the dividing line of the upper outer quadrant of the gluteal muscle

191. The advantage of leaving a small air bubble in the syringe before the needle is inserted into muscular tissue is

   1. to cleanse the needle of all medicine
   2. to help liquify the drug so that it will not be so hard to give
   3. to make sure all medication is injected into the muscle
   4. to replace the air lost when the needle is inserted

192. The nutritional state of the patient receiving an I.M. medication will determine

   a. the total amount of medicine given
   b. the length of the needle
   c. the position of the patient
   d. the depth the needle is inserted

   1. all of the above
   2. d only
   3. b and c
   4. b and d

193. The skin area to be injected is pinched or stretched for the purpose of

   1. keeping the procedure professional
   2. giving the nurse a better view of the injection site
   3. easing the penetration of the needle through the skin
   4. avoiding penetrating a blood vessel or a nerve

194. Any substance that is being injected directly into a vein must be

   1. sterile
   2. given with a doctor in attendance
   3. the same pH as the blood
   4. supplying some nourishment to the blood

195. Medication cannot be easily withdrawn from a vial unless

1. there is at least 10 c.c. of fluid in the bottle
2. the medicine bottle is held upright
3. air, equal to the amount of solution to be removed, is put in the bottle
4. the bottle is carefully tipped to one side while pressure is exerted on the plunger

196. The practical nurse must understand that in many work situations she will be allowed only

1. to observe the professional nurse set up for an I.V.
2. to sit with the patient who is getting an I.V.
3. to start an I.V. under the direction of a doctor
4. to give the patient an explanation of what is going to be done

197. The safest temperature for a solution that is to be given by I.V. is

1. normal body temperature
2. normal skin temperature
3. room temperature
4. 105°F

198. The I.V. needle can be kept sterile until the doctor is ready to start the treatment if it is

1. left on the sterile tray
2. wrapped in sterile gauze
3. covered with the sterile tube and fastened to the I.V. standard
4. inserted, full length, through the top of the bottle of solution

199. If the practical nurse is responsible for loosening the tourniquet after the needle is in the vein, great care must be taken

1. to keep the needle sterile
2. not to frighten the patient
3. not to upset the bottle of fluid
4. to avoid jarring the needle out of the vein

200. The importance of getting all the air out of the tubing before an I.V. solution is given is to prevent

1. a reaction to the fluid
2. an embolus
3. a thrombus
4. the "bends"

201. The practical nurse will recognize that the needle has slipped out of the vein when

1. fluid accumulates in the tissues
2. the patient gets restless
3. the bed linen is damp
4. the solution is leaving the bottle too rapidly

202. The practical nurse must know that symptoms of a reaction call for shutting off the flow of blood. Such warning symptoms include

a. nasal hemorrhage
b. cyanosis
c. hives
d. cold, clammy skin

    1. all of the above
    2. c only
    3. b and c
    4. d only

203. The organism that is responsible for causing a disease is described as

1. an exotoxin   3. pathogenic
2. a toxin   4. a fomite

204. If equipment is to be sterilized by boiling, the practical nurse must recognize the importance of

1. using distilled water
2. boiling it only the required length of time
3. having the articles covered with water
4. using a large kettle

205. It takes a longer and more complicated procedure (such as steam under pressure) to kill

1. pathogenic bacteria   3. endotoxins
2. viruses   4. spores

206. Equipment and supplies are sterilized because of the necessity for

    1. providing aseptically clean equipment
    2. destroying all microorganisms and their spores
    3. protecting hospitalized patients from germs
    4. preventing the spread of infection

207. If one student had an uncovered, draining abscess on the palm of her hand, the infection could be transferred to another student by way of a <u>fomite</u> such as

    1. a wet wash cloth   3. Kleenex
    2. the toilet seat   4. the door knob

208. If a sterile rubber tube touches the patient's hospital gown, it

    1. is contaminated
    2. can be used only on this patient
    3. is returned to the tray
    4. is wiped off with an alcohol sponge before use

209. At the completion of nursing care of one patient and before starting the care of a second patient, it would be effective to wash the hands for

    1. 1/2 to 1 minute   3. 2 to 4 minutes
    2. 1 to 2 minutes   4. 4 to 5 minutes

210. Hands will not be considered thoroughly washed unless

    1. a brush is used
    2. surgical soap is available
    3. a disinfectant is used
    4. all four sides of each finger are washed

211. When a brush is used in the handwashing procedure, the practical nurse must be sure

    1. to avoid vigorous brushing that might break the skin surface
    2. it has been sterilized first
    3. it is not left in the sink for others to use
    4. only liquid soap is used for handwashing

212. If the nurse's hands are contaminated with mucus, pus, blood, etc., her hands should be washed for

    1. 1 minute   3. 5 to 10 minutes
    2. 2 to 3 minutes   4. 15 minutes

213. If the policy of the ward unit is to consider the handles of the water faucets contaminated, the nurse must remember

    1. to leave the water running until her hands are clean
    2. to get someone else to turn off the water
    3. to put on a rubber glove so she can touch the faucet handle
    4. to use a paper towel to turn off the water

214. After the hands have been washed and rinsed, they are held higher than the elbows

    1. so that the nurse will not touch anything
    2. so that excess water will not run from the soiled to the clean area
    3. until they are dry
    4. until they are air dried

215. If a cloth towel is used to dry the hands and arms after scrubbing, the order in which they are dried will be

    1. right hand, wrist and arm, then the left side
    2. hands first
    3. the arms first and work toward the hands
    4. both hands, both wrists, and both forearms

216. The techniques of surgical asepsis are for the purpose of

    1. keeping disease organisms isolated with the sick one
    2. keeping the entire patient unit free of germs
    3. protecting a patient from any disease germs in his environment
    4. protecting the nurse from any germs the patient has

217. Most disease-producing organisms grow best in the presence of

    1. dirt and soil
    2. warmth, moisture, and food
    3. moisture, oxygen, and blood
    4. red and white blood cells

218. Surgical asepsis considers any article or area contaminated if

    1. it is not sterile
    2. it has been touched by anyone
    3. it is not used in the operating room
    4. anyone is in that area

219. A sterile article becomes contaminated as soon as

    1. it is removed from the autoclave
    2. the package is exposed to air
    3. it touches an unsterile area
    4. it is exposed to people

220. When equipment is sterilized after it has been used on one patient but is not handled as sterile when it is used on the second patient, the sterilization is considered one form of

    1. prophylaxis   3. pathogenesis
    2. medical asepsis   4. disinfection

221. Most articles used in the hospital can best be sterilized by

    1. boiling   3. autoclaving
    2. airing   4. chemical soaking

222. If a piece of equipment must be boiled for 10 minutes, the counting of time will begin

    1. from the beginning of the procedure
    2. when steam becomes visible
    3. as soon as brisk boiling starts
    4. after the water has begun to bubble furiously

223. Unless the nurse has on sterile gloves, it will be necessary to touch all sterile articles

    1. carefully
    2. by their wrapping
    3. with a sterile forceps
    4. after the hands are scrubbed

224. Sterile forceps cannot be safely removed from the sterile container unless the nurse remembers

    1. to get all equipment within reach first
    2. to keep the forceps closed to remove them from the jar
    3. how easy it is to contaminate them
    4. to work quickly so that they can be returned to solution

225. The level of the solution in a sterile forceps container should

    1. fill the container completely
    2. come to 1 inch of the rim
    3. be one-half full
    4. be one-fourth full

226. The parts of the forceps and the forceps container that are not considered sterile include the

    a. rim of the container
    b. prongs cf the forceps
    c. handle of the forceps
    d. area of the jar not covered with solution

       1. all of the above
       2. c only
       3. a and c
       4. a, c, and d

227. Even though the forceps are held in the correct position, it is not considered safe technique

    1. to hold them below the waistline
    2. to talk with your hands
    3. to use them to move sterile equipment
    4. to hold the prongs separated

228. It is difficult, if not impossible, to keep forceps sterile if

    1. both professional and practical nurses use the same ones
    2. they are autoclaved only once a day
    3. two forceps are kept in one jar
    4. they are used frequently

229. A common fault in the use of sterile forceps, which can easily result in contamination of the forceps, is

    1. emotional unsteadiness
    2. lack of study and concentration on the principles of aseptic technique
    3. holding them too close to the rim of the jar to shake off excess solution
    4. laying them down on an unsterile surface to do something else

230. As the practical nurse uses sterile forceps, she must constantly be aware that the forceps will become contaminated if she

    1. fails to wash her hands before using them
    2. shares them with another nurse
    3. holds the prongs upward
    4. touches the cotton ball after it is removed from a container

231. If the practical nurse sees someone else returning contaminated forceps to the container, she should realize that it will be necessary to

    1. use them as they are
    2. return them to Central Supply
    3. cancel all sterile treatments
    4. sterilize the jar and forceps

232. To keep the inside of the sterile wrapper sterile while the tray is opened in the Service Room, the work surface must be

    1. dry
    2. sterile
    3. covered with newspapers
    4. protected from unsterile equipment

INFORMATION FOR THE NEXT THREE QUESTIONS: The drawing below indicates a work table in the Service Room with a sterile wrapped tray already opened to expose the items on it. Each corner of the sterile wrapper has been numbered.

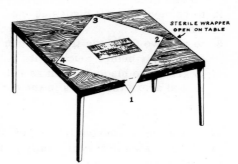

233. Which corner of this wrapper is most likely to be contaminated?

    1. #1   3. #3
    2. #2   4. #4

234. Which corner of this wrapper will be most sterile?

    1. #1   3. #3
    2. #2   4. #4

235. To cover the tray to carry it to the bedside, the corners are brought over the tray in the following order:

    1. #1, 2, 3, and 4
    2. #2, 4, 3, then 1
    3. #4, 1, 3, then 2
    4. #3, 4, 2, then 1

236. The information on a package of wrapped, sterile gloves should tell the nurse

    a. the name of the person who last wore the gloves
    b. the size of the gloves
    c. the date of sterilization
    d. the date on which the gloves were checked out to the ward

        1. all of the above
        2. a and d
        3. a, b, and c
        4. b and c

237. To keep a complete container of tongue blades sterile when only one is being removed, it will be important for the nurse

1. to place the one tongue blade on a sterile area
2. to remove several blades at one time
3. to remove the blade from the can completely before touching it
4. to grasp the blade as soon as it is raised above the others in the can

238. The nurse must constantly keep in mind that a sterile tray is easily contaminated by

1. placing it on a bedside stand
2. reaching over the sterile equipment
3. moving articles with a sterile forceps
4. keeping it covered too long

239. Any sterile item on a sterile tray can be touched if

1. the hands have been thoroughly washed
2. it is necessary to arrange it conveniently for use
3. sterile forceps are used
4. she does not use her hands

240. The nurse can determine whether a wrapped tray in the sterile cupboard is still safe to use by

1. the amount of dust on the wrapper
2. the signature of the person who wrapped it
3. the date on which it was autoclaved
4. the length of time it was kept in the autoclave

241. As the nurse moves from the hand-scrubbing sink to the bedside of the patient, she should remember that thoroughly scrubbed hands should be held

1. folded in the lap
2. relaxed, behind the back
3. relaxed, stretched out in front of the body
4. higher than the elbows

242. A disinfectant effective in the coagulation of germ protoplasm would

1. coagulate protoplasm of skin cells
2. be safe for a hand soak
3. sterilize most body surfaces
4. not be strong enough for the germs normally on the skin surface

243. The usual position of the patient who is to be given an enema is the

1. dorsal recumbent   3. jacknife
2. Sim's   4. Trendelenburg

244. A Sim's position is intended to expose the

1. vaginal os.   3. spinal area
2. abdominal wall 4. anal os

245. If the patient is to assume a dorsal lithotomy position in bed, the nurse would place the patient's

1. body across the bed, hips at the side edge, knees flexed and soles on the bed
2. hips high in the bed, feet in stirrups
3. feet on the lower bed frame and hips toward the end of the mattress
4. hips in the center of the bed, knees flexed, and soles on the mattress

246. Most of the nursing treatments of the female sex organs require the patient to be placed in the

1. dorsal position
2. dorsal recumbent position
3. Sim's position
4. knee-chest position

247. When an arm or leg must be bandaged, it is important

a. to use a figure-eight turn
b. to use an Ace bandage
c. to leave the fingers or toes exposed
d. to bandage toward the trunk

1. none of the above
2. c and d
3. b and d
4. a and c

248. The diagonal method of draping a patient for examination or treatment is most often used because it

1. is the best procedure known
2. prevents chilling
3. exposes the patient the least
4. is preferred by the patients

249. The diagonal draping procedure allows the drape to be held in place by

1. safety pins
2. the stirrups on the examining table
3. the weight of the patient's feet
4. the patient

250. The one bandage most useful in a variety of first-aid situations is the

1. Scultetus bandage
2. triangular bandage
3. circular bandage
4. Ace bandage

251. When several fingers of one hand must be bandaged, special attention must be given to prevent

1. a bulky appearance
2. two skin surfaces from touching
3. use of porous material
4. any pressure from the bandage

252. A leg bandage will be most effective when the nurse uses the bandaging turn known as

1. the roller
2. a figure eight
3. circular
4. spiral-reverse

253. Montgomery straps are most comfortable for the patient and easiest for the nurse when

1. profuse drainage makes the change of dressings frequent
2. it is necessary to put rectal dressings on a male patient
3. adhesive tape irritates the skin
4. gas places pressure on the stitches

254. Straight binders are used to hold dressings in place

1. over the vagina
2. on the chest or abdomen
3. after rectal surgery
4. over a joint

255. When support is needed to relieve tension on an abdominal incision, the binder of choice will be

1. the circular
2. the Scultetus
3. the Montgomery
4. the T-binder

256. The circular bandage turn is most frequently used

1. to support a joint
2. to hold a dressing over a joint
3. to anchor the bandage before starting another turn
4. to cover the scalp or the end of a finger

257. Dressings will be held in place over the anus or perineum of the male patient by use of

1. adhesive tape
2. a T-binder
3. a straight abdominal binder
4. a double T-binder

258. The procedure for admission to the hospital gives the nurse a good opportunity

1. to get the patient clean
2. to list carefully all the patient's clothing
3. to observe objective and subjective symptoms
4. to notify the nutritionist so that meals will not be omitted

259. The nurse's notes on a newly arrived patient, to be complete, must always indicate

1. the age of the patient
2. the sex of the patient
3. the seriousness of the patient's condition
4. the degree of ambulation on admission

260. The reason the efficient practical nurse takes time at the beginning of the day to estimate the amount of time it will require to care for each patient is

1. to insure each patient the care he needs
2. to get her work done before the doctor visits
3. to gain time for necessary housekeeping duties
4. to get a good evaluation report as a rapid worker

261. A well-organized plan of care will be helpful to the practical nurse because

1. her work can be done systematically with less frustration
2. she can get off duty on time
3. she will be in a position to solve the patient's emotional problems
4. she has definite, written proof of her organizational ability

262. The well-organized practical nurse will make out her plan of care

1. as soon as she reports for duty
2. after consulting the physician about the needs of the patient
3. after she has cared for the patient several days
4. after observing her patient

263. If a patient must have strong medicines to take at home, the practical nurse may need to teach him

a. the method of administration
b. the symptoms of overdose
c. the importance of accuracy
d. the importance of safe storage

   1. none of the above
   2. a only
   3. a, b and d
   4. all of the above

264 If normal urine is tested with Benedict's solution, the color will change to

1. green   3. blue
2. orange   4. yellow-green

265. A practical nurse can be most helpful to the patient going home from the hospital if she knows her community well enough to recommend

1. where special dressings and equipment can be obtained
2. the best trained specialist
3. a private duty nurse
4. an economical pharmacy

266. One of the greatest services the practical nurse can do the chronically ill or convalescent patient going home is

1. to stress the need for recreation
2. to emphasize the value of a hobby
3. to stress the importance of the patient doing for himself
4. to inform the family of the need to keep up morale

267. Tes-Tape can be used to tell the degree of sugar in the urine—from 1+ to 4+—by matching it to

1. a color chart on the tape container
2. a ward description of the color change
3. the color of normal urine
4. a color diagram posted on the wall in the Service Room

268. Urine that tests positive for acetone will change the color of the tablet or powder to

1. brick red   3. blue
2. green   4. purple

269. Urine that contains acetone will have an odor described as

1. the smell of new mown hay
2. ammonia
3. fruity
4. sour

270. The presence of sugar in the urine would be indicated if the color of Tes-Tape became

1. red or orange
2. blue or green
3. yellow or green
4. orange or blue

271. Urine that is properly tested with Benedict's solution must be boiled for

    1. 1 minute   3. 5 minutes
    2. 2 minutes   4. 10 minutes

272. A 4+ urine that is tested with Benedict's solution will change to a color described as

    1. green-yellow   3. blue
    2. brick red   4. purple

273. A 24-hour urine specimen has been ordered on a diabetic patient. The nurse must know that the first specimen to be saved is

    1. the 12:00 noon voiding
    2. the 8:00 A.M. voiding
    3. the first A.M. voiding after the bladder has been emptied of the night's collection
    4. the 6:00 A.M. voiding

274. Unless the nurse has other specific instructions concerning the 24-hour collection of urine, she can expect that the laboratory will want

    1. four ounces of the total specimen
    2. the total collection of urine
    3. a sample of urine q.4.h.
    4. a urine specimen each time the patient voids

275. The stomach will best accept a tube feeding that is poured into the stomach at a temperature of

    1. 90°F
    2. 100°F
    3. 105°F
    4. a degree that will allow it to be poured freely

276. A gavage tube should never be lubricated with mineral oil because of the danger of

    1. aspiration that will cause a lung complication
    2. rotting the rubber tubing
    3. destroying some of the vitamins in the feeding
    4. causing a diarrhea

277. The tube feeding is never poured into the gavage tube until the nurse has

    1. restrained the patient
    2. given the patient a chance to drink the feeding
    3. made sure the tubing is in the stomach
    4. enough help to keep the patient from pulling out the tube

278. It is evidence that the gavage tube is not in the stomach as desired when a precautionary check indicates

    1. the presence of fecal material
    2. the patient is becoming cyanotic
    3. belching sounds coming from the end of the tube
    4. bubbles in the bowl of water

279. Precautions to prevent any of the gavage feeding from getting into the respiratory system include

    a. checking the location of the tube before feeding is poured
    b. pouring water through the tube at the end of the feeding
    c. pinching off the tube before removing it
    d. stimulating the gag reflex so that the epiglottis will cover the opening into the trachea

        1. all of the above
        2. a only
        3. a, b, and c
        4. b, c, and d

280. Nausea, followed by emesis of the gavage feeding, can be prevented by

    a. placing pressure over the abdomen and the mouth
    b. having the feeding the right temperature
    c. removing the tube slowly
    d. keeping the patient quiet for 1/2 hour

        1. all of the above
        2. b, c, and d
        3. b and c
        4. c only

281. If the gastrostomy patient is allowed to chew and then expectorate favorite foods, it is desirable because

    a. the patient will accept his tube feeding more readily
    b. the flow of gastric juices will be stimulated
    c. the flow of saliva is increased
    d. the patient does not feel so sorry for himself

        1. all of the above
        2. a and c
        3. b and c
        4. a and d

282. As soon as the gastrostomy feeding has been placed in the stomach, oozing of the feeding from the end of the tube is prevented by

    1. clamping off the tube
    2. placing a rubber band around the tube
    3. folding the tube over on itself and tying
    4. placing a sterile gauze dressing over the entire opening

283. The skin around the gastrostomy opening can be protected from irritating gastric juices by application of

    1. talc powder   3. aluminum paste
    2. mineral oil   4. boric acid

284. A daily irrigation of the bowel through the colostomy opening is done in an attempt

    1. to keep the rectum free of fecal material
    2. to establish a habit of bowel control that will last all day
    3. to prevent the cut edges of the colostomy from growing together
    4. to prevent the development of an infection in the abdominal opening

285. If the colostomy irrigation must be given while the patient is confined to bed, the best position is

    1. dorsal recumbent   3. knee-chest
    2. prone   4. on the left side

286. The practical nurse who is responsible for irrigation and dressing of a colostomy must always keep in mind

    1. the need for a constant stream of conversation directed away from the treatment and the patient's condition
    2. the patient's resentment of the procedure
    3. the need to teach some member of the family to do the procedure
    4. that her attitude toward the procedure will influence the patient's acceptance of his condition

287. After the irrigating solution has been introduced into the colon, the colostomy patient can speed up defecation by

    1. deep-breathing exercises
    2. lying quietly in a prone position
    3. rubbing the abdomen, from the appendix upward
    4. straining, accompanied by massage of the descending colon

288. The term "soapsuds enema" is misleading because if such an enema is correctly given

    1. the suds will be removed from the solution
    2. a liquid soap will be added to the water
    3. the soap and water must be carefully measured
    4. soda bicarbonate must be added to create a suds

289. When the doctor has not written a specific order for the amount of solution to be used in an enema, the nurse must make this decision by considering

    1. the age of the patient
    2. the R. N.
    3. the reason for giving the enema
    4. the condition of the colon

290. The amount of solution usually given when the purpose of the enema is lubrication of feces is

    1. 100 to 150 c.c.   3. 250 to 300 c.c.
    2. 150 to 200 c.c.   4. 300 to 400 c.c.

291. If the bottom of the enema can is placed higher than 12 inches above the rectum, it will cause

   1. the solution to cool off too quickly
   2. injury to the colon as a result of the great pressure of the flow
   3. the solution to flow in drop by drop
   4. the colon to distend rapidly and the patient to expel the solution

292. When the nurse leaves a bed patient alone to expel an enema, it is most important to remember

   1. to elevate the head of the bed
   2. to wash the patient's face and hands
   3. to cleanse the anal area thoroughly
   4. to place the signal cord within reach

293. A carminative enema is ordered for the purpose of

   1. soothing the mucous membranes of the intestines
   2. stimulating expulsion of flatus
   3. killing intestinal worms
   4. softening feces in preparation for a cleansing enema

294. As soon as the enema tube is removed from the rectum, it should be placed

   1. in the enema can
   2. in the bedpan
   3. in the waste basin
   4. on the tray

295. The suppository should be inserted beyond the internal anal sphincter because this will

   1. increase its effect
   2. be done by the doctor
   3. decrease the desire to expel it
   4. lessen the effect of the treatment

296. It is easier for the patient to retain a suppository if the nurse will

   1. tell the patient he must not expel it
   2. exert slight pressure over the anus
   3. allow the patient to insert it
   4. insert it 8 to 10 inches into the rectum

297. The materials used as the suppository base stay best if they are stored in

   1. a cool, damp cupboard
   2. the locked part of the medicine cupboard
   3. a warm, dry cabinet
   4. the refrigerator

298. If the nurse is to obtain an uncontaminated specimen of feces, the patient must be instructed

   1. to take a cathartic the night before
   2. to void first in a separate container
   3. to take a soapsuds enema first
   4. to stimulate peristalsis by using a soap suppository

299. Preparation of a fecal specimen for the laboratory must be done with the greatest care to avoid

   1. contaminating the tongue blades
   2. labeling the container incorrectly
   3. alarming the patient
   4. contaminating the outside of the container

300. An emesis that would be described as projectile would mean

   1. regurgitation
   2. emesis with a fecal odor
   3. fluid with the appearance of coffee grounds
   4. forceful emesis

NURSING ARTS
PART II

(Answer sheet p. 309)

1. Hematemesis following hemorrhage from a stomach ulcer would be described as

   1. bleeding from the mouth
   2. coffee ground emesis
   3 . emesis of undigested food
   4. a thick, rusty colored emesis

2. An important fact to chart regarding an emesis, if the information is to be of value to the doctor, is

   1. the time of the emesis
   2. a statement that a specimen was sent to the laboratory
   3. the fact that the emesis was followed by oral hygiene
   4. the types of food the patient had eaten

3. The temperature of the water for a Sitz bath will be

   a. higher if application of heat is the purpose
   b. tepid, regardless of purpose of the treatment
   c. adjusted according to the age of the patient
   d. lower if the purpose is to promote healing

      1. c only
      2. a and d
      3. b and c
      4. all of the above

4. Following a hemorrhoidectomy, a Sitz bath will increase the supply of blood to the part and

   1. relieve swelling
   2. soak away necrotic tissue
   3. bring more white blood cells to the area
   4. stimulate peristalsis

5. One of the most important reasons for applying hot wet dressings to infected tissue is to speed the process of

   1. suppuration   3. sloughing
   2. necrosis   4. phagocytosis

6. Following a 30-minute Sitz bath procedure, the patient's circulation should gradually be returned to normal by insisting that he

   1. be active enough to stimulate circulation
   2. cool off slowly
   3. go to bed for at least 1 hour
   4. keep the feet warm

7. Hot wet dressings that are applied to an open wound must be

   1. clean
   2. sterile
   3. put on every 15 minutes
   4. made of wool flannel

8. The patient can tolerate hot wet dressings best if the nurse

   1. lets him apply the dressings himself
   2. allows a layer of air between the skin and the dressing
   3. covers the dressing with a rubber protector
   4. applies a hot water bottle to a dry dressing

9. If dry dressings are placed over a wound and then moistened, the solution will be placed in a sterile

   1. pitcher
   2. hypodermic syringe
   3. kidney basin
   4. Asepto syringe

10. The safest way to lubricate the suction tube for easy passage is

    1. to wipe it with mineral oil
    2. to place the tube in chipped ice
    3. to run hot water through the tube
    4. to ask the patient to drink water while the tube is being passed

11. The position of the patient's head that will allow the suction tube to be inserted more easily is one of

    1. hyperextension   3. supination
    2. hyperflexion   4. pronation

12. If the patient understands the reason for the suction procedure and knows how he can help, it will

    1. make the treatment more effective
    2. make passage of the tube easier
    3. prevent nausea and vomiting
    4. be easier for the nurse

13. If suction siphonage equipment is working properly, the patient will be relieved of

    1. vomiting and dizziness
    2. nausea and distention
    3. gas pains
    4. constipation

14. Alkalosis can complicate the condition of a patient who needs Wangansteen suction because

    1. the right mixture of fluids is not ordered
    2. of the accumulation of soda bicarbonate used to flush out the tube
    3. the loss of too much acid upsets the acid-base balance
    4. irrigation of the tube dilutes the gastric juices

15. The nurse would suspect that the suction was not working properly if

    1. nothing was suctioned from the stomach in a 20-to-30-minute period
    2. the patient complained of pain
    3. the red light stayed on too long
    4. the fluid coming from the stomach was dark green

16. The tube must be irrigated at stated intervals with

    1. lemon juice   3. water
    2. distilled water   4. ginger ale

17. When the Wangansteen tube is being irrigated,

    1. the patient must be given plenty of fluids by mouth
    2. the suction must be turned off
    3. the tube must be removed from the stomach
    4. all openings at the tip of the tube must be checked to avoid any clogging

18. Adequate oral hygiene for the patient with Wangansteen suction in operation will require care

    1. q. h   3. q. 4 h
    2. q. 2 h   4. q. 8 h

19. The usual reason for sending a sputum specimen to the laboratory is

    1. to determine the kind of bacteria present in the lungs
    2. to determine the symptoms of the patient
    3. to find out whether bacteria are present in the nose and throat
    4. to help the doctor decide which medicine will help the patient

20. The greatest amount of sputum will probably be coughed up

    1. after the noon meal
    2. at bedtime
    3. early in the morning
    4. after all medications have been given

21. The patient is asked to rinse his mouth with clear water before coughing up sputum that is to be examined in the laboratory. Such a rinse is important in order

    1. to wash away all traces of medicines
    2. to remove food particles and mouth bacteria
    3. to keep the collecting container free of contamination
    4. to keep bacteria from the various parts of the respiratory system from mixing

22. If accurate information regarding a lung disease is to be obtained from a sputum specimen, the patient must be instructed to

    1. expectorate in an emesis basin
    2. clear the throat with each cough
    3. collect the first secretions in a paper tissue
    4. cough up secretions from the bronchi

23. Observations the nurse will make on sputum to go to the laboratory will include

    1. temperature of the specimen
    2. color and consistency of the specimen
    3. condition of the patient
    4. position the patient was in at the time the specimen was collected

24. The patient will be positioned for postural drainage to help

    1. secretions drain from the bronchi
    2. increase the blood supply to the lungs
    3. clear the chest for an X-ray
    4. rest the affected part

25. Postural drainage can be effective only if it is based on the principle of

    1. getting the lungs lower than the trunk of the body
    2. the emotional outlook of the patient
    3. the physical condition of the patient
    4. changes in the color of the patient

26. The first time the patient is placed in position for postural drainage, the nurse must recognize how important it is that

    1. bleeding may occur
    2. cold compresses be placed on the forehead
    3. the treatment last only a few minutes
    4. the temporal pulse be checked every 15 minutes

27. The success of the postural drainage procedure is determined by

    1. the reaction of the patient
    2. the amount of drainage collected
    3. the laboratory reports
    4. the changes in temperature, pulse, and respiration

28. The effects of postural drainage can be increased if the nurse will encourage the patient

    1. to remain in position at least 1 hour
    2. to keep talking during the procedure
    3. to roll from side to side
    4. to breathe deeply or cough

29. When the purpose of throat irrigation is to apply heat to inflamed tissues, the amount of solution used will be

    1. 500 c.c.
    2. 500 to 1000 c.c.
    3. 1000 to 1500 c.c.
    4. more than 2000 c.c.

30. Steam inhalations are ordered for the purpose of

    a. soothing inflamed mucous membrane
    b. relieving swelling
    c. loosening secretions
    d. lubricating the sinuses

       1. a only
       2. a and b
       3. a and c
       4. all of the above

31. A croup tent must be set up to prevent condensation of hot steam which will drip on the patient. This is best done by using

    1. screens around the bed
    2. a spout extending into the tent
    3. bed sheets that can be easily laundered
    4. sheet blankets or bath blankets

32. One of the uses of the throat irrigation procedure is

    1. to warm the sputum so that a specimen can be obtained
    2. to prepare the patient for oral surgery
    3. to loosen and remove throat secretions
    4. to prepare the patient for postural drainage

33. When a throat irrigation is given to encourage the formation of pus, the temperature of the solution will be

    1. 98 to 100°F   3. 115°F
    2. 110°F   4. 120°F

34. When a throat irrigation is given to soften sticky mucus, the temperature of the solution will be

    1. 98 to 100°F   3. 115°F
    2. 110°F   4. higher than 120°F

35. The best position for a patient during a throat irrigation is

    1. prone, with the head turned to one side
    2. sitting
    3. supine
    4. modified Sim's

36. Before a throat irrigation is started, the patient must be instructed

    1. to breathe through his nose
    2. to breathe through his mouth
    3. to hold his breath as long as the solution is running
    4. to cough frequently during the procedure to distribute the solution evenly

37. The best cooperation is obtained from the patient during a throat irrigation if it is possible

    1. to check the pulse frequently during the procedure
    2. to allow the patient to hold the irrigating nozzle
    3. to paint the throat with an antiseptic solution
    4. to have the patient void before the procedure begins

38. The first time nose drops are instilled, the nurse should explain that

    1. the treatment will be painful
    2. the patient must learn to do this treatment himself
    3. some of the medicine will run back into the throat
    4. relief will be immediate

39. To protect the nares of an infant or an irrational patient when nose drops must be instilled, the nurse can

    1. cover the end of the dropper with gauze
    2. use an atomizer
    3. use a syringe
    4. cover the end of the dropper with rubber tubing

40. Medicine that is left in the dropper after nose drops have been instilled should be

    1. returned to the bottle
    2. saved for the next treatment
    3. washed out with soapy water
    4. thrown away

41. When the same bottle of nose drops must be used for several patients, the nurse must be sure that

    1. an adequate record is made so that the patient can be charged
    2. it is properly labeled
    3. it is put back in the medicine cabinet
    4. the dropper is not returned to the bottle after use

42. Cleaning of the medicine dropper will be difficult or impossible if the nurse allows

    1. hot water to reach the rubber tip
    2. medicine to stand in the dropper
    3. medicine to run back into the rubber tip
    4. the dropper to remain in the medicine bottle

43. The supplies collected for the oxygen therapy procedure must, for the safety of the patient, include

    1. a heavy woolen blanket
    2. a fire extinguisher
    3. "No Smoking" signs
    4. an electric fan

44. The humidifier needs water to function effectively. The nurse responsible for the care of the patient in an oxygen tent must know that

    a. the humidifier must be full at all times
    b. distilled water must be used
    c. the humidifier must be half full
    d. it is preferable to use distilled water

       1. a and b
       2. b and c
       3. c and d
       4. a and d

45. To know how many "liters per minute" of oxygen are flowing from the oxygen tank, the nurse must check

    1. the gauge
    2. the valve
    3. the flow indicator gauge
    4. the regulator inlet

46. The patient will be _less upset_ with the oxygen procedure if the practical nurse remembers to "crack" the oxygen tank

   1. before it is unloaded from the truck
   2. before it is taken to the patient's room
   3. after the gauge is attached
   4. after the tank is in the patient's room

47. The procedure for "cracking" an oxygen tank consists of

   1. opening the valve outlet full force
   2. allowing 1 liter to flow through the valve
   3. opening the valve slightly and closing it quickly
   4. removing dust from the valve by suction

48. The advantages of giving oxygen through the oropharyngeal catheter instead of by mask or tent include

   a. greater ease in giving nursing care
   b. less strain on lung tissue
   c. less danger of explosion
   d. less cost

      1. a, b, and c
      2. a and d
      3. c and d
      4. b, c, and d

49. The nurse can determine how far the nasal catheter must be inserted into the nose by

   1. measuring off 10 inches on the catheter
   2. the age of the patient
   3. checking the passage of the tube while the patient keeps his mouth open
   4. checking the distance from the tip of the nose to the tip of the ear

50. In the administration of nasal oxygen the nurse is instructed to start the flow of oxygen

   1. before the catheter is inserted
   2. while the catheter is being inserted
   3. after the catheter is in the nose
   4. after the catheter is in the correct position

51. If the nasal catheter is in the position necessary for greatest efficiency, the nurse should be able

   1. to notice improvement in the patient's color
   2. to regulate the flow of oxygen
   3. to adjust the equipment to the comfort of the patient
   4. to see the tip when the patient opens his mouth

52. The _first step_ in the process of cleaning a nasal catheter is

   1. the removal of mucus from the lumen
   2. washing it in hot soapy water
   3. letting it drip dry
   4. soaking it overnight before rinsing it

53. The patient receiving oxygen through a nasal mask must be instructed

   1. to breathe through the mouth to get an adequate supply of oxygen
   2. to watch the oxygen gauge to keep an even concentration
   3. to gargle frequently to keep the mucous membrane moist
   4. to breathe through the nose

54. The oxygen mask may be preferred to the oxygen tent because

   1. the oxygen concentration is better
   2. less oxygen is wasted
   3. the patient is less fearful of the equipment
   4. the nurse has greater control of the patient

55. After the oxygen flow has been regulated to 6 to 8 liters per minute, the oxygen mask will be put in place when

   1. the patient inhales
   2. the patient exhales
   3. the patient can assist
   4. it has been thoroughly lubricated

56. _As soon_ as the oxygen mask is in place, the flow of oxygen is

   1. increased
   2. decreased
   3. stabilized
   4. regulated according to the patient's need.

57. If the oxygen flow has been correctly regulated, the breathing bag

    1. can be removed
    2. will almost collapse during inhalation
    3. will need to be lubricated frequently
    4. will almost collapse during exhalation

58. The responsibilities of the practical nurse in the care of the patient receiving oxygen by mask include

    a. keeping the patient warm
    b. keeping the mask clean and dry
    c. washing and powdering the face frequently
    d. keeping windows and doors closed

        1. d only
        2. all of the above
        3. a and b
        4. b and c

59. The patient who is to get oxygen per tent must have a thorough explanation of the procedure before the equipment is brought into the room because

    1. fear makes the oxygen useless
    2. the cooperation of the patient is necessary for its effective use
    3. the noise of the machine will be disturbing
    4. the oxygen cylinder will fall if not handled properly

60. Once the patient adjusts to the oxygen tent, he will find it is easy to carry out such activities as

    1. elimination
    2. breathing
    3. eating and taking fluids
    4. perspiration

61. Excess oxygen will not escape from the oxygen tent while the patient is being given a bed bath if the nurse remembers

    1. to tuck the canopy under the patient's chin and shoulders
    2. to shut off the oxygen supply
    3. to omit care of the face
    4. to reduce the flow of the oxygen at the cylinder gauge

62. To keep from wasting oxygen when the patient is in an oxygen tent, it will be important for the nurse

    a. to cover a cotton mattress with a rubber sheet
    b. to tuck the canopy under the mattress
    c. to tuck the edge of the tent under the blankets
    d. to shut off the oxygen each time she opens the tent

        1. d only
        2. a and b
        3. a, b, and c
        4. all of the above

63. To get the concentration of oxygen into the tent as quickly as possible, the nurse is instructed

    1. to open the valve wide
    2. to "flood" the tent
    3. to give the patient no care until the desired concentration is reached
    4. to observe the gauge closely

64. The patient in an oxygen tent must be able to get the attention of the nurse. This is done by

    1. placing the call-bell cord in the tent
    2. leaving the tent open so that the patient can call her
    3. placing a hand bell in the tent
    4. providing pencil and paper or a "magic" slate so that the patient can write his requests

65. Only oxygen given by tent will require the nurse to check frequently and to control

    1. temperature and humidity
    2. fluid intake and output
    3. use of matches and electrical appliances
    4. wool blankets and visitors

66. The concentration of oxygen given to any patient should be

    1. regulated by prescription, just as the dosage of any medicine
    2. decreased as the flow increases
    3. higher in a tent than in a mask
    4. regulated according to the atmosphere

67. Oxygen will increase any flame near it. Recognizing this fact, the nurse will

    a. protect the exposed skin with oil
    b. remove any source of outside air
    c. remove electrical equipment
    d. take away matches and cigarettes

        1. d only
        2. a, c, and d
        3. c and d
        4. all of the above

68. Fluids by mouth are generally restricted postoperatively until

    1. the second postoperative day
    2. nourishing fluids can be tolerated
    3. nausea and vomiting have stopped
    4. the swallowing reflex has been regained

69. Intravenous fluids are often given the postoperative patient

    1. to keep the mouth from becoming dry
    2. to help the kidneys function better
    3. to replace body fluids lost in surgery
    4. to stimulate the circulation

70. Complications involving the lungs and the circulation can be prevented postoperatively if

    1. the respiration is checked often
    2. the position is changed often and deep breathing is carried out
    3. the blood pressure is checked often until it is stable
    4. I.V. fluids are not allowed to run too fast

71. The postoperative patient should not be placed in the Fowler's position for long periods of time because

    1. it may tire the patient
    2. it will be more difficult to turn him
    3. it will interfere with return flow of venous blood
    4. there is great danger that muscle contractures will develop

72. The amount, the type, and the frequency of vomiting during the postoperative period are important to record because

    1. it is proof the patient is nauseated
    2. it shows the physician the nurse is alert
    3. it tells the doctor something about the patient's fluid balance
    4. it is an early sign of shock that should be corrected quickly

73. Gas pains will be a more common complaint in a patient who has had

    1. lung surgery
    2. rectal surgery
    3. kidney surgery
    4. abdominal surgery

74. If a rectal tube has been inserted to aid in expelling gas, it will not be left in place longer than

    1. 1 hour   3. 30 minutes
    2. 45 minutes   4. 15 minutes

75. Stimulation of the skin surface before alcohol or tepid water is applied will

    1. dilate the surface blood vessels
    2. contract the surface blood vessels
    3. increase muscle contraction
    4. prepare the patient for the shock of the application

76. To reduce temperature effectively by use of a tepid sponge bath, the treatment must be continued at least

    1. 10 minutes   3. 30 minutes
    2. 15 minutes   4. 45 minutes

77. Cold cloths placed in the axillary and groin regions will help reduce an elevated temperature more quickly because

    1. the skin is thinner in these places
    2. large blood vessels come near the surface at these points
    3. they are closer to the heart
    4. the patient will begin to shiver

78. Cold compresses to the head will prevent headache due to congestion because

1. the patient is more comfortable
2. cold prevents edema
3. cold slows up circulation
4. the nerve endings are less sensitive

79. A hot water bottle at the feet during a tepid sponge bath will prevent

1. congestion in the head
2. further danger of the effects of cold
3. a state of shock
4. a feeling of fatigue

80. An alcohol sponge is used more often than a tepid sponge when the temperature is

1. over 101°F
2. over 104°F
3. constantly rising
4. fluctuating above and below normal

81. The catheterization procedure is one that the nurse can never do unless

1. the doctor refuses to do it
2. the condition of the patient makes it an emergency
3. the patient is free of all venereal disease
4. there is a written order by the doctor

82. The nurse must know the reason why the urine is being removed by catheterization because this will influence

1. the reassurance the patient needs
2. the assignment to a practical nurse
3. the kind and amount of equipment needed
4. the orders for fluid intake

83. The catheter must be discarded and a sterile one substituted if the first catheter used

1. seems to be defective
2. touches anything but the meatus
3. touches anything in the sterile field
4. is not long enough

84. The nurse who is doing a catheterization shows a poor understanding of aseptic technique when she

1. reaches over sterile equipment
2. fails to make an adequate explanation to the patient
3. places a sterile tray on the patient's bed
4. fails to wear sterile gloves to do a sterile procedure

85. The sterile technique required in the catheterization procedure always includes

a. preparation of equipment
b. preparation of the patient
c. insertion of the catheter
d. collection of the urine

1. a only
2. all of the above
3. a and c
4. a, c, and d

86. If the urethra is not inflamed or the area swollen, the nurse can safely assure the patient that the only discomfort of catheterization will be

1. the force needed to push the catheter into the bladder
2. some pain as the catheter is pushed through the meatus
3. pressure of the catheter as it reaches the ureters
4. the pressure of the catheter against the mucous membrane of the urethra

87. The catheterization procedure will be easier to do if the patient is relaxed and cooperative. This can be accomplished by

a. keeping the patient warm and comfortable
b. giving the patient an understandable explanation
c. respecting the modesty of the patient
d. keeping the patient's attention on diverting conversation

1. b only
2. b and c
3. a, b, and d
4. all of the above

88. The purpose of lubricating the catheter is

    1. to make the procedure easier
    2. to reduce friction against the mucous membrane of the urethra
    3. to protect the catheter
    4. to lessen the amount of pressure needed to push the catheter into the bladder

89. The number of inches the catheter is inserted will depend on

    1. the reason for the catheterization
    2. the physical condition of the patient
    3. the length of the urethra
    4. the length of the ureters

90. The ease with which infection can spread throughout the urinary system demands that sterile technique be maintained until

    1. the catheter tip is through the meatus
    2. the catheter reaches the bladder
    3. all urine has been drained from the bladder
    4. the equipment is removed from the room

91. The male catheterization procedure describes the position of the patient for the procedure as

    1. supine
    2. prone
    3. dorsal recumbent
    4. Sim's

92. When the flow of urine through the catheter decreases to a "drip-drip," the flow can be speeded up by

    1. pulling the catheter back 3 inches
    2. pulling the catheter back 1 inch
    3. pushing the catheter farther into the bladder
    4. pushing the catheter into the urethra

93. Catheterization of the female patient requires her to be placed in

    1. the supine position
    2. the prone position
    3. the knee-chest position
    4. the dorsal recumbent position

94. Sterile technique will be broken in catheterization of the female patient if

    1. the folds of the labia touch the meatus before the catheter is inserted
    2. the catheter is inserted more than 4 inches into the bladder
    3. the tray is left in the patient's room while the nurse scrubs her hands
    4. more than one person tries to carry out the procedure

95. A retention catheter stays in the bladder because

    1. one end is taped to the patient's thigh
    2. one end is attached to a drainage bottle
    3. of its special construction
    4. one part of the catheter is inflated

96. The nurse will know how much solution is needed to blow up the retention catheter by

    1. checking the capacity as determined by the size French
    2. reading the orders on the doctor's order sheet
    3. the size of the syringe on the catheterization tray
    4. reading the directions printed on each catheter

97. Pain associated with inflation of the retention catheter should warn the nurse

    1. that the patient's anatomy is not normal
    2. that the catheter tip is still in the urethra
    3. of the dangers of rupturing the bladder
    4. of the need to remove the catheter and call the doctor

98. Frequent irrigation of the retention catheter is necessary

    1. to stimulate the flow of urine
    2. to keep the tube free of mucus plugs
    3. to wash out blood clots
    4. to keep the tube free of obstructing particles

99. Irrigation of a <u>retention catheter</u> requires the nurse to be very certain that

    1. the solution is the correct temperature
    2. the patient is not uncomfortable
    3. all the solution has been returned
    4. the irrigating fluid is placed in the correct catheter opening

100. Irrigating solutions that would not irritate the bladder would be

    1. 10% saline or glucose
    2. 10% Lysol or 5% mercurochrome
    3. surgical soap or sterile water
    4. normal saline or boric acid

101. The temperature of the solution placed into the bladder for purpose of irrigation should be about

    1. 90°F   3. 105 to 107°F
    2. 100°F   4. 110°F

102. The amount of irrigating fluid placed in the bladder at one time will vary from

    1. 120 to 250 c.c.   3. 500 to 750 c.c.
    2. 250 to 500 c.c.   4. 750 to 1000 c.c.

103. The <u>label</u> on the urine specimen bottle should always be completed

    1. in pencil
    2. in ink
    3. before the specimen is collected
    4. by laboratory personnel

104. An adequate amount of urine for most laboratory tests is

    1. 50 c.c.   3. 250 c.c.
    2. 100 c.c.   4. 500 c.c.

105. A urine specimen for "routine examination" is best obtained

    1. at bedtime
    2. after breakfast
    3. in the early A.M.
    4. before medications are given

106. If the laboratory report form indicated the specific gravity of a urine specimen was 1.055, the nurse would know that this urine was

    1. normal   3. concentrated
    2. dilute   4. highly acid

107. The procedures for collection of fractional urine and 24-hour urine specimens have <u>in common</u> the facts that

    a. the first voided A.M. urine is discarded
    b. the urine is collected for a 24-hour period
    c. all the urine collected is sent to the laboratory
    d. a record of total intake must accompany the specimen to the laboratory

        1. all of the above
        2. a only
        3. b and c
        4. a and b

108. A urine specimen collected at 8:00 P.M. and left at the nurses' desk until the laboratory opened at 8:00 A.M. could not be accurately tested because

    a. the urine would be cold
    b. any evidence of diseased kidneys or bladder would be changed by standing
    c. the reaction of the urine would be alkaline
    d. the urine would become more concentrated on standing and the specific gravity would be incorrect

        1. d only
        2. b and c
        3. b and d
        4. all of the above

109. When the vaginal irrigation is given to cleanse the vagina of a discharge the amount of solution prepared will be

    1. 500 c.c.   3. 2 liters
    2. 1 liter   4. 1 gallon

110. Unless the neck of the cervix is open and there is danger of forcing infected materials into the uterus, the equipment for a vaginal irrigation is used as

1. disposable
2. sterile
3. clean
4. the property of the patient

111. When a solution 110°F or hotter is used to irrigate the vagina, preparation of the patient for the treatment includes

1. sterile equipment
2. extra precaution in the preparation and testing of the solution
3. protection against chilling
4. protection of the labia and perineum with oil

112. If a vaginal irrigation were ordered, following vaginal surgery or delivery, the presence of stitches in the perineal area would indicate that irrigation must be

1. sterile
2. for the purpose of deodorizing
3. to apply heat
4. to prevent infection

113. To allow enough pressure for effective cleansing yet not force the mucus plug out of the cervix, the base of the irrigating can must be

1. 8 inches above the cervix
2. 12 inches above the vagina
3. 16 inches above the uterus
4. 16 inches above the foot of the bed

114. If the flow of solution into the vagina is under great pressure, the result can be

1. severe pain
2. spread of infection to the pelvic cavity
3. rupture of the cervix
4. rapid dilatation of the vaginal walls

115. The patient who must take a daily medicated douche at home to treat a vaginitis should be directed to lie in the bath tub because

1. in this position the vaginal canal can be more completely cleansed
2. it is more comfortable
3. the pressure of the flow of solution can be better controlled
4. the medicated solution can be split into smaller particles

116. In most cases of vaginitis the procedure is clean rather than sterile. It would not be poor technique if the nurse allowed the patient

1. to sit up on the toilet
2. to use her personal douche equipment
3. to use disposable equipment
4. to insert the douche tip

117. If there were any danger of infectious discharge getting from the vagina into the eyes of the nurse, protection should be provided in the form of

1. penicillin injections
2. glasses and gown
3. a shield
4. rubber gloves

118. Clean up of the vaginal irrigation equipment calls for setting up the tray, wrapping it, and autoclaving it. This is done because

1. it is good aseptic technique
2. the irrigating can may be needed for other purposes
3. the next patient may require a sterile vaginal irrigation
4. the tube may contain vaginal discharge

119. A perineal irrigation is done to cleanse stitches in the perineal area. It is important that this procedure be carried out following

1. A.M. care
2. each voiding and defecation
3. the daily bath
4. application of heat to the stitches

120. If the patient is not encouraged to void before the vaginal irrigation begins, the nurse can expect that

1. pressure from the bladder will prevent dilatation of vaginal walls
2. the warm solution will stimulate the desire to void
3. severe cramps will start as soon as the fluid reaches the cervix
4. the irrigating fluid will be retained

121. When the condition of the patient permits, the patient should sit upright on the bedpan following a vaginal irrigation for the purpose of

1. keeping the solution out of the uterus
2. duplicating the technique used at home
3. keeping the return flow away from the urinary meatus
4. providing more complete drainage of the solution

122. The solution for perineal care must not exceed a temperature of

1. 90°F   3. 100°F
2. 98°F   4. 104°F

123. The temperature of a sterile irrigating solution must be checked with

1. a thermometer
2. the back of the hand
3. a sterile solution thermometer
4. the bath thermometer

124. Following a perineal irrigation, the vulva is dried with cotton balls. This technique instructs the nurse

a. to use each cotton ball once
b. to start the stroke at the urinary meatus and wipe toward the anus
c. to discard the cotton balls in the bedpan
d. to leave one cotton ball in the vaginal opening

    1. all of the above
    2. a only
    3. a and b
    4. b, c, and d

125. The doctor tells the nurse to prepare the patient and the equipment for a pelvic examination. The doctor will expect

a. rubber gloves and lubricant
b. vaginal specula
c. the patient in dorsal recumbent position
d. the patient draped

    1. a and c
    2. b and d
    3. a only
    4. all of the above

126. Five hundred c.c. of 5% sodium bicarbonate solution is to be prepared for perineal irrigation. The nurse will do this by

1. dissolving 2 1/2 c.c. of sodium bicarbonate in 500 c.c. of water
2. adding 25 grams of sodium bicarbonate to 475 c.c. of water
3. dissolving 25 c.c. of sodium bicarbonate in enough sterile water to make 500 c.c.
4. dissolving 250 c.c. of sodium bicarbonate in 250 c.c. of sterile water

127. Potassium permanganate, 1-2000 strength, is ordered for deodorizing vaginal irrigations. The nurse is expected to make up enough solution for these irrigations. The drug on hand is in crystal form. The amount of drug needed is

1. 3 c.c.   3. 30 minims
2. $\frac{3 \div}{3 \: 1}$ 4. 300 grams

128. Unpleasant sensations in the patient's head will be prevented if the <u>preparation</u> of ear drops for instillation <u>includes</u>

1. removing ear wax
2. sterilizing the irrigating can
3. warming the solution
4. turning the patient on one side

129. The solution used for sterile hot compresses applied to the eyes should be kept at a temperature of

1. 120°F   3. 110°F
2. 115°F   4. 105°F

130. The effectiveness of ear drops will be prolonged if, as soon as the drops are instilled, the nurse remembers that the procedure directs her

1. to dry the inside of the ear with an applicator
2. to place a small amount of loosely packed cotton in the ear
3. to give the patient a hot water bottle to keep the drops warm
4. to insert a well-packed plug of cotton into the ear

131. The amount of solution to use for an ear irrigation will

1. always depend on the amount ordered
2. depend on the reason for the treatment
3. depend on the strength of the solution used
4. depend on the temperature of the solution ordered

132. The nurse must know the reason for the order to irrigate an eye. The reason will determine

1. the concentration of the solution ordered
2. the type of equipment to assemble
3. the condition of the patient
4. the length of the treatment

133. An eye irrigation is most commonly ordered

1. before an eye examination
2. before eye surgery
3. in the treatment of glaucoma
4. when there is excessive purulent drainage

134. The purpose of the eye irrigation is the application of heat. It will be necessary to prepare and use

1. 8 gtts. of solution
2. 30 c.c. of solution
3. 100 c.c. of solution
4. 1000 c.c. of solution

135. In any eye treatment the nurse is warned to do the procedure in such a way that she can avoid

1. cooling the solution
2. conversation with the patient
3. infecting the other eye
4. overheating the eye

136. Ointment is applied to the eye after the nurse

1. irrigates the eye
2. instructs the patient to close his eyes
3. everts the lower lid
4. places a sterile gauze sponge over the untreated eye

137. Injury to the eye must be avoided during the application of an ointment. The nurse is instructed to avoid

1. touching the eye with the tip of the tube
2. squeezing the ointment into the inner canthus
3. applying the ointment while it is cold
4. failing to put on sterile gloves

138. To permit the full benefit from the solution instilled in the eye, the patient should be instructed

1. to look upward
2. to keep the eyes closed for 2 minutes
3. to hold a sponge over the outer angle of the eye
4. to rotate the position of the eyes

139. The size of the catheter used to suction the outer tube of the tracheotomy set must be carefully selected because

1. secretions will not be pulled through a small catheter
2. only one size will fit the suction pump
3. the number of openings in the end will determine its effectiveness
4. the supply of oxygen to the lungs will be shut off by a large catheter

140. The inner tube of the tracheotomy set can be kept clean by

1. boiling the tube
2. autoclaving
3. suctioning
4. disinfectants

141. It will be dangerous to use cotton or gauze to clean the inner canula of the tracheotomy tube because

1. they do not clean effectively
2. loose particles may be aspirated
3. the technique will not be sterile
4. these materials are too expensive

142. The <u>emergency treatment</u> necessary if the tracheotomy tube becomes dislodged by coughing or vomiting is

1. to clean and reinsert the tube at once
2. to administer oxygen into the incision
3. to hold the incision open until the doctor arrives
4. to observe the patient closely for respiratory distress

143. The nurse must know a tracheotomy patient is in need of suctioning when she hears

1. Cheyne-Stokes respiration
2. a hissing sound with each inspiration
3. sterterous breathing
4. apnea

144. The mask gives the nurse in a communicable disease unit the greatest protection when

1. the patient has respiratory symptoms
2. the incubation period is over
3. the cause of the disease is a virus
4. the diagnosis is uncertain

145. The nurse on a communicable disease unit must put many good personal hygiene habits into practice. One of the most important of these is careful attention

1. to a high calorie diet
2. to supplementary vitamins
3. to her hands
4. to general body cleanliness

146. In a communicable disease unit the hands of the nurse require frequent attention. To protect her hands this care must include

1. use of a hand brush to cleanse them
2. use of a germicidal soap
3. special attention to the cuticle
4. thorough drying and application of lotion

147. Ward A houses only 8 patients, all with a diagnosis of measles. The nurse assigned to this unit will find it is not necessary

1. to wear a mask
2. to sterilize the thermometers after each use
3. to put on a gown before she enters the unit
4. to change gowns between patients

148. The nose and throat discharges of a communicable-disease patient often contain the causative organism. To avoid spreading the disease the nurse will

a. give the patient oral hygiene often
b. supply paper tissues
c. collect tissues in a sack pinned to the bed
d. wear a cap

1. a, b, and c   3. a and d
2. b, c, and d   4. b and c

149. Scarring will result if the eruptions of some communicable diseases are scratched. To keep a small child from scratching such lesions, the nurse will be instructed

1. to apply ointment to the irritated areas
2. to apply elbow restraints
3. to use a sheet restraint
4. to give a medicated bath

150. Cleaning of a room or unit after the child with a "childhood disease" has been dismissed can be effectively done by

1. closing the room for a week
2. fumigating with sulfur candles
3. exposing the room to sun and air for several weeks
4. washing the furniture and airing the room 24 hours

NURSING ARTS
PART III
INTEGRATED EXAMINATION

(Answer sheet p. 310)

INSTRUCTIONS

This set of questions refers to nursing responsibilities in the care of Mrs. X, from preadmission procedures to postmortem care.

Throughout the test descriptive information is given in capital letters. Read this material carefully, for it is background information needed to answer correctly the questions that follow.

ABOUT THE PATIENT

AGE 80, WIDOW.
LIVES WITH TWO UNMARRIED DAUGHTERS, AGES 55 AND 60.
SHE HAS FALLEN DOWN 20 CELLAR STEPS.
SHE IS BEING ADMITTED, PER AMBULANCE, FOR EXAMINATION AND DIAGNOSIS.
HER DAUGHTERS ACCOMPANY HER.
MRS. X IS TO BE ADMITTED TO A PRIVATE ROOM ON THE SURGICAL SERVICE.

THE ADMITTING OFFICE NOTIFIES THE SURGICAL SERVICE OF THE EXPECTED ARRIVAL OF MRS. X AND INDICATES THE ROOM SHE WILL OCCUPY. THE CLINICAL INSTRUCTOR ASSIGNS MISS SMITH, STUDENT PRACTICAL NURSE, TO PREPARE TO ADMIT THE PATIENT.

151. The admission of Mrs. X on a stretcher will be faster and smoother because Miss Smith has prepared for her arrival by

1. getting all her charting materials in order
2. assembling all the equipment that will be needed in the care of this patient
3. loosening the top bedding and fan folding them to the foot of the bed
4. finding out all she can about her new patient

152. The room to which Mrs. X will be admitted was cleaned by the Housekeeping Department yesterday, following the dismissal of Mr. A. Miss Smith has been taught that embarrassment and delay in patient care can be prevented if in her preliminary preparation of the room she also

1. checks dresser drawers, bathroom, and bedside stand for essential equipment and supplies
2. checks out complete equipment for this unit from the Central Supply
3. asks the housekeeping employee to check this unit for occupancy
4. asks the head nurse to O.K. the unit for occupancy

153. The ambulance driver, accompanied by the admitting nurse, brings Mrs. X. to her room on the stretcher. Miss Smith first tries to put the patient, and her daughters, at ease by

a. asking the patient what happened to her
b. calling the patient Mrs. X
c. introducing herself as Miss Smith
d. asking the patient where she hurts

1. c only	3. a, b, and d
2. b and c	4. all of the above

THE DOCTOR HAS NOT YET EXAMINED THE PATIENT; THUS THE EXTENT OF HER INJURIES IS STILL UNKNOWN. MISS SMITH WILL CONSIDER THE AGE OF THE PATIENT AND THE SEVERITY OF THE FALL AND WILL SUSPECT THAT MRS. X HAS SOME BROKEN BONES.

154. Mrs. X must be moved from the stretcher to the bed without increasing the extent of her injuries. Correct movement in this situation will require

1. Miss Smith, with the patient assisting
2. the help of the two daughters
3. the help of an orderly who is strong enough to lift Mrs. X easily
4. a minimum of three from nursing personnel

AFTER MRS. X IS PLACED ON THE BED, MISS SMITH MUST GET THE PATIENT UNDRESSED AND INTO A HOSPITAL GOWN. SHE RECOGNIZES HOW FRIGHTENED BOTH THE PATIENT AND HER DAUGHTERS ARE OF THIS HOSPITAL EXPERIENCE.

155. Miss Smith could best lessen these fears by asking the daughters

    1. to wait in the lobby until their mother is ready for visitors
    2. to come back during the evening visiting hours
    3. to stay in the room and assist with the admission procedure
    4. what financial arrangements they intend to make for their mother's care

MISS SMITH NOTICES THAT THE RIGHT ANKLE IS WRAPPED WITH AN ACE BANDAGE. THE DAUGHTER TELLS MISS SMITH THAT IT COVERS A CHRONIC, DRAINING ULCER, A COMPLICATION OF VARICOSE VEINS.

156. It will be easier for Mrs. X to have her temperature taken orally. The oral thermometer will be left in place for

    1. 1 minute   3. 3 minutes
    2. 2 minutes   4. 4 minutes

157. The pulse is taken by applying slight pressure with the index, middle, and third fingers on the thumb side of the patient's wrist. The artery in this location is called

    1. the carotid artery   3. the brachial artery
    2. the temporal artery   4. the radial artery

158. Next, Miss Smith checks the blood pressure. She places the stethoscope

    1. over the pulse
    2. above the sphygmomanometer cuff
    3. over the brachial artery
    4. in the crook of the elbow

159. The blood pressure reading is 180/100. Miss Smith is not too disturbed about this reading because she understands that

    1. older people usually have high blood pressure
    2. fear and nervousness increase the blood pressure
    3. the daughters are making their mother excited
    4. this is within the normal range for an 80-year-old

THE ADMISSION PROCEDURE HAS BEEN COMPLETED AND MRS. X HAS BEEN MADE AS COMFORTABLE AS POSSIBLE. MISS SMITH'S NEXT RESPONSIBILITY IS TO RECORD THE ADMISSION ON THE PATIENT'S CHART.

160. The admission chart on this patient would correctly include

    a. the time of admission
    b. admission per stretcher
    c. the extent of the patient's injuries
    d. the presence of the varicose ulcer on the right leg

        1. all of the above
        2. d only
        3. a and d
        4. a, b, and d

ABOUT 4:30 MISS SMITH BEGINS TO PREPARE MRS. X FOR SUPPER.

161. To avoid an interruption after the tray has arrived, Miss Smith knows it is good procedure

    1. to wash the patient's face and hands
    2. to elevate the head of the bed
    3. to ask the patient if she needs to use the bedpan
    4. to give oral hygiene

162. Before the tray arrives, Miss Smith will make it possible for Mrs. X

    1. to change her position
    2. to wash her hands
    3. to use a room deodorant
    4. to rest

THE FAMILY DOCTOR HAS NOT YET BEEN LOCATED. THE HOUSE DOCTOR HAS WRITTEN AN ORDER FOR A SOFT DIET FOR THIS MEAL ONLY.

163. The extent of injury has not yet been determined. Miss Smith feels it will be safest to feed her patient. The patient will not feel quite so helpless if she is allowed

    1. to hold a piece of bread
    2. to express her likes and dislikes
    3. to sit up on the edge of the bed
    4. to eat all of one food before starting on another

164. Mrs. X will enjoy her meal more if Miss Smith keeps telling her

1. what is happening to other patients on the service
2. the amount of time she has to feed the patient
3. which food she is offering her next
4. various hospital rules and regulations

MISS SMITH WILL USE THIS FIRST MEAL-TIME TO GET SOME INFORMATION FROM THE PATIENT.

165. During the meal it would be appropriate for Miss Smith to get her patient to talk about

1. her life at home
2. her food likes and dislikes
3. her subjective symptoms
4. any fears about her condition and the period of hospitalization

VISITING HOURS 7:00 to 8:00 P.M. THE DAUGHTERS AND SEVERAL NEIGHBORS ARRIVE. THE ROOM BUZZES WITH NEIGHBORHOOD GOSSIP. MISS SMITH NOTICES HER PATIENT IS TENSE, HER HANDS GRIPPING THE BEDSPREAD. SHE KEEPS TURNING HER HEAD FROM PERSON TO PERSON AS THEY TALK AROUND HER.

166. Miss Smith recognizes her patient's discomfort. It would be most helpful to Mrs. X if Miss Smith would tactfully

1. remind the visitors that this IS a hospital
2. request all visitors to leave
3. hand all visitors a copy of the hospital regulations
4. call the daughters' attention to the mother's fatigue and suggest that they all leave

SHORTLY AFTER 8:00 P.M. THE FAMILY DOCTOR ARRIVES TO DO A THOROUGH PHYSICAL EXAMINATION.

167. The examination will begin with the patient in the

1. dorsal recumbent position
2. prone position
3. supine position
4. Fowler's position

168. Miss Smith recognizes the need to respect the modesty of this 80-year-old woman, as well as to avoid exposure. To accomplish both, the draping will consist of

a. leggings
b. face towel
c. draw sheet
d. full-sized sheet

   1. all of the above
   2. d only
   3. b and d
   4. a, b, and d

169. It will not be possible to keep the patient completely covered throughout the examination. To avoid any unnecessary embarrassment to Mrs. X, Miss Smith will

a. close the windows
b. close the door
c. screen the bed
d. turn out the ceiling light

   1. b and c
   2. a and b
   3. c only
   4. all of the above

X-RAYS INDICATE A BROKEN HIP. SURGERY WILL BE NECESSARY AND A CAST WILL BE APPLIED. THE DOCTOR EXPLAINS THE NEED FOR THE SURGERY AND TRIES TO PREPARE MRS. X FOR THE DISCOMFORTS TO COME. SURGERY IS SCHEDULED FOR 9:00 A.M. THE NEXT DAY. THE DOCTOR WRITES THE PREOPERATIVE ORDERS.

AS MISS SMITH MAKES HER LAST ROUNDS AT 10:45 P.M., SHE FINDS MRS. X STILL AWAKE. SHE DISCOVERS THE PATIENT IS WORRIED ABOUT GOING TO SURGERY WITHOUT SEEING HER DAUGHTERS FIRST. SHE PLEADS FOR SPECIAL RELAXATION OF VISITING HOURS, JUST THIS ONCE.

170. From the tone of the patient's voice, Miss Smith might rightly conclude that Mrs. X is

1. worrying about her daughters' welfare
2. planning to die
3. afraid of the outcome of surgery
4. trying to avoid the surgery

MISS SMITH SITS DOWN AT THE
BEDSIDE AND REASSURES MRS. X
THAT HOSPITAL RULES ALWAYS
ALLOW THE FAMILY TO VISIT
BEFORE THE PATIENT GOES TO
SURGERY.

171. Miss Smith is aware that the
preoperative attention to the
emotional problems of the patient will be rewarded by

1. smoother postoperative
   recovery
2. satisfied relatives
3. a shorter rehabilitation
   period
4. a sedative effect on the
   patient

TIME: 7:00 A.M. — DAY OF SURGERY.

THE DOCTOR READS MISS SMITH'S
DESCRIPTIVE CHARTING OF MRS. X'S
EMOTIONAL OUTBURST.

172. The doctor visits Mrs. X to evaluate
her attitude toward surgery after a
good night's rest. He may decide it
is necessary

1. to explain the surgery in
   detail
2. to consult a second surgeon
3. to postpone the surgery
3. to ask the family to remain
   in constant attendance

173. Miss Smith checks her day's assignment and makes out a plan that will
make it possible for her

1. to talk with the family
2. to make the ether bed correctly
3. to prepare Mrs. X without being
   rushed
4. to give the preoperative medication early

174. The only concern Mrs. X seems to
have this morning is a dread of "being
put to sleep." Miss Smith reassures her
that she will soon be given a medication
that will

1. make her too drowsy to care about
   the anesthetic
2. paralyze her senses
3. bring to mind many things that
   happened in her past
4. increase her alertness so she
   can see what happens to her

175. Miss Smith is aware of the legal hazards
of any surgery. Before she prepares the
preoperative medication, she checks the
patient's chart for the purpose of determining

1. postoperative orders
2. the presence of a signed surgical
   permit
3. when the patient last voided
4. when food and fluid were last given
   to the patient

THE PREOPERATIVE MEDICATION OR-
DERED IS MORPHINE gr. 1/6 AND
ATROPINE gr. 1/150. THE ONLY MORPHINE
AVAILABLE THIS EARLY IN THE MORN-
ING IS gr. 1/2.

176. Under supervision, Miss Smith works
the mathematical problem and discovers
that gr. 1/6 of the medication can be
given if she

1. dissolves 1 tablet gr. 1/2 in m. 30
   of sterile water, discards m. 15,
   gives the patient m. 15
2. dissolves 1 tablet gr. 1/2 in m. 24,
   discards m. 22, gives the patient
   m. 2
3. dissolves 1 tablet gr. 1/2 in m. 30
   of sterile water, discards m. 20,
   and gives the patient m. 10
4. dissolves 3 tablets gr. 1/2 in m. 20
   of sterile water and gives the patient
   m. 20

177. Miss Smith gives the preoperative medication hypodermically, inserting the needle into the skin at a

1. 30° angle
2. 45° angle
3. 75° angle
4. 90° angle

MISS SMITH ACCOMPANIES HER PATIENT TO SURGERY, THEN RETURNS TO THE ROOM TO MAKE AN ANESTHETIC BED AND SET UP THE UNIT FOR POSTOPERATIVE CARE

178. Miss Smith knows that the equipment needed to follow her patient's progress must include

a. sphygmomanometer
b. stethescope
c. tourniquet
d. catheterization tray

1. a, b, and c
2. a only
3. a and b
4. all of the above

179. Miss Smith knows that a patient in a full body cast must be kept in good body alignment. To accomplish this postoperatively, she will prepare the bed with

1. an air mattress
2. foam rubber pillows
3. side rails
4. a bedboard

180. Postoperatively, Miss Smith has been instructed to check

1. T.P.R. q. 15 minutes
2. pulse and respiration q. 15 minutes until the patient is conscious
3. the incision for bleeding
4. the degree of consciousness

181. Shock is suspected when Miss Smith obtains a blood pressure reading

1. 30 points lower than the preoperative reading
2. of 120/90.
3. that was decreased
4. that was higher than normal

182. Miss Smith puts in the call bell to get some assistance. She also begins to counteract the process of shock by

1. application of additional heat
2. applying cold compresses to the forehead
3. putting the patient in Fowler's position
4. elevating the foot of the bed

183. As soon as the blood pressure is stabilized and Mrs. X is well oriented, Miss Smith adds to her comfort by

1. stopping all I.V. fluids
2. giving a partial bath, back rub, and oral hygiene
3. giving her warm milk to relieve the nausea
4. covering her with a bath blanket and leaving her alone

184. Mrs. X is encouraged to take deep breaths and move about as much as the cast will allow to help

1. her to regain her strength more rapidly
2. prevent unnecessary fatigue
3. avoid onset of gas pains
4. prevent pulmonary and circulatory complications

THE CAST EXTENDS FROM THE WAIST TO THE TOES OF THE LEFT LEG AND TO JUST BELOW THE KNEE ON THE RIGHT LEG.

185. Miss Smith finds it necessary to give Demerol, I.M., in

1. the gluteal muscle
2. the anterior thigh
3. the radial artery
4. the arm

186. Miss Smith's chart must tell the next nurse on duty all about Mrs. X's medications. Therefore, Miss Smith must be very sure

1. to chart the exact location of the injection
2. to fill out the drug book completely
3. to give a full oral report
4. to explain to the family the reasons for the various procedures

AFTER SUPPER OF BROTH AND TEA, MRS. X
COMPLAINS OF A HEADACHE. HER TEM-
PERATURE ORALLY IS 100°F. ON HIS
EVENING ROUNDS THE DOCTOR ORDERS
ASPIRIN gr. XV AND AN ICE CAP.

187. Aspirin gr. XV is equivalent to

   1. 0.1 gram   3. 1.0 gram
   2. 0.5 gram   4. 1.5 grams

188. In the medicine room the nurse remembers
    that her previous teaching had stressed
    the importance of

   1. checking the label on the medicine
      bottle three times
   2. using sterile water to dissolve the
      aspirin
   3. crushing the aspirin into a powder
      and placing it in a capsule
   4. using a paper rather than a plastic
      medicine glass

189. If the ice cap is to be comfortable on
    the patient's forehead, careful prepara-
    tion will provide for

   1. using only ice cubes
   2. using only crushed ice
   3. chilling the filled ice bag in the
      refrigerator
   4. smoothing off sharp corners under
      running water

190. To keep the ice cap as light as possible,
    the nurse fills it

   1. 1/2 full   3. 2/3 full
   2. 1/3 full   4. 3/4 full

IT IS THE THIRD POSTOPERATIVE DAY.
MISS SMITH IS ON THE 3 to 11 SHIFT.
AFTER VISITING HOURS SHE IS GETTING
MRS. X READY FOR SLEEP. MRS. X
ASKS FOR THE BEDPAN.

191. This procedure can be done with less
    strain on the patient and nurse if

   a. the bed is left flat
   b. the patient is first rolled to one side
      and the pan placed in position
   c. the nurse places her hands under the
      buttocks and lifts the hips
   d. the patient helps as much as she can

      1. c only
      2. a and b
      3. d only
      4. b and d

192. The patient will be more comfortable
    after Miss Smith

   1. tightens the bottom linen and brushes
      out any crumbs
   2. elevates both the head and the foot
      of the bed
   3. puts the side rails in place
   4. puts on a clean sheet and draw sheet

193. During the back rub the bedding will be
    protected by

   1. using a spray can of lotion
   2. placing a bath towel the length of
      the patient's back
   3. protecting the linens with newspaper
   4. moving the patient to the far edge of
      the bed

194. Miss Smith will clean Mrs. X's dentures
    by

   1. rinsing them with mouthwash
   2. placing them in a salt solution
   3. using a specially prepared toothpaste
   4. brushing them under cold, running
      water

195. Mrs. X does not sleep with her dentures
    in her mouth. Miss Smith will place them
    in a denture cup that contains
   a. mouthwash
   b. soda solution
   c. salt solution
   d. 70% alcohol

      1. any of the above
      2. only b or c
      3. a, b, or c
      4. all except a

196. Mrs. X states she is quite comfortable.
    Before Miss Smith leaves the room she
    will be sure it is easy for Mrs. X to reach

   1. her glasses
   2. the water pitcher
   3. the call bell
   4. the bedpan

WHEN MISS SMITH CHECKS ON HER PA-
TIENTS AT 10:00 P.M., SHE FINDS MRS. X
WEEPING SOFTLY. SHE COMPLAINS OF
MULTIPLE ACHES AND PAINS WHICH KEEP
HER AWAKE. MISS SMITH KNOWS THAT
A SEDATIVE HAS BEEN ORDERED P.R.N.

197. Miss Smith feels safe giving Mrs. X the ordered sedative because a P.R.N. medication is intended to be given

1. at bedtime
2. whenever the patient requests it
3. when the nurse feels the patient needs it
4. on the appearance of pain.

198. Miss Smith's other patients are asleep. Her charting is complete up to 10:00 P.M. After the sedative has been given, Miss Smith hopes to comfort Mrs. X by

1. talking about the treatments scheduled for tomorrow
2. asking about her plans to go home
3. turning the radio on to a musical program
4. sitting quietly by the bedside holding her hand

199. Before Miss Smith reports off duty at 11:00 P.M., she does not fail to chart

1. the patient's complaints
2. the effect of the sedative
3. her intention of going off duty
4. the medication she has given

200. On the fourth postoperative day, Mrs. X finds she must share Miss Smith with two other patients. With such an assignment, it is most essential that Miss Smith

1. get one patient done before breakfast
2. leave one bath until after lunch
3. organize an effective work plan
4. do the hardest patient first

201. Mrs. X cannot move about freely in bed because of the restricting cast. The daily bed bath becomes a valuable way

1. to promote sleep
2. to learn the patient's complaints
3. to stimulate circulation
4. to occupy the patient's time

202. Because of the type of cast placed on Mrs. X, Miss Smith will find it necessary to modify her bath procedure. She will eliminate

1. the back rub
2. the foot soak in the bath basin
3. oral hygiene
4. nail care

203. Mrs. X's hair is very fine and becomes snarled easily. Tangled hair is more easily combed if the nurse uses

1. a small amount of alcohol or vaseline
2. a vinegar rinse
3. a coarse toothed comb
4. a wire brush

MRS. X HAS SLID TOO FAR DOWN IN BED. MISS SMITH ARRANGES FOR ANOTHER NURSE TO HELP HER GET THE PATIENT BACK INTO A MORE COMFORTABLE POSITION.

204. The cast is heavy. There will be less strain on the patient and on the nurses if they move her by first

1. elevating the foot of the bed and pulling on the mattress
2. joining hands under the buttocks and shoulders
3. grasping her under each arm and pulling upward
4. standing on the same side of the bed

205. Muscle strain will be decreased if the nurses practice good body mechanics. For this procedure it is recommended both nurses stand

1. at the head of the bed
2. facing the head of the bed
3. with toes pointed toward the foot of the bed
4. with knees flexed and feet widely separated

THE VARICOSE ULCER ON THE RIGHT LEG REQUIRES DAILY CHANGE OF DRESSING.

206. Before Miss Smith handles the sterile forceps or the dressings, her first action is

1. to sterilize the skin surface
2. to burn the soiled dressings
3. to wash her hands thoroughly
4. to protect the bedding with a sterile sheet

207. When Miss Smith removes the sterile forceps from the solution container, she is especially careful

    1. to shake off all the excess moisture from the forceps
    2. to avoid touching the sides or the top of the container
    3. to keep the forceps blades widely separated
    4. to keep her arm directly over the container opening

208. Miss Smith has the sterile forceps in one hand and uses the other hand to remove the lid of the sterile dressing container. It is essential that she remember to hold the sterile forceps

    1. over the container opening
    2. with the tips pointing downward
    3. with the tips pointing upward
    4. in her left hand

209. The location of the varicose ulcer makes it necessary to apply the Ace bandage by using turns described as

    1. circular   3. figure eight
    2. recurrent   4. spiral reverse

210. Miss Smith will need to chart the fact that the dressing was changed. It is important to describe

    a. the number of stitches in the incision
    b. the appearance of the wound
    c. the degree of gangrene present
    d. the amount, color, and consistency of the drainage

        1. all of the above   3. b and d
        2. a and c   4. a, b, and c

IT HAS BEEN THREE WEEKS SINCE MRS. X HAD HER HAIR WASHED. SHE ASKS MISS SMITH TO WASH IT DURING THE BATH PROCEDURE.

211. Miss Smith is aware that a bed shampoo cannot be given unless

    1. the procedure is explained to the patient
    2. all the supplies are available
    3. it is possible to get the patient into a comfortable position
    4. the doctor has given permission

212. An acceptable rinse usually available in a hospital unit is

    1. soda water
    2. boric acid
    3. vinegar
    4. lemon and glycerine

213. The rinse for the hair will be <u>prepared</u> in the Service Room at a temperature of

    1. 95°F   3. 110°F
    2. 105°F   4. 115°F

MRS. X IS COMFORTABLE ONLY ON HER BACK. SHE WILL REMAIN ON HER SIDE FOR ONLY SHORT PERIODS. IN SPITE OF CAREFUL BACK CARE, PRESSURE AREAS BEGIN TO DEVELOP OVER THE SHOULDER BLADES.

214. Miss Smith wishes to move the accumulation of waste products from weakened cells of the pressure area. To do this she will

    1. put Mrs. X on an air cushion
    2. place sponge rubber pads under this area
    3. stimulate muscle contraction by application of alcohol
    4. massage lightly and frequently away from the pressure center

215. Sandbags and a footboard will be used on the right leg to prevent the complication known as

    1. ankylosis
    2. gangrene
    3. foot drop
    4. paralysis

216. This type of cast must be considered as a form of restraint. Miss Smith knows that any patient in restraint must be checked often for evidence of

    1. circulatory disturbance
    2. cyanosis
    3. inflammation
    4. pressure sores

MRS. X MUST RETURN TO X-RAY FOR A CHECK ON THE DEGREE OF HEALING THAT HAS TAKEN PLACE. THREE NURSES, USING GOOD BODY MECHANICS, WILL MOVE MRS. X TO THE STRETCHER.

217. These nurses will work together more smoothly if they are all

1. about the same size
2. past 20 years of age
3. strong physically
4. graduates of the same school

218. These nurses will recognize that the heaviest part of Mrs. X is her

1. head   3. buttocks
2. shoulders   4. extremities

219. In order for the nurses to have to carry the patient the shortest distance, the stretcher should be placed

1. parallel to the bed
2. at right angles to the head of the bed
3. at right angles to the foot of the bed
4. at the foot of the bed

MRS. X HAS BEEN IN THE HOSPITAL THREE WEEKS AND SHE IS GETTING HOMESICK. SHE OVERHEARS THE DOCTOR TELL HER DAUGHTERS THAT SHE WILL NEED CHEAPER NURSING HOME CARE FOR SEVERAL MONTHS. THE TOTAL COST OF HER ILLNESS BECOMES A MAJOR CONCERN TO HER. HOW CAN IT EVER BE PAID?

220. Miss Smith checks Mrs. X before she goes off duty. Her facial expression and unwillingness to talk to the nurse suggest her mood is one of

1. depression
2. irritability
3. resignation
4. hostility

221. If Mrs. X could talk about these feelings, they could be traced to her idea that she is

1. a hopeless case
2. not loved by her daughters
3. a financial burden
4. never going to see her home again

222. Miss Smith gets some hint of Mrs. X's problem when she asks, "Isn't there something I can do for you?" and Mrs. X replies

1. "I don't need a thing."
2. "Please put me on the bed pan. I need a drink of water. I'm not comfortable in this position."
3. "Go away."
4. "Don't waste your time on an old lady that can't pay you."

MISS SMITH HAS BEEN OFF DUTY FOR TWO DAYS. SHE FINDS MRS. X ON THE CRITICAL LIST WITH HYPOSTATIC PNEUMONIA. THE DAUGHTERS ARE EACH STAYING A 12-HOUR SHIFT WITH HER. SHE SEEMS TO BE IN A STUPOR.

223. The daughter tries to tell Miss Smith how bad off her mother is. Miss Smith warns her that

1. she cannot be of any help if she continues to worry so
2. Mrs. X might well understand their conversation
3. it is not wise to have such a hopeless attitude
4. the patient could not benefit by such an attitude of hopelessness

224. The doctor brings samples of a new drug to try on Mrs. X. Before Miss Smith gives this medicine, she will be wise

1. to look through the magazines for more information
2. to listen to the conversation of the professional nurses
3. to ask the pharmacist for more information about the drug
4. to say nothing until the pharmacist sends around pertinent information.

225. While Mrs. X is unconscious, Miss Smith cleanses her mouth

    1. before and after each feeding
    2. only when she can be aroused
    3. with a refreshing alcohol solution
    4. using a gauze sponge

BECAUSE MRS. X DOES NOT SEEM TO HAVE THE WILL TO LIVE, HER DOCTOR FEELS SHE WILL BE MORE COMFORTABLE WITH THE HEAVY CAST REMOVED.

226. Once the cast is removed, Miss Smith places her patient in the position that will make breathing easier. For the dying patient, this position will be

    1. dorsal recumbent
    2. prone
    3. modified Sim's
    4. knee-chest

227. Wangansteen suction is started to relieve abdominal distention. Miss Smith prepares the tube for insertion by

    1. lubricating it with vaseline
    2. pouring hot water through the tube
    3. giving the patient orange juice to drink
    4. placing the tube in chipped ice

228. Since the suction tube will be left in for several days, Miss Smith secures it in place by

    1. pinning the tube to the pillow
    2. placing a weight on the end of the tube
    3. using adhesive tape to fasten the tube to the forehead
    4. taping the tube to the head of the bed

229. Mrs. X does not understand the reason for the suction procedure. In her stuporous condition she often tries

    1. to get out of bed
    2. to pull out the tube
    3. to get a drink of water
    4. to change her position

230. The swallowing reflex is absent. To prevent aspiration of saliva, Miss Smith will keep her patient's head

    1. in good body alignment
    2. elevated
    3. turned to the left side
    4. turned to one side

231. Each time Miss Smith turns the patient's head from side to side, she makes sure there is no pressure on

    1. the eye
    2. the heart
    3. the respiratory organs
    4. the mouth

232. Miss Smith carefully records the symptoms and behavior of Mrs. X. The major criticism doctors make of nurses' notes is

    1. the poor spelling
    2. the illegible writing
    3. the many erasures
    4. the habit of recording only routine care

233. Mrs. X expires while her daughters are out to lunch. In consideration for the family, Miss Smith will

    1. call them from the dining room
    2. delay postmortem care until the family has seen the patient
    3. notify all the other relatives
    4. take care of calling the mortician and making funeral arrangements

234. Postmortem care will be easier if, as soon as the patient dies, the nurse will

    1. remove all dressings and drains
    2. remove the false teeth
    3. fasten identification tags on the ankle and wrist
    4. place the body in good alignment

235. Miss Smith's ability to maintain an objective attitude toward her dead patient will depend on

    1. her fears
    2. her past experiences with death
    3. her age
    4. how long she has been in nursing

236. The hospital procedure states that a wide bandage is to be placed under the chin of the corpse and tied on top of the head. This bandage must not be too tight or the result will be

   1. contractures
   2. edema
   3. discoloration of the face
   4. stiffness of the jaw

237. Miss Smith cannot remove Mrs. X's wedding ring. To be sure it will not be lost, she will

   1. note on the chart the fact that the ring was left on
   2. tell the daughters they must be responsible for it
   3. place a strip of gauze under the ring and fasten the gauze at the wrist
   4. make the mortician sign a statement that the ring was on the body when he accepted it

238. Information that Miss Smith must record on Mrs. X's chart includes

   a. the time the patient died
   b. the time respirations ceased
   c. the time the doctor pronounced the patient dead
   d. the reaction of the relatives to the death

      1. b only
      2. b and c
      3. a and b
      4. all of the above

239. The daughters will not be thinking clearly enough to give instructions regarding the things Mrs. X had brought with her to the hospital. Miss Smith will assemble and check her belongings and

   1. mail them to the relatives
   2. give them to the mortician
   3. give them to the Business Office until the bill is paid
   4. leave them at the nurses station until after the funeral

240. The doctor would like to have an autopsy performed on Mrs. X. This can be done only if

   1. the coroner approves
   2. a pathologist is employed
   3. the patient or her daughters have given written consent
   4. the medical staff can testify that the cause of death is not known.

241. The undertaker has removed the body. Miss Smith must prepare the chart for storage in the Medical Record Room by

   1. filling in all the vacant lines
   2. placing it in a cardboard file folder
   3. placing the pages in the order recommended
   4. sending it to the Supervisor's Office

AN EMERGENCY ADMISSION IS COMING IN. THE ONLY PRIVATE ROOM EMPTY IS THE ONE SO RECENTLY OCCUPIED BY MRS. X. WILL MISS SMITH PLEASE GET THIS UNIT READY FOR THE NEW PATIENT? THE HOUSEKEEPING STAFF IS OFF DUTY.

242. The cleaning that is done in a patient unit after the patient has been discharged is correctly called

   1. fractional   3. bacteriostasis
   2. terminal   4. concurrent

243. The bath basin, emesis basin, and the bedpan from the unit occupied by Mrs. X can be most efficiently freed of any disease-producing germs by

   1. boiling
   2. soaking in a strong disinfectant
   3. airing for 24 hours in the sun
   4. autoclaving

244. After the bed, mattress, and springs have been thoroughly cleaned, a closed bed will be made. This procedure directs Miss Smith

   1. to make one side of the bed completely before moving to the opposite side
   2. to tuck all the covers under the mattress starting at the food of the bed and working toward the top
   3. to tuck the bottom sheet under on both sides before putting on the top linen
   4. to fan fold the top covers to the foot of the bed

ANATOMY AND PHYSIOLOGY
PART I

(Answer sheets pp. 311-312)

The anatomy and physiology questions are divided into two parts: an introductory and an applied section.

A factual knowledge of anatomy and physiology is of little value unless the student is able to apply it to an understanding of the reasons for a patient's symptoms and for the treatment that has been ordered. The student should understand the effect of medications on the physiology of the system. Such questions are included in this section rather than in the medical and surgical sections.

INTRODUCTORY ANATOMY AND PHYSIOLOGY

1. The study of the functioning of the organs and systems of the body is called

    1. hygiene
    2. anatomy
    3. physiology
    4. psychology

2. When we study about the location of the various parts of the body, this is a study of

    1. hygiene
    2. anatomy
    3. physiology
    4. growth and development

3. The word DORSAL describes

    1. normal posture
    2. those body parts farthest from the heart
    3. the internal organs
    4. the back of an organ or the body

4. The blood vessels that lie closest to the surface of the skin are described as

    1. dorsal
    2. peripheral
    3. ventral
    4. visceral

5. The FUNCTIONAL UNIT of any body system can be identified as

    1. a group of similar cells working together
    2. a group of organs working together to get a job done
    3. an individual cell responsible for doing the important work of the system
    4. the structural organization of cells which do the major work of the system

6. The VENTRAL CAVITY is divided into two main parts which are named

    1. peripheral and ventral
    2. proximal and distal
    3. thoracic and peritoneal
    4. dorsal and pelvic

7. An example of a body part that would be described as DISTAL is

    1. the lungs
    2. the skull
    3. the shoulder
    4. the big toe

8. The FUNCTIONAL UNIT of the entire body is

    1. the blood
    2. the nerves
    3. the cell
    4. the oxygen

9. A characteristic of a functional unit that will help the student to identify it in future questions is

    1. the name of the unit that describes the system
    2. the size, which allows it to be seen without the help of a microscope
    3. the importance of the unit when disease affects the job it does
    4. the size, which is so small it can be seen only with the help of a microscope

10. The body makes continuous adjustments to keep the internal environment almost constantly at the same temperature and of the same chemical composition. This process is called

    1. metabolism
    2. digestion
    3. homeostasis
    4. protection

11. Another characteristic of the functioning units of any system that is aimed to keep the part doing its job is

    1. the very large number available
    2. the ability to increase in number when more work must be done
    3. the ability to cooperate with other parts of the system
    4. the principle of work and rest used by these units

12. The nucleus is an important part of any cell because it

    1. nourishes the cell
    2. produces body energy
    3. stimulates elimination of cell wastes
    4. is responsible for cell growth and reproduction

13. When a group of several different tissues work together to do a job it is known as

    1. homeostasis   3. an organ
    2. a gland   4. a system

14. When identical cells are grouped together to do the same job, they are called

    1. a tissue
    2. an organ
    3. a system

15. A group of organs working together to get a complicated process done will be called

    1. a system   3. a gland
    2. a tissue   4. an organ

16. Tissue fluid can be found

    1. in the cytoplasm of the cell
    2. only in the blood stream
    3. around each cell
    4. in all body fluids

17. The life of the cells depends on the tissue fluid because

    a. food substances are absorbed from it
    b. foods are broken down for cell use here
    c. bacteria-fighting forces are located here
    d. wastes are discharged into it

        1. a and d
        2. b, c, and d
        3. a only
        4. all of the above

18. Heat can be used to kill a cell because it will

    1. coagulate the protein of the protoplasm
    2. widen the pores of the cell membrane
    3. increase the effect of soap and water
    4. increase the activity of the nucleus

19. The SEMIPERMEABLE cell membrane makes it possible for the cell

    1. to filter out invading bacteria
    2. to select the food materials it needs and cast off all others
    3. to allow food and oxygen to enter and waste products to leave
    4. to control the size of the cell pores

20. If a fluid put into the vein of a person is to have no effect on the body cells, it must be

    1. a neutral solution
    2. a hypotonic solution
    3. an isotonic solution
    4. a hypertonic solution

21. A HYPERTONIC solution is described as one that is

    1. less concentrated than intracellular fluid
    2. more concentrated than intracellular fluid
    3. of the same concentration as tissue fluid
    4. too dangerous to give to a human

22. The combination of food substances and oxygen within the cell will produce

    1. fatigue
    2. a feeling of hunger
    3. fever and dehydration
    4. heat and energy

23. Food substances required for oxidation are

    1. the protein group
    2. carbohydrates and fats
    3. minerals and carbohydrates
    4. vitamin C and protein

24. The entire activity of a cell is carried on by

    1. its nucleus   3. its cytoplasm
    2. its protoplasm   4. its tissue fluid

25. Each cell can produce energy when

    1. it digests the right food
    2. oxygen burns the absorbed food substances
    3. it is stimulated
    4. it receives enough carbohydrate foods

26. Cell growth and reproduction require an adequate amount of

    1. water   3. oxygen
    2. vitamins   4. protein

27. Metabolism depends on balanced cooperation of

    a. the respiratory system
    b. the circulatory system
    c. the glandular system
    d. the skeletal system

       1. all of the above
       2. a and d
       3. a, b, and c
       4. b only

28. Cartilage is different from bone because of its decreased amount of

    1. osseous tissue   3. protein
    2. mineral deposits   4. protoplasm

29. The role of the skeletal system in HOMEOSTASIS is noted when the bones

    1. manufacture calcium in the absence of adequate nutrition
    2. give up their calcium to keep the blood calcium level constant
    3. remove calcium from other cells to strengthen the skeleton
    4. leave needed calcium in the blood stream instead of using it

30. Bony tissue containing a large amount of red bone marrow is important to body welfare because it produces

    1. energy   3. white blood cells
    2. red blood cells   4. bone marrow

31. The bones that carry the greatest body weight must have a greater amount of tissue called

    1. dense or compact 3. red bone marrow
    2. spongy   4. periosteum

32. The greatest amount of red bone marrow can be found in

    a. the dense bony tissue
    b. the periosteum
    c. the epiphyses of long bones
    d. the ribs

       1. all of the above
       2. c and d
       3. b only
       4. a and c

33. Materials needed to build bone include

    a. carbohydrates
    b. water
    c. protein
    d. calcium and phosphorous

       1. all of the above
       2. d only
       3. c and d
       4. b, c, and d

34. The bones of the skull protect

    a. the brain
    b. the eyes
    c. the spinal cord
    d. the ears

       1. a and b
       2. all of the above
       3. a, b, and d
       4. a only

35. The longest bone of the human body is

    1. the tibia   3. the femur
    2. the humerus   4. the vertebra

36. After an injury to the bone, it is the function of the periosteum

    1. to produce new bone cells
    2. to supply the calcium necessary for repair
    3. to bridge the span of the injury
    4. to replace the lost proteins

37. Bone containing a large per cent of spongy tissue will be those that

    1. bend easily
    2. store the most calcium and phosphorous
    3. are not responsible for carrying much weight
    4. have the largest nerve and blood supply

38. The human body continues to increase in height as long as bone growth continues in

   1. the red bone marrow
   2. the yellow bone marrow
   3. the epiphyses
   4. the diaphyses

39. The best example of a flat bone in the human body is

   1. the humerus
   2. the femur
   3. the rib
   4. the vertebra

40. If we had long bones in those places where we now find short bones, we would be limited in our ability

   1. to perform fine movements
   2. to move quickly
   3. to step up or down
   4. to move from side to side

41. The chief jobs performed by the long bones include

   a. carrying the body weight
   b. providing for growth of the skeleton
   c. increasing our elasticity
   d. movement

      1. a and b
      2. a only
      3. a, b, and c
      4. all of the above

42. The kind of joint located between two bone ends will determine

   1. the work the part can do
   2. the efficiency of the part
   3. the amount of movement possible for the part
   4. the amount of body weight the part can carry

43. The kind of joint that will allow the greatest range of motion for the part is

   1. the hinge joint
   2. the ball and socket joint
   3. the pivot joint
   4. the synovial joint

44. The end of one bone can move smoothly over the end of another bone because the joint lining produces

   1. tissue fluid
   2. a lubricating oil
   3. a smooth cartilage
   4. synovial fluid

45. The bones connected by a hinge joint have movement limited to

   1. circular motion
   2. forward or backward action
   3. up or down action
   4. extension

46. Ligaments have the job of

   1. attaching muscles to bone
   2. attaching one bone to another bone
   3. contracting to allow movement
   4. supporting muscle tissue

47. Skeletal muscles are attached to bones by

   1. ligaments
   2. nerve fibers
   3. fascia
   4. tendons

48. Skeletal muscle cells perform their work

   1. individually
   2. with the help of one nerve cell
   3. as a group, in bundles
   4. only if the nutrition supply is at a high level

49. Skeletal muscle tissue is chiefly composed of the nutrient

   1. calcium
   2. carbohydrate
   3. fat
   4. protein

50. Movement, as required in walking, is the result of

   1. the relaxation of smooth muscles
   2. energy produced by the cardiac muscle
   3. the contraction of the skeletal muscles
   4. food burned by the skeletal muscles

51. Muscle cells get their energy to contract from the oxidation of

    1. simple sugar such as glucose
    2. digested food substances
    3. protein in the cells
    4. fat around the cells

52. Blood vessels contract and relax because of the action of

    1. the skeletal muscles surrounding them
    2. the cardiac muscle tissue
    3. oxidation
    4. the smooth muscles in their walls

53. The ability of a stretched muscle to return to its normal length is known as

    1. contractibility   3. extensibility
    2. elasticity   4. irritability

54. As soon as one muscle of a pair of muscles contracts, the opposing muscle must

    1. also contract
    2. relax
    3. produce more energy
    4. rest, waiting its turn to contract

55. Smooth muscle cells make up the walls of

    1. the skeleton   3. the heart
    2. the stomach   4. the mouth

56. Smooth muscle cells function

    1. involuntarily
    2. at our will
    3. at regular intervals
    4. only in time of emergency

57. The most important nutrient needed by the teeth that should be supplied in the diet is

    1. fat   3. protein
    2. carbohydrate   4. calcium

58. The crown of the tooth can be described as that part which

    1. is below the gum line
    2. is above the gum line
    3. protects the pulp
    4. provides nourishment to the tooth

59. The tooth will begin to give warnings of decay as soon as the decay reaches

    1. the enamel   3. the dentin
    2. the cementum   4. the root

60. The blood and nerve supply of the tooth is located in

    1. the enamel   3. the cementum
    2. the pulp   4. the crown

61. If we compare the enamel of the tooth with other body tissues, it can be described as

    1. the tissue nearest the surface
    2. the most useful
    3. the tissue requiring the most nourishment
    4. the hardest tissue in the body

62. The shape of the front teeth best fits them for the job of

    1. grinding
    2. cutting and dividing
    3. chewing
    4. cutting food into tiny particles

63. The flat edges of the back teeth enable us to rub the teeth back and forth in

    1. a grinding action
    2. a scissors action
    3. a rotary motion
    4. a protective motion

64. Teeth are benefited by the addition of chewy foods to the diet because they help

    1. to increase the enjoyment of food
    2. to stimulate an increased flow of saliva
    3. to increase circulation by massaging the gums
    4. to add to the necessary taste of the food

65. In the process of metabolism, each living cell is able

    1. to contract
    2. to produce heat
    3. to absorb food rapidly
    4. to receive stimulation from sensory organs in the skin

66. The combination of oxygen and digested food substances in the cells is necessary to supply the body with

1. heat and energy
2. a feeling of warmth
3. heat
4. energy

67. Man can adjust to the climates of the many parts of the world because

1. his intelligence is superior to that of animals
2. he can control the amount of his clothing
3. the type of energy foods eaten is controlled by the appetite
4. homeostasis allows the cell environment to remain constant

68. A greater amount of body heat will be lost into the environment when the surface blood vessels

1. contract
2. dilate
3. increase the production of sweat
4. help the skeletal muscles to relax

69. An artery that can be used to count the pulse must be located

1. close to the heart
2. close to the skin surface, over a bone
3. near an important organ
4. in the upper part of the body

70. A psychosomatic disease is one in which

1. the real cause cannot be found
2. the patient has serious symptoms requiring treatment by a psychiatrist
3. the damage done to the organs produces emotional tensions and fears
4. emotional tensions finally result in a change in cells or organs that can be found by physical examination

71. Swelling occurs with an inflammation when an increase of intercellular fluid floods the part. This fluid comes from

1. toxins of the bacteria
2. tissue fluid
3. phagocytosis
4. blood plasma

72. The pain that follows the swelling is caused by

1. application of cold
2. pressure of fluid on nerve endings
3. activity of the part
4. toxins produced by pathogenic bacteria

73. The dilatation of the capillaries in an inflamed part is responsible for the symptom of

1. pain   3. redness
2. heat   4. swelling

74. The increased flow of blood to the inflamed part will cause the symptom of

1. pain   3. redness
2. heat   4. swelling

75. The enzyme ptyalin, contained in the saliva, begins the digestion of

1. carbohydrate   3. fatty acids
2. protein   4. cooked starch

76. The digestive action of ptyalin stops as soon as it is mixed with

1. mucin   3. pancreatic juice
2. chyme   4. hydrochloric acid

77. Food is normally kept out of the respiratory tract during the process of swallowing because of the "shutterlike" action of

1. the oropharynx   3. the pharynx
2. the larynx   4. the epiglottis

78. Food that has been chewed, mixed with saliva, and is ready for swallowing is called

1. segmentation   3. a bolus
2. mastication   4. peristalsis

79. Mechanical digestion of food requires tongue action because the tongue

1. supplies a lubricating secretion
2. provides taste stimulations
3. moves food around to the various grinding surfaces and mixes food with saliva
4. breaks foods into small pieces against the hard palate so that saliva can cover each particle

80. The muscle layers of the stomach and the intestines go in several directions for the purpose of

   a. moving the food forward
   b. mixing the food with the digestive juices
   c. muscle strength for straining
   d. better absorption of food materials

   1. d only
   2. a and b
   3. a and c
   4. a, b, and c

81. The peristaltic movements of the stomach normally begin in

   1. the esophagus and work toward the fundus
   2. the pylorus and work toward the cardiac sphincter
   3. the fundus and work toward the pylorus
   4. the duodenum and work toward the cecum

82. The stomach contents must reach the correct consistency and degree of acidity before

   1. peristalsis carries the material through the pyloric valve to the small intestine
   2. the pyloric valve opens and allows some of the material to enter the duodenum
   3. the cardiac valve opens to release material into the fundus
   4. the gall bladder is stimulated to produce more bile

83. The churning and mixing of food in the stomach prepares a semisolid liquid that is called

   1. chyme   3. pylorus
   2. cecum   4. ptyalin

84. Protein digestion in the stomach begins with the action of

   1. pepsin   3. mucin
   2. saliva   4. secretin

85. The speed with which foods move through the stomach and intestines is referred to as

   1. peristalsis   3. rugae
   2. motility   4. villi

86. Movements in the small intestine that are stimulated by the presence of food materials include

   a. mastication
   b. salivation
   c. peristalsis
   d. segmentation

   1. all of the above
   2. c only
   3. c and d
   4. b and c

87. As the highly acid chyme moves from the stomach to the small intestine it stimulates

   1. carbohydrate digestion
   2. the production of secretin in the duodenum
   3. the movements of the villi
   4. the first steps in the digestion of fats

88. The digestive juices that are either produced in the small intestine or flow into the small intestine include

   a. hydrochloric acid
   b. pancreatic juice
   c. intestinal juice
   d. bile

   1. all of the above
   2. a and b
   3. a, b, and c
   4. all except a

89. Pancreatic juice is so important because it aids in the digestion of

   1. all food substances
   2. fatty acids
   3. amino acids
   4. carbohydrate

90. Bile is necessary for the complete digestion of fats because it

   1. supplies the coloring material of feces
   2. breaks fats into smaller particles for action by lipase
   3. stimulates the flow of insulin
   4. stimulates the flow of pancreatic juices

91. The end products of carbohydrate and protein digestion are absorbed by

    1. the blood stream
    2. the blood vessels in the villi
    3. the lymphatic system
    4. the lymph vessel in the villi

92. When fat digestion has been completed in the small intestine, the fat has been changed to

    1. lipase
    2. maltose
    3. fatty acids and glycerol
    4. steapsin

93. Enzymes from the pancreatic and intestinal juices complete protein digestion in the small intestine and change the protein into

    1. glycogen
    2. incomplete proteins
    3. amylopsin
    4. amino acids

94. The solid part of the blood consists of

    a. proteins
    b. gamma globulin
    c. red and white blood cells
    d. platelets

       1. all of the above
       2. c only
       3. c and d
       4. a, b, and d

95. The oxygen carrying part of the blood is contained in

    1. the red blood cells
    2. the monocytes
    3. the plasma
    4. the hemoglobin

96. Worn out red blood cells are removed from action by

    1. the bone marrow
    2. the liver and spleen
    3. the lymph nodes
    4. the monocytes

97. Hormones such as the sex hormones are carried from their place of production to the organs they will stimulate in

    1. the red blood cells   3. the plasma
    2. the white blood cells   4. the lymph vessels

98. A normal red blood count would vary from

    1. 5000 to 10,000 cells per cubic millimeter of blood
    2. 4-1/2 to 5-1/2 million cells per cubic millimeter
    3. 1 to 2 million cells of each type per cubic millimeter
    4. 7 to 10 million cells per cubic millimeter

99. A normal white blood count would average

    1. 5000 to 9000 cells per cubic millimeter of blood
    2. 4-1/2 to 5-1/2 million cells per cubic millimeter
    3. 1 to 2 million cells of each type per cubic millimeter
    4. 7 to 10 million cells per cubic millimeter

100. Materials that must be supplied in the diet to produce red blood cells include

    1. CHO and fats
    2. minerals and vitamins
    3. Iron and vitamin B_{12}
    4. Calcium and phosphorus

101. The white blood cells that are most important in the system of body defense and protection are

    1. granular and nongranular
    2. the lymphocytes and phagocytes
    3. the monocytes and lymphocytes
    4. phagocytes and basophils

102. Lymph is a material that is obtained from

    1. the diet
    2. blood plasma
    3. fluid absorbed from the large intestine
    4. the breakdown of red and white blood cells

103. Blood is forced out of the left ventricle and into the blood vessels in the following pattern:

    1. arteries, veins, capillaries
    2. arteries, capillaries, veins
    3. veins, capillaries, arteries
    4. capillaries, arteries, veins

104. The inside of the heart is divided into

1. two parts
2. three parts
3. four parts
4. equal sections

105. The rate of flow of blood is the fastest in

1. the heart
2. the arteries
3. the capillaries
4. the veins

106. The rate of flow of blood is the slowest in

1. the heart
2. the arteries
3. the capillaries
4. the veins

107. Blood that flows into the right side of the heart is going to

1. the brain
2. the lungs
3. the parts of the body
4. the heart

108. The blood that is pumped out of the left ventricle contains

1. a full supply of oxygen
2. impurities that must be removed by the liver
3. a high per cent of carbon dioxide
4. all the wastes to be delivered to the organs of excretion

109. The blood carrying the highest possible per cent of oxygen is delivered to the heart muscle because

1. the first branch of the aorta supplies the coronary blood vessels
2. blood flows directly from the lungs to the heart muscle
3. the heart muscle is able to select the purest blood
4. the heart muscle contains a higher per cent of red blood cells

110. The heart contracts in the following pattern:

1. right auricle, left auricle, then the ventricles
2. both auricles, then both ventricles
3. right auricle, right ventricle, then the left auricle, left ventricle
4. ventricles, rest, then auricles

111. Changes in the blood vessels affect the blood pressure. It is true that

a. the size of the blood vessel depends on the force of the heart beat
b. constricted blood vessels increase blood pressure
c. relaxed blood vessels decrease blood pressure
d. all body activities cause a change in the blood vessels

1. all of the above
2. a and d
3. b and c
4. a only

112. The valve that separates the top from the bottom section of the right side of the heart opens

1. into the pulmonary artery
2. from the auricle into the ventricle
3. from the ventricle into the auricle
4. to allow blood to enter from the inferior vena cava

113. The thickest part of the heart muscle is

1. the valve
2. the ventricle
3. the right auricle
4. the left ventricle

114. The inside membrane lining the heart and the valves is called

1. the endocardium
2. the myocardium
3. the pericardium
4. the epicardium

115. The blood in the right side of the heart normally is not mixed with the blood in the left side of the heart because of the intact (whole) dividing

1. cartilage
2. tendon
3. septum
4. cordae tendinae

116. Valve flaps prevent the back flow of blood from the pulmonary artery into

1. the lung
2. the right auricle
3. the right ventricle
4. the left auricle

117. The superior vena cava drains all the veins from the head and upper extremities and pours the blood into

1. the right auricle
2. the left auricle
3. the pulmonary artery
4. the pulmonary vein

118. If the blood oozes back through the valve separating the right ventricle from the right auricle, edema will be noticed in

1. the eyelids
2. the feet and ankles
3. the abdominal cavity
4. the face

119. The blood carrying a full supply of oxygen goes back to the heart through

1. the pulmonary artery
2. the pulmonary vein
3. the aorta
4. the bicuspid valve

120. The rest period for the heart muscle occurs

1. during sleep
2. while the blood is in the lungs
3. after the auricles contract
4. every 15 seconds

121. The smooth muscle walls of the veins are

1. the same thickness as those of the arteries
2. thicker than the artery walls
3. thinner than the artery walls
4. made of cardiac muscle cells

122. A vein is different in structure from an artery because

a. a vein is not so elastic
b. all veins go in the same direction
c. there are two major veins
d. the veins contain valves

    1. all of the above
    2. d only
    3. a and d
    4. b and c

123. Skeletal muscles help the veins with the upward movement of blood when they

1. dilate
2. contract
3. complain of fatigue
4. stimulate the nerve endings

124. Vasoconstriction of the veins will affect the flow of blood by

1. narrowing the lumen of the veins
2. irritating the nerve endings
3. increasing the force of the heart beat
4. dilating the lumen of the veins

125. The flow of blood through the veins would be slowed up when

1. the feet are elevated above the head
2. leg muscles need extra blood
3. the hemoglobin is loaded with CO_2
4. the arterial blood pressure is slow

126. The term "peripheral veins" refers to those veins located

1. at the surface of the body
2. deep in the abdominal area
3. in the brain
4. only in the legs

127. If a job requires a man to stand quietly in one place for 8 hours, day after day, damage to valves in the veins is the result of

1. nerve tension produced by a monotonous job
2. heavy lifting
3. increased pressure of the column of blood on the valves
4. fatigue which makes relaxation impossible

128. If too much blood collects in the veins, the result will be

1. edema
2. stretching of the venous walls
3. thrombosis
4. pitting edema and a feeling of heaviness

129. The greatest strain comes on those veins located in

1. the abdomen   3. the lungs
2. the kidney   4. the legs

130. Endocrine glands are different from exocrine glands because they

1. produce essential body secretions
2. pour their secretions directly into the blood stream
3. all regulate some area of growth and development
4. are necessary for life

131. The secretions produced by endocrine glands are called

1. estrogens   3. digestens
2. androgens   4. hormones

132. The pituitary gland is considered the most important endocrine gland because

1. its secretions stimulate other endocrine glands to produce
2. its secretions control the nervous system
3. it produces so many different secretions
4. its secretions circulate freely in the blood stream

133. An important function of a secretion of the anterior lobe of the pituitary gland is its regulation of

1. cell use of blood sugar
2. pregnancy
3. the rate and amount of growth
4. the fear mechanism

134. If the thyroid gland is to function adequately, it must have a sufficient supply of

1. calcium   3. iron
2. phosphorous   4. iodine

135. The amount of thyroxin produced by the thyroid gland determines

1. the growth of axillary and pubic hair
2. the quantity of milk produced by the breast
3. our muscle coordination
4. the speed of metabolism

136. If the calcium metabolism of the body is upset by the accidental removal of all the parathyroid glands, the result will be

1. convulsions   3. anoxia
2. muscle tetany   4. hyperpnea

137. The islands of Langerhans produce

1. bile   3. insulin
2. parathormone   4. adrenalin

138. Adrenalin is the hormone that prepares us

1. to metabolize sugar
2. to use our calcium reserves
3. to fight or run
4. to force a baby out of the uterus

139. An adequate supply of insulin is necessary for

1. body preparation in a fear situation
2. the cells to use the blood sugar
3. good bone and tooth development
4. skeletal development

140. In the female the endocrine glands known as the gonads are

1. the tubes
2. Bartholin's glands
3. the ovaries
4. the pituitaries

141. The vaginal wall is made up of many folds of mucous membrane to allow

1. for stretching during the menstrual flow
2. a greater surface to produce vaginal secretions
3. a place for the normal vaginal bacteria to grow
4. for stretching during childbirth

142. The FUNCTIONING UNIT of the female reproductive system is

1. the ovary   3. the ovum
2. the uterus   4. the meatus

143. If the doctor wrote on the patient's history sheet "menarche — age 13," he would be referring to

1. the appearance of the secondary sex characteristics
2. the first appearance of the menstrual flow
3. the onset of menopause
4. the onset of adolescence

144. Menstruation will occur if one ovary
and all or part of the uterus remain
and the Fallopian tubes are removed or
tied off. This can happen because

    1. the pituitary gland in the brain
directs the uterus to prepare for
pregnancy
    2. the hormones from the ovary
reach the uterus by way of the blood
    3. the uterus has its own cycle and
does not need the ovary
    4. the release of the egg from the
ovary is enough to stimulate the
uterus

145. The girl at puberty will need to be
reassured that her menstrual cycle will
probably

    1. occur every 28 days
    2. vary each month with her mental,
physical, and emotional condition
    3. be difficult until her first child
is born
    4. establish its own regular rhythm

146. An emotional state that frequently
precedes each menstrual period is
that of

    1. disorganization   3. lethargy
    2. irritability   4. fear

147. The mature egg is encouraged to enter
the Fallopian tube by

    1. the ovary
    2. the movements of the ends of the
tube
    3. movement of the cilia
    4. the presence of a motile sperm

148. The only purpose for the thickening of
and the increase in the blood supply of
the lining of the uterus each month
is

    1. to limit the girls activity
    2. to prepare for a fertilized egg cell
    3. to provide the necessary female
sex hormones
    4. to insure the continuation of the
human race

149. A peritonitis is possible when the infection begins in the vagina because

    1. the organisms may multiply rapidly
    2. any object placed in the vagina will
push the infection into the uterus
    3. the mucous membrane is continuous,
from the vagina through the
Fallopian tubes
    4. the blood supply to the part is
greatly increased during an
infection

150. The ovaries are responsible for

    a. producing estrogens
    b. fertilization of the ova
    c. maturing the ova
    d. pushing the ova into the pelvic
cavity

        1. all of the above
        2. b only
        3. a, c, and d
        4. b, c, and d

151. Menstrual bleeding that results from
the normal sloughing off of the uterine
lining cannot occur

    1. if ovulation has been painful
    2. after the woman has passed the
menopause
    3. during an infection of the uterus
    4. if the regular cycle has been
interrupted for any reason

152. Ovulation is defined as the process of

    1. freeing a mature egg from the ovary
    2. beginning the menstrual flow
    3. fertilization of a mature egg
    4. peristalsis that carries the mature
egg to the uterus

153. Ovulation normally occurs

    1. two days after the menstrual flow
stops
    2. immediately before the start of
menstruation
    3. at the mid-point of the menstrual
cycle
    4. after the egg has been fertilized

154. The function of the fringed edges of the Fallopian tubes (fimbriae) is

1. to guide the sperm to the tube carrying the mature egg
2. to free the mature egg from the ovary
3. to secrete a hormone that starts menstruation
4. to wave the mature egg from the peritoneal cavity into the Fallopian tube

155. Once the mature egg gets into the Fallopian tube, its progress is continued by the movement of

1. the egg under its own power
2. the tail of the sperm
3. the menstrual flow
4. the cilia and the peristalsis

156. Menstruation cannot continue in the premenopausal female unless her anatomy includes at least

1. the ovaries, and the Fallopian tubes
2. 1 ovary, 1 tube, and the cervix
3. 1 ovary and all or part of the uterus
4. the uterus and both Fallopian tubes

157. The word secretion means

1. the production of substances by some part of the body
2. the pouring out of substances into a part for use by the cells
3. passing waste substances out of the body
4. elimination

158. Materials for the production of urine come from

1. the kidney   3. the lymph vessels
2. the blood stream   4. the bladder

159. Urine is manufactured from

a. water from the blood
b. proteins
c. blood sugar
d. wastes from food metabolism
    1. all of the above
    2. a and d
    3. a, c, and d
    4. d only

160. The amount of fluid and other substances that leave the glomerulus is determined by

1. the fluid intake
2. the blood pressure
3. the salt intake
4. the physical condition of the patient

161. The role of the kidney in homeostasis is demonstrated by the fact that

1. sugar cannot accumulate in the blood stream
2. the kidney always returns useful materials to the blood stream
3. only small particles can get through the capillary wall
4. the greater the fluid intake, the greater the urine output

162. The urine leaving the collecting tubule is emptied into

1. the cortex   3. the kidney pelvis
2. the medulla   4. the urethra

163. The production and elimination of urine includes the organs of the system in the correct order of

1. cortex, urethra, bladder, ureter
2. kidney, urethra, bladder, ureter
3. kidney pelvis, ureter, bladder, urinary meatus
4. kidney, ureter, bladder, urethra, urinary meatus

164. Glomerular filtrate will be found in

1. the Bowman's capsule
2. the glomerulus
3. the collecting tubule
4. the loop of Henle

165. The glomerulus, Bowman's capsule, proximal, and distal tubules are located in

1. the cortex   3. the pyramids
2. the medulla   4. the capsule

166. The collecting tubule is found in

1. the cortex   3. the pyramids
2. the medulla   4. the capsule

167. The functioning unit of the urinary system is

1. the glomerulus
2. the cortex
3. the nephron
4. the afferent and efferent arteriole

168. The lumen of the ureter is about

1. 1 inch   3. 1/2 inch
2. 1-1/2 inches   4. 1/5 inch

169. Urine moves down the ureter because of

  1. blood pressure
  2. peristalsis
  3. gravity
  4. force due to an accumulation of urine in the kidney pelvis

170. If the proximal or distal tubules are affected by some disease condition, the result will be

  a. reabsorption of materials that should be eliminated
  b. hematuria
  c. anuria
  d. failure to reabsorb fluid and materials the body needs

    1. b and c
    2. b, c, or d
    3. a or d
    4. a only

171. The FUNCTIONING UNIT of the male reproductive system is

  1. the testicle   3. the penis
  2. the scrotum   4. the sperm

172. The testicles are located in

  1. the abdominal cavity
  2. the groin
  3. the scrotum
  4. the seminal ducts

173. Sperm are produced by

  1. the penis
  2. the lining of the seminiferous tubules
  3. the epididymis
  4. the Cowper's glands

174. Sperm are stored in

  1. the bladder
  2. the prostate gland
  3. the ejaculatory duct
  4. the seminal vesicles

175. The fluid carrying the sperm out of the body of the male is called

  1. semen   3. the male hormone
  2. mucus   4. the gonad

176. The FUNCTIONING UNIT of the male reproductive system is produced by

  1. the prostate
  2. the seminal vesicles
  3. the testes
  4. the seminiferous tubules

177. The one structure of the male anatomy that is used by both the urinary system and the reproductive system is

  1. the prostate gland   3. the urethra
  2. ureter   4. the glans penis

178. The sex hormone secreted by the testicle, an endocrine gland, is poured

  1. through ducts into the blood stream
  2. directly into the blood stream
  3. into the lymph vessels
  4. into the epididymis

179. The nurse can expect that any condition affecting the prostate gland will produce some urinary symptoms because

  1. the prostate surrounds the bladder
  2. the ureters will be affected
  3. the openings into the bladder are shut off
  4. the urethra passes through its center

180. The position of the prostate gland makes it possible to examine part of it through the

  1. cystoscope   3. fluoroscope
  2. rectum   4. Xray

181. In times of stress the nervous system sends messages to the adrenal glands directing them

  1. to protect themselves
  2. to increase the production of adrenalin so that the glucose supply to the blood stream and muscles can be increased
  3. to regulate their activities better
  4. to increase the output of urine so that the waste products of increased muscle metabolism can be carried off

182. The functioning unit of the nervous system is

  1. the neuron   3. the myelin sheath
  2. the nerve   4. the axon

183. Adequate protection in times of stress will require that the nervous system provide messages to increase the activities of

    a. the respiratory system
    b. the circulatory system
    c. the liver
    d. the muscular system

       1. a only
       2. a and d
       3. a, b, and d
       4. all of the above

184. A nerve cell will have one axon and

    1. a dendrite
    2. a myelin sheath covering
    3. one or more dendrites
    4. ganglia

185. It is the function of the neurons

    1. to carry messages to the brain
    2. to carry messages to the spinal cord
    3. to interpret the messages to the muscles
    4. to carry messages to and from the brain

186. A characteristic difference between a nerve cell body and other cells in the human body is its

    1. inability to repair or replace itself
    2. sensibility and irritability
    3. nonelasticity
    4. location in one concentrated section of the brain

187. The central nervous system is made up of

    1. the spinal cord and vertebrae
    2. the brain and cranial nerves
    3. the brain and spinal cord
    4. the white matter and gray matter

188. The anatomical structure of the human body attempts to protect nerve cell bodies by

    1. providing many more than the body needs
    2. locating them only in areas with a bony covering
    3. making them microscopic in size
    4. providing a cushion of spinal fluid

189. Cerebrospinal fluid is produced from materials supplied by

    1. the brain
    2. the spinal cord
    3. the meninges
    4. the circulatory system

190. Messages of touch or smell are carried to the brain by the nerves classified as

    1. motor   3. cranial
    2. sensory   4. peripheral

191. You would know something was burning if you SAW flames, HEARD a crackling noise, FELT a stinging in your eyes, and SMELLED smoke. This would be an example of the function of the brain known as

    1. control of stimuli
    2. receiving stimuli
    3. stimulating action
    4. coordination of stimuli

192. That function of the spinal fluid which would be described as protective is the one that provides for

    1. cushioning the brain and spinal cord against injury
    2. a source of food to the brain
    3. getting rid of the products of brain metabolism
    4. equalizing the pressures on the brain

193. The eye is able to focus on a near object and then immediately adjust to an object in the distance. The term for this ability is

    1. accommodation   3. myopia
    2. adjustment   4. strabismus

194. The number and intensity of light rays reaching the retina will depend on the size of the opening called

    1. the cornea   3. the lens
    2. Schlemm's canal 4. the pupil

195. The pressure of the aqueous humor will be measured with a tonometer placed on

    1. the pupil   3. the lens
    2. the iris   4. the cornea

196. Two sets of muscles control the size of the iris. Which set of muscles will contract to increase or decrease the size of the iris will depend on the

1. pressure within the eyeball
2. amount of tears produced
3. amount of light available
4. curvature of the cornea

197. The ciliary body is the muscle that surrounds and changes the shape of

1. the lens   3. the cornea
2. the pupil   4. the retina

198. The function of the firm, gelatinlike vitreous humor is

1. to screen the light rays
2. to hold the shape of the eyeball
3. to interpret colors
4. to supply food to the eye

199. Rods and cones pick up the light impulses and transfer them to the optic nerve. The rods and cones are located in

1. the pupil   3. the sclera
2. the cornea   4. the retina

200. A person will be nearsighted or far-sighted, depending on whether the light rays fall

1. in front of or behind the retina
2. in the rods or the cones
3. on the blind spot of the retina
4. directly or indirectly on an object

201. A continuous flow of tears across the eyeball not only protects the eye from environmental dusts but is also necessary

1. to destroy all body bacteria
2. to keep the eyeball moist
3. to filter the light rays
4. to permit light rays to focus on the retina

202. Tears leave the lacrimal gland and flow across the eye in the direction of

1. the temple   3. the conjunctiva
2. the nose   4. the cornea

203. Sound vibrations are first picked up by

1. the auricle
2. the external auditory canal
3. the tympanic membrane
4. the cilia in the ear

204. The external auditory canal of the small child is made up chiefly of material called

1. tendons   3. gristle
2. ligaments   4. cartilage

205. Another name for the eardrum is

1. the otitis media
2. middle-ear divider
3. ossicles
4. tympanic membrane

206. Vibrations pass from the outer eardrum across to the inner eardrum (oval window) by way of the

1. malleus   3. incus
2. ossicles   4. stapes

207. The external ear is separated from the middle ear by

1. the malleus   3. the ear drum
2. the stirrup   4. the cerumen

208. When the throat, Eustachian tubes, and middle ear are all in good health, the middle ear will be filled with

1. air   3. the ossicles
2. fluid   4. tympanites

209. The vibrations along the ossicles pass from the stirrup to the inner ear by stimulating vibrations of

1. the cochlea
2. the semicircular canals
3. the perilymph
4. the oval window

210. Sound vibrations are transferred to the brain by way of the auditory nerve. The auditory nerve picks up these impulses in the structure known as

1. the semicircular canals
2. cochlea
3. stirrup
4. olfactory nerve

211. The ability to maintain balance and to know our position in space are functions of

    1. the semicircular canals
    2. the cochlea
    3. the stirrup
    4. the hypothalmus

212. Most germs that are swept to the back of the nose by the cilia do not cause a disease because they are

    1. sources of infection in the upper respiratory tract
    2. paralyzed by the nasal secretions
    3. destroyed by the gastric juices
    4. helped to increase by the warmth in the nose

213. Nose breathing is important because the mucous membrane lining of the nose with its great blood supply is responsible for

    1. warming and moistening inspired air
    2. encouraging the spread of bacteria to other parts of the body
    3. producing a sticky substance
    4. keeping disease-producing bacteria out of the rest of the body

214. The secretion produced by the lining membrane of the respiratory tract is called

    1. cilia   3. mucous
    2. mucus   4. sputum

215. A middle ear infection can be caused by extension of a nasal infection by way of

    1. the sinuses   3. the oropharynx
    2. the tonsils   4. the Eustachian tube

216. The adenoids can be found in

    1. the frontal sinus 3. the nasopharynx
    2. the hard palate   4. the oropharynx

217. The lymph tissue, from which the two kinds of tonsils are made, make these parts important

    1. in filtering out bacteria
    2. producers of white blood cells
    3. points of cancer metastasis
    4. surgical emergencies

218. Food and fluids are kept out of the trachea by the action of

    1. the faucil tonsil   3. the hard palate
    2. the esophagus   4. the epiglottis

219. The two body systems that share the responsibility for supplying an adequate amount of oxygen to all the cells of the body are

    1. the muscular and respiratory systems
    2. the circulatory and respiratory systems
    3. the circulatory and skeletal systems
    4. the digestive and respiratory systems

220. The one important function of the entire respiratory tract is

    1. to serve as a passageway for air to the alveoli
    2. to supply oxygen to all the cells of the body
    3. to provide oxygen to the circulatory system
    4. to get rid of the cell waste products

221. The FUNCTIONING UNIT of the respiratory system is

    1. the lung   3. the alveolar duct
    2. the trachea   4. the alveolus

222. A hard, forceful blowing of the nose during a cold will

    1. hurt
    2. stimulate the production of more mucus
    3. spread the infection to other mucous membranes
    4. injure tissues and cause a hemorrhage

223. The use each body cell makes of its oxygen supply is described as

    1. breathing
    2. internal respiration
    3. external respiration
    4. combustion

224. An important responsibility of the FUNCTIONING UNIT of the respiratory system is

    1. to continue breathing activities
    2. external respiration
    3. to keep the oxygen level in the brain constant
    4. to pass O_2 from the respiratory system into the circulatory system

225. It would not be possible for oxygen to reach lung tissue if there were an obstruction in

    1. the left bronchus
    2. the trachea
    3. the esophagus
    4. the alveolar sacs

226. The exchange of oxygen and carbon dioxide in external respiration takes place in

    1. the lungs
    2. the bronchioles
    3. the capillaries and the body cells
    4. the alveoli and pulmonary capillaries

227. Paralysis of the diaphragm would cause respiratory difficulty because it would make it impossible

    1. for the intercostal muscles to contract
    2. to increase the up and down size of the chest cavity
    3. for the alveolar muscles to relax
    4. to prevent bronchial spasm

228. After the cells have used the oxygen supplied to them, the waste produced is called

    1. metabolism   3. carbon dioxide
    2. combustion   4. energy

229. Faster and deeper respirations are ordered by the respiratory center in the brain when

    1. the bronchioles go into spasm
    2. carbon dioxide accumulates in the blood stream
    3. activity is increased
    4. accumulated food supplies must be burned

230. The up and down (vertical) size of the chest cavity is increased by

    1. the contraction of the diaphragm
    2. the relaxation of the diaphragm
    3. the contraction of the lung tissue
    4. the relaxation of the lung tissue

231. The action that forces air out of the lungs is

    1. the contraction of the intercostal muscles
    2. the relaxation of the diaphragm
    3. the contraction of the abdominal muscles
    4. the filling of the alveoli with carbon dioxide

232. In addition to its role in respiration, the diaphragm is also important as

    1. a muscle type
    2. a part of the lung
    3. a division between the chest and abdominal cavities
    4. a muscle that controls the rate and depth of breathing

233. The spread of an upper respiratory infection through the Eustachian tube will cause

    1. tonsillitis   3. an ear infection
    2. laryngitis   4. pleurisy

234. When the cells of the body are not receiving any oxygen, the condition is called

    1. apnea   3. dyspnea
    2. anoxia   4. orthopnea

235. The nurse would recognize hemoptysis because the blood would be

    1. dark red and clotted
    2. dark brown
    3. bright red and frothy
    4. mucopurulent

236. The nutritive substances needed by the skin are available through

    1. the vitamins and proteins in the diet
    2. specially prepared formula creams
    3. adequate fat intake
    4. the blood supply

237. Local or systemic infection can follow squeezing of pimples and boils because

1. the pus spreads all over the skin surface
2. the pus is spread to other parts of the body through the lymph
3. the protective barrier around the infection is broken
4. the blood vessels are broken

238. The outer layer of the skin (the epidermis) consists of layers of

1. connective tissue
2. dead cells
3. sweat and oil glands
4. sensitive nerve endings

239. The epidermis will be thickest on

1. the soles of the feet
2. the cranial surface
3. the buttocks
4. the elbows

240. The sebaceous glands are also called

1. hair follicles   3. sweat glands
2. oil glands   4. nerve endings

241. The thinnest skin surface covers

1. the septum of the nose
2. the abdomen
3. the eyelid
4. the perineum

242. One of the important functions of the skin is protection. The skin is being protective when it

a. absorbs the shock of trauma
b. makes the body sensitive to its surroundings
c. keeps infection from entering the body
d. absorbs vitamins from the sun

1. all of the above
2. d only
3. b and c
4. a and c

243. The oil glands must get the oil they produce to the skin surface by way of

1. the oil ducts
2. the hair follicles
3. the sweat tubules
4. the dermis

ANATOMY AND PHYSIOLOGY

PART II

APPLIED ANATOMY AND PHYSIOLOGY

(Answer sheets pp. 313–314)

1. If a broken femur is not reduced and allowed to heal in correct alignment, the deformity that results will be caused by

1. failure to heal in the poorly aligned position
2. the strong upward pull of the tendons
3. the large muscles attached to the femur pulling the broken end out of line
4. delay of the healing process because of the age and the nutritional state of the patient

2. The longer the delay in reducing the ends of a broken bone, the more difficult it will be to accomplish because of

1. calcification of the ends
2. spasm of attached muscles
3. the patient's emotional attitude
4. inability to give an anesthetic

3. If a fracture is suspected, the nurse must discourage the patient from moving the injured part to prevent

1. forcing infection into the part
2. increase of muscle spasm
3. increased pain that might send him into shock
4. further damage to muscles, blood vessels, and nerves

4. If muscle, nerves, and blood vessels are trapped between the broken bone ends, healing will be

1. delayed
2. more rapid
3. impossible
4. accompanied by deformity

5. The calcium that settles in the clot between the broken bone ends comes from

   1. milk in the diet
   2. the nutritional intake
   3. the broken bone ends
   4. the periosteum

6. In the first aid care of the patient with a compound fracture the greatest effort will be made to prevent

   1. infection
   2. added trauma to the soft tissue
   3. contractures
   4. charges of malpractice

7. The diagnosis of a sprain informs the nurse that the injury has occurred to

   1. the ligaments
   2. long bone
   3. tendons
   4. muscles

8. Green-stick fracture occurs in children because

   1. of the play normal to this age group
   2. the bones are brittle
   3. children tend to be accident-prone
   4. calcification of the bones is incomplete

9. The patient has just had a leg cast applied. Any circulatory disturbance can be corrected early when the nurse makes a frequent check of

   1. blood pressure
   2. edges of the cast
   3. color and temperature of the affected part
   4. buttocks for evidence of pressure sores

10. The fingers or toes will not be covered by a cast on an extremity to make it possible for the nurse

    1. to stimulate passive exercise
    2. to recognize symptoms of inadequate circulation
    3. to take the pulse q.2.h.
    4. to take the blood pressure P.R.N.

11. Unless the patient with a dislocation remains immobilized long enough for healing to be complete, the individual can expect

    1. joint deformity
    2. future dislocation of the part following slight strain
    3. permanent loss of function
    4. production of excess granulation tissue

12. If constant attention is not given to the correct alignment of the stump in an amputation below the knee, the result will be

    1. ankylosis of the knee joint
    2. crutch paralysis
    3. pressure sores on the stump
    4. upward contracture of the stump below the knee

13. The amputee will be able to use a prosthesis more easily and smoothly if the leg has been removed

    1. below the knee joint
    2. above the knee joint
    3. mid-line of the femur
    4. at the knee joint

14. The amputated stump is bandaged with a pressure bandage for weeks after surgery for the purpose of

    1. controlling hemorrhage
    2. supporting new scar tissue
    3. aiding resistive exercises
    4. molding the stump for a better prosthesis fit

15. The pain of osteomyelitis is caused by the pressure of

    1. inelastic bone
    2. the pus in the bone marrow
    3. the cast
    4. long leg braces

16. The pain of rheumatoid arthritis is caused by

    1. the inflammation present in the joints
    2. the excessive weight the affected joints must carry
    3. the "freezing" of the joints
    4. the swelling caused by the accumulation of blood in the joint

17. Distention of the abdomen occurs after abdominal surgery because peristalsis is decreased or stopped as a result of

  1. the necessary handling of the intestines
  2. preoperative diarrhea
  3. muscle spasms
  4. exposure of the intestines to environmental air during the surgery

18. An obstruction to the movement of materials through the small intestine would produce a symptom such as

  1. rectal hemorrhage
  2. bleeding hemorrhoids
  3. vomiting of fecal material
  4. hematemesis

19. Intestinal obstruction will not occur when a cancer develops in the ascending colon because

  1. the growth of the cancer is into the lymph vessels
  2. peristaltic movements are strong in this area
  3. the feces are still fluid
  4. nausea and vomiting keep the nutrients from getting this far

20. The first 3 inches of the duodenum are susceptible to ulcer formation because of the membrane irritation from

  1. bile   3. acid chyme
  2. pancreatic juice 4. mucin

21. A patient will be placed in a Fowler's position for the purpose of

  a. localizing pus in the lower abdomen in peritonitis
  b. preventing distention
  c. increasing peristalsis
  d. relieving incision strain after a hernia repair

    1. a, b, and c
    2. a and d
    3. a only
    4. all of the above

22. Preparation for surgery on the bowel will include

  a. nothing by mouth for 3 days pre-operatively
  b. medications to stop peristalsis
  c. a diet that reduces the amount of a formed stool
  d. medications to lower the bacteria count in the bowel

    1. a only
    2. b and c
    3. c and d
    4. all of the above

23. The very structure of the stomach that allows for absorption of liquids also permits the rapid spread of cancer by way of the

  1. lymph vessels   3. liver
  2. blood stream   4. spleen

24. Relief from the pain of a stomach ulcer can be expected

  1. as soon as the chyme becomes alkaline
  2. as soon as the gastric juice is diluted or neutralized
  3. when the food substances pass into the duodenum
  4. only after an antacid medication is given

25. The temporary relief of stomach pains provided by baking soda or a commercial preparation such as Tums comes from their ability

  1. to coat the ulcer
  2. to put something in the stomach so that the lining walls cannot rub together
  3. to act on the pain center in the brain
  4. to neutralize the gastric juices

26. Bleeding, slow but steady, from a stomach ulcer or cancer should be suspected in the presence of

  1. bright red, frothy emesis
  2. black, tarry stools
  3. continuous abdominal cramping
  4. low blood pressure

27. An ulcer will perforate as a result of

    1. hemorrhage
    2. digestion of the three muscle coats
       in the area of the ulcer
    3. coarse, fibrous foods in the diet
    4. pressures from overeating

28. The symptoms accompanying perforation
    of an ulcer are

    a. hematemesis
    b. apnea
    c. abdominal rigidity
    d. sudden, sharp abdominal pains

       1. all of the above
       2. a, b, and c
       3. a and d
       4. c and d

29. When the stomach has been completely
    removed, the patient must be prepared
    for the inability of the intestines

    1. to provide any digestive juices
    2. to control hunger pangs
    3. to digest and absorb completely
       all types of food
    4. produce a formed stool

30. Diarrhea is the result of any intestinal
    disturbance that increases

    1. the absorption of fluid
    2. the breakdown of nutrients
    3. the peristaltic movements
    4. the desire for fluid intake

31. An excessive diarrhea will endanger
    the life of the patient because of

    1. the dehydration of body cells
    2. the rapid loss of essential nutrients
    3. exhaustion
    4. infection

32. Malnourishment and vitamin deficiencies
    will follow prolonged periods of
    diarrhea because

    1. passage of intestinal contents
       through the large intestines is too
       fast
    2. digested materials are incompletely
       absorbed by the villi
    3. the patient will not have strength
       enough to eat well
    4. there will be a shortage of
       digestive juices

33. A poorly fitted truss can be dangerous
    because of

    1. muscle relaxation
    2. constipation
    3. constant pressure that will rupture
       the bowel
    4. pressure that may cut off circulation
       to a loop of the bowel

34. The patient who has had a hernia repair
    will not be allowed to do any heavy
    lifting or straining

    1. for an indefinite period to avoid
       a recurrence
    2. unless a truss is worn
    3. until a strong scar tissue has
       developed
    4. for at least a year or two

35. Symptoms of appendicitis will contra-
    indicate prescribing a laxative because

    1. it may hide the true symptoms and
       result in a misdiagnosis
    2. the bowel should be at rest when
       surgery is performed
    3. it is poor preoperative preparation
       to dehydrate the patient
    4. increased peristaltic action in the
       bowel may cause rupture

36. The pain of diseases of the liver and the
    gallbladder would be expected to begin
    in

    1. the epigastrium
    2. the sternum
    3. the right inguinal region
    4. the right upper quadrant

37. A bacterial inflammation of the gall-
    bladder may spread to produce

    1. peritonitis   3. gallstones
    2. a liver abscess   4. an ileitis

38. If the patient with ascites is placed in
    a Fowler's position, it would increase
    his symptom of

    1. backache   3. dyspnea
    2. dizziness   4. distention

39. The body's attempt to put the gall-bladder at rest during an attack of cholecystitis is evidenced by the symptoms of

1. gaseous distention
2. collateral circulation
3. nausea and anorexia
4. a distaste for meats

40. The patient with a disease of the gallbladder may have clay-colored stools because of the absence in the intestines of

1. hemoglobin   3. bile pigments
2. vitamin K   4. prothrombin

41. If inflammation of the common bile duct follows gallbladder surgery, the flow of bile into the intestine will be

1. increased   3. continuous
2. irregular   4. blocked

42. After the gallbladder is removed, bile still reaches the small intestine through

1. the blood stream
2. the cystic duct
3. the pancreatic duct
4. the hepatic and common bile duct

43. Bile can produce gallstones whenever it becomes

1. concentrated enough to crystallize
2. deficient in prothrombin
3. overloaded with bile pigments
4. thin and watery

44. The patient will bleed easily and form clots slowly when a gallstone prevents drainage of bile through the common bile duct because

1. vitamin K is not being absorbed in the absence of bile
2. bile circulating in the blood interferes with the clotting process
3. the blood is lacking in calcium
4. the red blood cell count is too low

45. The severe pain associated with biliary colic is produced by

1. pressure of accumulated bile
2. the inflammation
3. pressure on nerve endings in the bile duct
4. twisting of the bile duct

46. Gallbladder X-rays could not be taken if the patient ate breakfast before going to the X-ray department because

1. the food would interfere with the picture
2. the X-ray procedure would cause a gastric upset
3. the bile in the gallbladder would be too dilute
4. the gallbladder would be emptied of bile and the opaque medicine

47. The breathing difficulty in atelectasis is the result of the poor exchange of oxygen and carbon dioxide because

1. the alveoli are filled with fluid
2. the bronchi are plugged
3. there is a tracheal obstruction
4. the alveoli are collapsed

48. Steam inhalations lessen the symptoms of bronchitis because

1. the humidity of the air is raised
2. the cough stops
3. the bronchi relax
4. the irritated pleura are treated

49. The cyanosis of the pneumonia patient is caused by

1. destruction of oxygen carrying red blood cells
2. a decrease in the amount of oxygen reaching the blood
3. lessened activity and therefore poor circulation
4. carbon dioxide accumulating in the body cells

50. Stuffiness in the nose during a cold is caused by

1. mouth breathing
2. swelling and congestion of the mucous membranes
3. inflammation of the sinuses
4. anemia of the part

51. The administration of oral medications to an unconscious patient can produce an aspiration pneumonia because

1. the epiglottis allows material to pass into the trachea
2. they flood the sinus cavities
3. the pleura become filled with the fluid
4. the epiglottis directs the food or fluid into the esophagus

52. Epistaxis may be controlled by the application of ice compresses to the nose because

1. the capillaries constrict
2. the capillaries dilate
3. the return of venous blood to the head is slower
4. the blood clots more easily

53. The pain in sinusitis is greatest when

1. drainage is prevented by swollen nasal mucous membrane
2. the infection is caused by a virus
3. fluid fills the pleural cavities
4. air is replaced with pus

54. Deafness results from prolonged hypertrophy of the adenoids because

1. the ears become infected by extension through the Eustachian tube
2. the eardrum ruptures with the pressure
3. the pharyngeal opening of the Eustachian tube is closed
4. mental dullness slows the child

55. Tonsils and adenoids are not removed unless they are enlarged or are foci of infection because

1. they are lymphoid tissue with a protective function
2. the person is protected from poliomyelitis
3. the quality of the voice is affected by their removal
4. they prevent swelling of the glands in the neck

56. When a patient has a respiratory disease, an <u>accurate</u> temperature must be taken

1. orally
2. in the axilla
3. per rectum
4. with a skin thermometer

57. When the dry pleura rub back and forth, as in pleurisy, the nurse can expect that pain will cause the patient's breathing to be

1. deep but slow 3. orthopneic
2. shallow 4. intermittent

58. Any time a patient has pain so great he will not do deep breathing exercises or allow his position to be changed, atelectasis may follow because

1. stretching of the bronchi increases the accumulation of secretions
2. the intercostal muscles and the diaphragm lose elasticity
3. alveoli in the lowest part of the lung are not filled with air on shallow inspiration
4. pressure of fluid in the pleural cavity contracts the alveoli

59. Irritation of the mucous membrane lining the bronchi will result in

1. elevation of temperature
2. rapid pulse
3. a cough
4. hemoptysis

60. The chronic, forceful cough of the asthma patient may produce an emphysema because

1. infected material has been aspirated
2. chronic stretching of the alveoli lessens the force of exhaling
3. of chronic atrophy of the diaphragm
4. the plugged bronchioles decrease the oxygen intake

61. The symptoms of angina pectoris result when the coronary arteries are in a condition described as

1. dilated 3. plugged
2. relaxed 4. constricted

62. Normal speech is not possible after a laryngectomy because

   1. the connection between the pharynx and the trachea has been closed
   2. the larynx is raw and irritated
   3. there is an opening into the trachea from the outside
   4. inspired air must now come in through the mouth

63. The patient with bronchiectasis can expect that coughing and expectoration of sputum will be increased

   1. when the bronchi collapse
   2. when the carbon dioxide supply in the blood stream is excessive
   3. when the bronchial arteries rupture
   4. as the patient changes from supine to an upright position

64. Edema of the feet and ankles in the cardiac patient will follow the inefficient functioning of

   1. the right ventricle
   2. the left ventricle
   3. the pulmonary vein
   4. the inferior vena cava

65. The location of the heart will enable the nurse to describe the pain of a coronary thrombosis as in the area

   1. above the stomach
   2. below the stomach
   3. behind the sternum
   4. behind the diaphragm

66. The nurse should know that the diagnosis of congestive heart failure will explain the patient's symptoms on the basis that

   1. the heart does not function
   2. the heart is unable to carry out its function efficiently
   3. the arteries have become hardened
   4. the total amount of circulating blood has decreased

67. The dyspnea that accompanies left-ventricle inefficiency is caused by

   1. decreased hemoglobin
   2. interference with inhaled air
   3. back-flow of blood through the valves
   4. pulmonary edema

68. The administration of oxygen to the patient with a heart attack is helpful to the heart because

   1. the blood is supplied with pure oxygen
   2. oxygen stimulates deep breathing
   3. the heart does not have to work so hard to supply the tissues with enough oxygen
   4. oxygen under pressure is more effective than the oxygen in the environment

69. An acute carditis accompanies rheumatic fever. The heart involvement makes "complete bed rest" important

   1. to lessen the work of the heart
   2. to prevent the spread of the disease to others
   3. to allow for the best nursing care
   4. to allow the medicine to work more effectively

70. "Vegetations" interfere with the work of the heart because they

   1. do not allow the ventricles to contract as forcefully
   2. prevent the flow of blood through the pulmonary artery
   3. slow up the coronary circulation
   4. do not allow the valves to close completely

71. A coronary occlusion blocks a blood vessel supplying food and oxygen to

   1. the left ventricle
   2. the periosteum
   3. the heart valves
   4. the myocardium

72. The severity of symptoms of a coronary thrombosis or occlusion will depend on

   a. the age and sex of the patient
   b. the size of the blood vessel involved
   c. the importance of the muscle area cut off from blood
   d. the presence or absence of collateral circulation

   1. b only
   2. a, b, or d
   3. b, c, and d
   4. all of the above

ANATOMY AND PHYSIOLOGY

73. The swollen cervical glands in the patient with Hodgkin's disease may be responsible for symptoms such as

    1. polyuria and albuminuria
    2. dyspepsia and anxiety
    3. anorexia
    4. dysphagia and dyspnea

74. Leukemia is complicated by anemia because the white blood cells

    1. surround and kill the red cells
    2. crowd the red cells out of the bone marrow
    3. take nourishment away from the red cells
    4. are polymorphynuclear

75. The patient with leukemia is always in danger of a fatal hemorrhage if he is injured because in this disease

    1. every red blood cell is needed
    2. the platelet count is reduced
    3. the diet does not provide materials for clotting
    4. clotting materials are not produced in the liver

76. The symptoms of anemia will be present if

    a. the total number of red blood cells is decreased
    b. there is a decrease in the amount of hemoglobin
    c. the white blood cells are lacking in iron
    d. the total number of platelets is increased

       1. a and c
       2. d only
       3. a and b
       4. all of the above

77. When anemia has been produced as the result of chronic, bleeding hemorrhoids, the cause is

    1. loss of calcium from the body
    2. loss of protein from the body
    3. loss of iron from the body
    4. loss of phosphorous from the body

78. The anemic patient has dyspnea as a result of

    1. pressure from enlarged lymph glands
    2. decreased hemoglobin
    3. nasal obstruction
    4. overeating

79. The anemic patient will complain of being cold because

    1. the dietary intake is inadequate
    2. fat pads break down in the absence of iron
    3. a decreased oxygen supply slows metabolism
    4. a decreased oxygen supply wastes blood sugar

80. The anemic patient is chronically tired because

    1. foodstuffs are burned more slowly
    2. too little protein is available
    3. there is too little pancreatic juice for good digestion
    4. the absorption of all foods is decreased

81. The patient with anemia so often has symptoms of gastric distress because

    1. the liver extract upsets him
    2. the consistency of the diet is nauseating
    3. the hydrochloric acid is decreased or absent
    4. iron tablets by mouth irritate the lining of the stomach

82. The pallor of the anemic patient is the result of

    1. vitamin deficiency
    2. reduced hemoglobin content
    3. vasoconstriction of the surface blood vessels
    4. chronic fatigue

83. Drowsiness and an inability to concentrate are an indication that the patient with anemia has

    1. a low metabolic rate
    2. not digested all foods eaten
    3. symptoms of fatigue
    4. an anemia of the brain

84. Moderate blood loss over a period of several months will produce an anemia because

1. the iron intake is not high enough to produce an extra supply of red blood cells
2. gastric irritation prevents the absorption of nutrients
3. the hemoglobin count is low
4. red blood cells have been lost faster than they were replaced

85. A chronic fatigue in the patient with anemia has been produced by

1. the shortage of oxygen-carrying material
2. the inability to absorb energy foods
3. the inability of the liver to store glucose
4. the excessive use of the energy material for respiratory purposes

86. When hydrochloric acid is decreased or missing from the stomach, the anemic patient has symptoms of

1. indigestion
2. heart burn
3. gastritis and headache
4. sore tongue and anorexia

87. The anemic patient's sense of balance and his ability to walk will be disturbed in the presence of symptoms such as

1. anemia of the brain
2. eye disturbances
3. numbness and tingling of the feet
4. muscle weakness

88. Bone marrow activity may be decreased as a result of

a. stunted growth
b. hormone deficiencies
c. inadequate iron intake
d. inadequate iron assimilation

1. all of the above
2. c only
3. c and d
4. a, b, and d

89. In the absence of the intrinsic factor it is not possible

1. to absorb iron taken orally
2. to digest food
3. to change gastric contents to alkaline consistency
4. to heal wounds rapidly

90. The number of red blood cells can be decreased as a result of

1. sickness
2. rapid death of the hemoglobin
3. destruction of the cells or the area of their production
4. failure to get rid of the wastes they are carrying

91. If the amount of hemoglobin in the blood is quite low, the nurse should expect to notice symptoms of

1. cyanosis and bradycardia
2. shortness of breath and pallor
3. dyspnea
4. dehydration

92. A diagnosis of myocarditis would mean that the inflammation would be located in

1. the sac around the heart
2. the heart valves
3. the heart muscle
4. the blood supply to the heart

93. When the arteries and arterioles are sclerosed, the blood pressure will be

1. increased
2. decreased
3. difficult for the nurse to read
4. responsible for the development of specific symptoms

94. Hypertension causes headaches. If these headaches are not relieved, the result is

1. death
2. increased blood pressure due to increased tension
3. exhaustion as a result of insomnia
4. mental confusion resulting from the intense, lasting pain

95. The danger of atherosclerosis lies in the fact that the cholesterol deposits on the lining wall of the arteries and arterioles make it possible for

    1. platelets to rupture and cause blood clots
    2. toxic effects to occur when the cholesterol level is high
    3. the death rate to increase
    4. the heart to compensate for overweight

96. Continued high blood pressure caused by arteriosclerosis increases the chance of

    1. rupture of a blood vessel
    2. phlebitis
    3. deformity
    4. emotional explosions

97. The middle, elastic layer of the artery may be in a state of continued constriction as the result of

    1. an overactive glandular system
    2. emotional excesses
    3. limelike deposits in the arteries
    4. muscle hypertrophy

98. Hypertension places an extra strain on both the heart and the arteries because

    a. the heart must beat with increased force
    b. less blood leaves the capillaries for cell use
    c. the return flow of blood to the heart is slowed up
    d. blood must move through the arteries under increased pressure

        1. all of the above
        2. a and d
        3. a only
        4. a, b and c

99. In order for the heart to push the blood around the blood vessel network in the presence of arteriosclerosis, or hypertension, it will need to

    1. contract twice as often
    2. rest more often
    3. use less blood itself
    4. hypertrophy

100. Hypertension occurs when the spasm of the muscles of the blood vessels makes it difficult for the blood to get through

    1. the arterioles   3. the venules
    2. the capillaries   4. the aorta

101. The doctor will look for evidence of arteriosclerotic blood vessels by

    1. checking the blood pressure
    2. feeling the radial pulse
    3. checking the fatigue tolerance
    4. looking at the arteries that supply the eyes

102. "Pipestem" arteries result from

    1. fatty deposits in the blood vessels
    2. spasm of the middle muscle layer of the arteries
    3. the pressure of blood in the artery
    4. emotions

103. Veins need valves for the purpose of

    1. pumping blood through the veins
    2. filtering out any blood clots that might be headed in the direction of the heart
    3. keeping venous blood flowing in the direction of the heart
    4. preventing the escape of fluid from the veins and edema as the result

104. The chief job of the veins is

    1. to filter out foreign materials in the blood
    2. to return unoxygenated blood to the heart
    3. to carry oxygenated blood to the cells
    4. to permit the exchange of oxygen and carbon dioxide between the cells and the blood stream

105. When the blood vessels in the leg are contracted, the tissues of the leg cannot get enough blood. The patient can bring about dilation of the veins by

    1. sitting with the feet higher than the heart
    2. alternately standing for 30 minutes and then sitting for 30 minutes
    3. putting the leg in hot water
    4. staying in bed to relieve the pain

106. A patient with a peripheral vascular disease will require an amputation when

1. there is danger of a thrombus becoming an embolus
2. the cells die of starvation
3. the part can no longer be used by the patient
4. destructive organisms are poured into the general circulation

107. If the patient with abdominal surgery is left in the Fowler's position for an extended period of time, thrombosis may result because

1. motion in limited in this position
2. the return flow of blood to the heart is speeded up
3. the patient becomes emotionally tense and irritated in such a position
4. the pressure on the large veins behind the knee slows up circulation in the legs

108. When it is necessary to stand quietly for long periods of time, circulation can be stimulated by

1. elevating one foot at a time
2. taking deep breaths
3. doing bicycle exercises
4. wriggling toes and bending ankles

109. If the blood vessels in the leg are diseased, muscle cramping results when

1. the nerve endings are fatigued
2. emotional tension becomes too great
3. circulation is rapid
4. waste products accumulate in the tissue fluid

110. The veins at the surface of the body are more likely to be affected by varicosities than the deeper veins because

1. they receive a greater supply of blood
2. the blood flow is slower
3. the protection and support of the muscles around them is less
4. clot formation occurs where the blood pressure is higher

111. A person who has had surgery on varicose veins should be carefully instructed to avoid

1. a low protein diet
2. anything that will slow up the peripheral circulation
3. any activity lasting longer than 30 minutes
4. tight clothing

112. The characteristic appearance of varicose veins is caused by the

a. stretched walls of the veins
b. stagnating blood which is high in CO_2
c. constriction of the blood vessels
d. sclerosis of blood vessels

1. b only
2. a, b, and d
3. a and b
4. all of the above

113. Varicose veins result from any pressures that prevent

1. circulation of tissue fluid
2. uninterrupted return of venous blood to the heart
3. sufficient exercise of a part
4. the exchange of oxygen and carbon dioxide in the lungs

114. After an 8-hour day as a checker in a supermarket, a person with varicose veins should be encouraged to spend some time in

1. a supine position with feet elevated (about 10 minutes)
2. a prone position with head elevated
3. a supine position with feet hanging over the edge of the bed
4. a dorsal recumbent position

115. The insulin which the body produces is chiefly responsible for

1. preventing the body from changing so much sugar into glucose
2. slowing up the appetite for sugar
3. helping the body use up its glucose
4. making the digestive juices effective

116. When the blood sugar level in the normal person gets too high, the process of homeostasis stimulates

1. an urge to exercise and work it off
2. the intake of enough fluid to dilute the sugar
3. the kidneys to work harder to get the extra sugar out of the body
4. the bone marrow to speed up the manufacture of red blood cells so that there will be storage space for the extra glucose

117. The untreated diabetic loses weight and tires easily because

1. he is not hungry
2. his diet is high in carbohydrate
3. his food is being eliminated before it is completely digested
4. he lacks the substance needed to change blood sugar to energy

118. The untreated diabetic will find that cuts and other wounds will heal slowly because

1. the excess sugar in the blood decreases the healing properties
2. the excess of insulin interferes with the healing process
3. the blood is slow to clot
4. the person does not take proper care of himself

119. The diabetic patient has a HOLD BREAKFAST order. The nurse gives the insulin at the usual prebreakfast time. The patient will have a reaction because

1. the blood sugar gets too high
2. the blood sugar gets too low
3. in the absence of food the pancreas produces insulin
4. the insulin is absorbed faster than sugar is released from the liver

120. Acidosis, or diabetic coma, is produced when the body is in a condition described as

1. hypoglycemia   3. glycosuria
2. hyperglycemia   4. polyuria

121. Even in the absence of a family history of diabetes, the obese person may develop the disease because

1. the accumulation of fatty tissue increases the blood sugar
2. the pancreas gets exhausted trying to supply insulin for the excessive food intake
3. the liver cannot store all the extra sugar taken into the system and tries to eliminate it in the urine
4. overweight occurs only when other health habits are poor

122. In acidosis the blood becomes less able to combine with carbon dioxide. The result is noticed as

1. rapid, shallow breathing
2. sterterous respirations
3. polypnea
4. air hunger

123. If the diabetic sharply restricts his CHO intake, the body may use the stored fats for energy. If an excess of fatty acid piles up in the blood, a complication occurs, known as

1. acidosis   3. coma
2. alkalosis   4. convulsions

124. The first change that occurs when the pancreas fails to provide enough insulin to use or to store sugar is indicated by the term

1. hypoglycemia   3. polyuria
2. hyperglycemia   4. polydipsia

125. Polyuria is a symptom of diabetes. This is the result of the body's attempt

1. to get the sugar to the body areas that need it
2. to replace fluids lost through the kidneys
3. to get rid of the excess sugar in the blood
4. to dilute the blood

126. The symptom of polyuria makes it necessary for the body cells to complain. The result is the symptom known as

1. polydipsia   3. polyglycemia
2. dysphagia   4. uremia

ANATOMY AND PHYSIOLOGY

127. Even though the untreated diabetic eats quantities of food, he will still complain of

a. easy fatigue
b. muscle weakness
c. constipation
d. anorexia

    1. a and b
    2. b, c, or d
    3. a only
    4. all of the above

128. The body attempts to get rid of the substances that accumulate in the blood stream and produce an acidosis. This is indicated by the presence of

    1. albuminuria
    2. acetone in the urine
    3. hematuria
    4. glycosuria

129. When the diabetic has more insulin available to his cells than he has food materials to be burned, the complication that results is

    1. diabetic coma   3. insulin shock
    2. convulsions   4. hypoglycemia

130. The diabetic who complains of pruritus vulvae can be reassured that this condition will

    1. respond to proper habits of personal cleanliness
    2. disappear after menopause
    3. disappear when sugar is no longer spilled out in the urine
    4. be bothersome only during menstruation

131. Insulin shock may be caused by

a. too much insulin
b. too little food
c. a high carbohydrate intake
d. vomiting or diarrhea

    1. all of the above
    2. a and b
    3. c only
    4. a, b, and c

132. A simple goiter is produced as the body makes an effort to compensate for

    1. the increased rate of growth during adolescence
    2. the increased thyroxin production
    3. inadequate intake of iodine
    4. a calcium imbalance

133. The hyperthyroid patient will lose weight as the result of

a. increased perspiration
b. increased peristalsis
c. overactivity
d. exaggerated emotions

    1. a and c
    2. b or c
    3. a and d
    4. all of the above

134. If the hyperthyroid patient does not get treatment that will lessen the symptoms, death will be due to

    1. physical exhaustion
    2. heart failure
    3. muscle fatigue
    4. toxemia

135. The increased production of thyroxin which produces the symptoms of hyperthyroidism is the result of

    1. hypertrophy of the gland
    2. dietary excesses
    3. hyperplasia of the gland
    4. a decrease in colloid

136. Surgery for the removal of a simple goiter would be necessary only when

a. great pressure is placed on the esophagus
b. an increased amount of thyroxin is produced
c. its size interferes with the growth of a child
d. pressure is placed on the trachea

    1. d only
    2. a, b, and d
    3. a and d
    4. all of the above

137. The decreased metabolism of the myxedema patient is responsible for sensitiveness

    1. to coffee and tea
    2. to criticism
    3. to most medications
    4. to cold

138. Dysmenorrhea will be increased in the presence of

    1. constipation and a full bladder
    2. a discharge
    3. leukoplakia
    4. nonpathogenic bacteria

139. Amenorrhea in the adolescent girl may be due to a deficiency of

    a. ovarian hormones
    b. thyroid hormone
    c. insulin production
    d. pituitary hormone

        1. a and c
        2. a, b, or d
        3. a only
        4. all of the above

140. Amenorrhea would be normal following

    1. a subtotal hysterectomy
    2. a bilateral oophorectomy
    3. amputation of the cervix
    4. placement of a pessary

141. The application of heat to the abdomen, a hot bath, or foot soak may relieve dysmenorrhea that is caused by

    1. uterine congestion
    2. uterine muscle spasm
    3. emotional rejection of the menstrual process
    4. inability to expel the mucus plug in the cervix

142. Infection with the trichomonads may not be limited to the vagina; it may also attack

    1. the bladder
    2. the rectum
    3. the small intestine
    4. the skin of the inner thighs

143. A cystitis often adds to the discomfort of a cystocele. The inflammation is produced by

    1. the presence of red blood cells in the urine
    2. excess multiplication of bacteria in stagnant urine
    3. the increased acidity of stagnant urine
    4. the relaxation of the bladder wall

144. A symptom commonly found in the patient with a rectocele is that of

    1. bloody diarrhea   3. leukorrhea
    2. hemmorrhoids   4. constipation

145. Leukorrhea will be present when there is a prolapse of the uterus, first, second, or third degree. It is the result of

    1. an infection
    2. irritation of the cervix
    3. congestion of blood in the vaginal mucosa
    4. increased acidity of vaginal secretions

146. Cancer of the cervix can spread by extension to the

    a. bladder
    b. large intestine
    c. pelvic bones
    d. rectum

        1. all of the above
        2. a or d
        3. a, b, and d
        4. a, c, and d

147. Cancer cells discovered by the "Pap" test appear in the vaginal secretions as the result of

    1. biopsy techniques
    2. flushing out by the menstrual flow
    3. stimulation by the estrogens
    4. normal sloughing away of cervical cells

148. Sterility can be a complication of fibroid tumors that are large enough

    1. to prevent dilatation of the cervix
    2. to stretch the walls of the uterus
    3. to block entrance to the Fallopian tubes
    4. to put pressure on the ovaries

149. Menstrual bleeding is increased when a fibroid tumor, or tumors, arises from the mucous membrane lining of the uterus. This results from

1. increased membrane surface to slough off
2. increased hormone production by the tumor
3. irritation of the mucous membrane lining
4. the tumor blocking the cervical neck

150. The extreme pain associated with any inflammation of the Fallopian tubes can be explained anatomically because

1. the ends open directly into the peritoneal cavity
2. the peristaltic movements are painful
3. the lumen is only 1/16 inch across
4. the tubes twist so easily

151. A pyogenic infection in the Fallopian tubes may be the cause of sterility when the accumulation of pus

1. seals off the fimbriated ends
2. produces a peritonitis
3. produces a tumor mass in the tube
4. kills the mature ovum

152. Menopause is complete when

a. sweating and hot flashes cease
b. ovulation stops
c. menstruation ceases
d. production of the maturing hormone increases

   1. b and c
   2. a and c
   3. b or d
   4. all of the above

153. The amount of residual urine in the patient's bladder will be discovered when the nurse is given an order

1. to catheterize the patient every 8 hours
2. to measure all urine output
3. to insert a Foley catheter and allow the urine to drain out every 4 hours
4. catheterize the patient after each voiding

154. The postoperative care of the patient who has just had a kidney removed will require the nurse to be constantly alert for the symptoms of herorrhage. Such a complication is dangerous because

1. the loss of blood during surgery has been excessive
2. pressure in the renal artery may be responsible for a fatal hemorrhage
3. postoperative low blood pressure decreases clotting ability
4. the patient does not complain of any symptoms

155. Uremia is a symptom rather than a diagnosis. It may occur as the result of a variety of causes that produce

1. visual disturbances
2. damage to the functioning units that greatly decreases kidney function
3. overactivity of the functioning unit of the urinary system
4. an inability of the kidney to reabsorb essential elements

156. The appearance of "uremic frost" indicates an attempt on the part of the body

1. to decrease the total white blood cell supply
2. to overpower any germs in the kidney
3. to eliminate protein wastes through perspiration
4. to get rid of an accumulation of fluid in the tissues

157. Stones in the kidney or bladder are most often formed when

1. bile becomes concentrated in the bladder
2. the mucous membrane lining of the kidney pelvis is constantly irritated
3. the specific gravity of the urine decreases
4. substances normally in solution in urine crystallize

158. The tubule damage in nephrosis will produce the objective symptom of

1. jaundice   3. polyuria
2. edema   4. glycosuria

159. The tubule damage in nephrosis is responsible for a dangerous decrease in urine output because

    1. the kidney pelvis is plugged with casts
    2. too much fluid is trapped in the tissues
    3. the acid-base concentration of the blood is alkaline
    4. most of the glomerular filtrate is reabsorbed

160. If the kidney damage in nephrosis results in anuria, the fluid intake must be

    1. restricted
    2. increased
    3. stimulated by Sitz baths
    4. given by I. V. method

161. The smoky urine of an acute nephritis is produced when

    1. the kidney pelvis is irritated
    2. kidney stones damage the mucous membrane of the ureter
    3. red blood cells are pushed into Bowman's capsule
    4. bladder distention progresses to an inflammation

162. In chronic nephritis the kidneys progressively become unable to function as the result of

    1. replacement of damaged nephrons with scar tissue
    2. reabsorption of waste products into the blood
    3. destruction of the kidney pelvis due to swelling
    4. plugging of the nephrons with pus

163. Infection in the bladder (cystitis) may occur as the result of

    a. extension up the urethra
    b. descent from the kidney
    c. irritation from kidney stones
    d. upward extension through the ureters

        1. all except a
        2. a or b
        3. a or c
        4. b, c, and d

164. Cystitis caused by the colon bacillus is a disease more common in

    1. females
    2. men
    3. children
    4. the senile individual

165. Pyelitis that follows introduction of pathogenic bacteria during the catheterization procedure is the result of extension by way of

    1. the catheter
    2. the urethra
    3. the ureter
    4. the urinary meatus

166. When the prostate gland is increased in size, the urinary symptoms are the result of

    1. drainage of the prostate into the bladder
    2. pressure around the neck of the bladder
    3. decreased secretion of urine
    4. complications of the inflammation

167. The condition of the prostate gland can be determined by the doctor following

    1. a series of X-ray pictures
    2. special examinations of the urine
    3. digital examination through the rectum
    4. percussion and auscultation

168. The first part of the functioning unit of the kidney to be damaged in acute nephritis is

    1. the glomerulus
    2. Bowman's capsule
    3. the proximal tubule
    4. collecting tubule

169. The albumin in the urine of the patient with nephrosis comes from

    1. the kidney tubules
    2. the medulla of the kidney
    3. lymph
    4. blood plasma

170. Albuminuria that occurs for several days or weeks will probably be accompanied by the symptom of

1. chills and fever
2. nausea and vomiting
3. edema
4. hematuria

171. When albumin and red blood cells appear in the urine, something has interfered with the semipermeability of

1. the capillaries
2. the tubules
3. the kidney pelvis
4. glomeruli

172. The hematuria that accompanies cystitis will be recognized as urine that is

1. smoky   3. brown
2. bright red 4. black

173. The pain of otitis media is caused by an accumulation of pus. Such pain begins when pressure increases on

1. the brain
2. the eardrum
3. the semicircular canal
4. the Eustachian tubes

174. An ear infection that follows a cold has passed from the throat through the Eustachian tube to

1. the eardrum
2. the inner ear
3. the semicircular canals
4. the middle ear

175. A common type of chronic, progressive deafness is the result of mineral or bony deposits

1. in the middle ear
2. in the fluid part of the semi-circular canals
3. on the cochlea
4. around the foot plate of the stirrup

176. The ear condition that will have the most serious effects on the patient's hearing is located in

1. the external auditory canal
2. the tympanic membrane
3. the middle ear
4. the inner ear

177. The nurse must appreciate that the child who has both ears covered with dressings following a double mastoidectomy will

1. be confused and dizzy
2. demand a lot of attention
3. have difficulty understanding a normal tone of voice
4. be very uncomfortable and need sedation

178. Any infection in a repair of a cleft lip is dangerous because

1. the whole repair will break down and it will be more difficult to do it again
2. a systemic infection will require extensive antibiotic therapy
3. the extension of the infection is fatal
4. there is no known therapy to stop the spread of the infection

179. High protein, high vitamin C foods are given the child with cleft palate repair because they

1. stimulate the appetite
2. stimulate healing
3. are easily digested
4. can be readily eaten, even with the stitches in place

180. A pipe cleaner or bottle brush is best for cleaning the inner part of the tracheotomy tube. Cotton or gauze are not used because of the danger of

1. leaving mucus in the tube
2. aspirating loose particles of lint
3. forgetting sterile techniques
4. wasting expensive materials

181. The size of the catheter used to suction the outer tube of the tracheotomy set must be carefully selected because

1. secretions will not be pulled through a small catheter
2. only one size will fit the suction pump
3. the number of openings in the end will determine its effectiveness
4. the supply of oxygen to the lungs will be shut off by a large catheter

182. A steam inhalator is often kept running in the room of a tracheotomy patient. Steam is helpful because

1. moistened air gets through the tube easier
2. the air is more comfortable
3. the warm air relaxes the lungs
4. it warms and moistens the air in preparation for direct inhalation

183. Diseases of the middle and inner ear must, because of their anatomical structure, be treated with medications that

1. produce direct effects
2. circulate in the blood stream
3. affect the nerve endings in the ear
4. can be placed in the external auditory canal

184. The patient with untreated glaucoma will become blind because the increased pressure in the eye causes

1. blocking of tear ducts
2. bulging of the cornea
3. atrophy of the retina and optic nerve
4. weakening of the muscles holding the lens

185. A routine eye examination aimed at finding early signs of glaucoma makes use of the tonometer to check the pressure of

1. the lens
2. the vitreous humor
3. the pupil
4. the aqueous humor

186. In glaucoma the increased pressure within the eyeball is produced when

a. solution is produced faster than it is drained away
b. the pupil is contracted
c. the drainage system is decreased in size
d. the lens cannot accommodate

1. a and c
2. c and d
3. b only
4. all of the above

187. The only reason for covering both eyes when just one has been operated on is that

1. the patient is more relaxed in complete darkness
2. it is easier for the nurse to do the necessary treatments
3. one-sided vision is blurred
4. the use of one eye causes movement of the other eye

188. Conservative treatment for a crossed eye includes

1. eye drops that contract the pupil
2. exercises for the tightened muscle
3. corrective glasses
4. all efforts to accommodate quickly

189. The use of a local anesthetic and all aspects of the postoperative care following cataract removal are aimed at preventing

1. excitement or worry
2. any increase of intraocular pressure
3. detaching of the retina
4. a corneal infection

190. In glaucoma vision is first lost in the field described as

1. pupillary   3. refractive
2. "straight"   4. peripheral

191. When a cataract has been removed, the nurse knows that the anatomical parts removed are

1. the iris and pupil
2. the lens and vitreous humor
3. the lens and its capsule
4. the cornea and conjunctiva

192. An incision through the cornea is necessary to remove the lens. If the incision is opened postoperatively, as a result of jolting or movement of the head, the result would be

1. hemorrhage
2. loss of aqueous humor
3. collapse of the eyeball
4. injury to the optic nerve

193. The patient who has had a cataract removed will be up the day after surgery. He must be patiently instructed and reminded

   a. to remain quietly where he is seated
   b. keep the head in an upright position
   c. make all movements slowly
   d. keep the unaffected eye quiet

      1. b only
      2. all except a
      3. b and c
      4. all of the above

194. The retina is deliberately irritated after it has become detached in the hope that

   1. as the inflammation heals the retina will stick to the choroid
   2. collateral circulation will be stimulated
   3. other nerve cells will take over the function of the rods and cones
   4. an increase in vitreous humor will place added pressure on the retina

195. When the bandages are removed following surgery on a unilateral detached retina, smoked glasses with only a pin point of clear place are supplied. Such glasses force the patient

   1. to rest
   2. to look only at a distance
   3. to move the entire head instead of the eyes
   4. to remember that all tension increasing activities are harmful

196. If a patient has convulsions because of a brain tumor or a scar, the pattern of the seizure would be indicated by the term "Jacksonian." The nurse would recognize that such a seizure always

   1. begins in the same group of muscles
   2. can be cured with surgery
   3. is severe enough to cause injury
   4. can be stopped with an emotional attack

197. The cyanosis produced while the patient is in a grand mal seizure is the result of

   1. low hemoglobin
   2. excessive muscle activity
   3. paralysis of the diaphragm
   4. spasm of the respiratory muscles

198. Indications that a convulsion is a grand mal seizure and not a hysterical convulsion include

   a. presence of the corneal reflex
   b. a positive Babinski sign
   c. inability to swallow saliva
   d. presence of an aura

      1. all of the above
      2. b and c
      3. a only
      4. a, b, and d

199. The symptoms of a stroke occur as the result of

   1. hemorrhage
   2. a blood clot
   3. blood-vessel spasm
   4. shutting-off the blood supply to a part of the brain

200. <u>Predisposing</u> causes of a stroke include

   a. hypertension
   b. atherosclerosis
   c. advancing age
   d. rheumatic carditis

      1. a only
      2. a or b
      3. a, b, or d
      4. all of the above

201. The nurse is advised to put external heat on a paralyzed part with extreme caution. The patient cannot feel the heat because

   1. the nerves carrying motor neurons are malnourished
   2. sensory messages do not get through to the brain and spinal cord
   3. the heat-regulating center in the brain does not work
   4. the brain patterns for heat and cold are confused

202. Tension of the muscles of the neck and scalp is sufficient to cause a headache. Such tension is the result of

1. a need for emotional release
2. an accumulation of lactic acid in the blood
3. pinching off blood vessels and reducing blood supply to the brain
4. eye strain

203. If the patient cannot see following a stroke, it is evident that the blood vessel involved is located in

1. the occipital lobe of the brain
2. the temporal lobe of the brain
3. the frontal lobe of the brain
4. the parietal lobe of the brain

204. The seriousness of a stroke will depend on

a. the size of the blood vessel affected
b. the location of the blood vessel affected
c. personality problems
d. medical efficiency

1. all of the above
2. a only
3. a and b
4. all except c

205. The eye symptoms that precede a migraine headache are produced by

1. constriction of cerebral arteries
2. psychosomatic lesions
3. relaxation of eye muscles
4. distention of arteries in the brain

CONDITIONS OF ILLNESS

(Answer sheets pp. 315-316)

This section concentrates on symptoms that may be found in a large number of diseases or as complications in illness or surgery. The questions are general in nature. An understanding of the material in this section will enable the student to make specific applications in the area of medical and surgical nursing.

1. When a child is born with a deformity that is the result of some illness of the mother during pregnancy, the deformity is known as

   1. latent
   2. chronic
   3. acquired
   4. congenital

2. When a disease has an exact cause, the cause is listed as

   1. inherited
   2. idiopathic
   3. congenital
   4. specific

3. To be correctly listed as inherited, a disease must be present

   1. at birth
   2. from the time of conception
   3. prenatally
   4. before the end of the neonatal period

4. If no physical cause for the patient's symptoms can be found after a thorough examination, the disease is described as

   1. idiopathic
   2. chronic
   3. acute
   4. functional

5. Regardless of the age of the child, or adult, measles would be considered an example of

   1. an acquired disease
   2. an idiopathic disease
   3. a latent disease
   4. a functional disease

6. If the child has an inherited disease that does not show any symptoms for a number of years after birth, the disease is described as

   1. acute
   2. functional
   3. latent
   4. congenital

7. A psychosomatic disease is one in which

   1. the real cause cannot be found
   2. the patient has serious symptoms requiring treatment by a psychiatrist
   3. the damage done to the organs produces emotional tensions and fears
   4. emotional tensions finally result in a change in cells or organs that can be found by physical examination

8. If a postnatal brain injury forms scar tissue and is followed by convulsions, or "fits," it would not be correct to call this condition

   1. idiopathic
   2. acquired
   3. postnatal
   4. organic

9. The pattern of a disease in which the symptoms are present for a while, then go away completely, only to return at some later time, is described as characterized by

   1. excoriations and regressions
   2. fluctuations
   3. exacerbations and remissions
   4. attitudes of hopelessness

10. If a man complained of severe stomach pains and physical examination could not find the cause, medications did not help, but the symptoms went away when his wife "returned to mother," it would be correct for the doctor to consider the cause as

    1. functional
    2. organic
    3. psychosomatic
    4. idiopathic

11. The swelling of an inflammation is the cause of

    1. the pain
    2. the heat
    3. the redness
    4. the edema

12. Loss of function of a part as a result of an inflammation may be due to a combination of

    a. heat
    b. redness
    c. swelling
    d. pain

        1. all of the above
        2. a and c
        3. b and c
        4. c and d

13. Chemicals applied to the skin can produce an inflammation if they are strong enough

        1. to cause the skin to toughen
        2. to change its color
        3. to irritate the tissues
        4. to increase the blood supply to the part

14. Swelling occurs with an inflammation when an increase of <u>intercellular</u> fluid floods the part. This fluid comes from

        1. toxins of the bacteria
        2. tissue fluid
        3. phagocytosis
        4. blood plasma

15. The pain that follows the swelling is caused by

        1. applications of cold
        2. pressure of fluid on nerve endings
        3. activity of the part
        4. toxins produced by pathogenic bacteria

16. The nurse must understand that the suffix "itis" means inflammation but that it can be present without

        1. a cause
        2. an infection
        3. the typical symptoms
        4. any cell reaction

17. The pain of an inflammation in the extremities will be relieved by

        1. I.V. medications
        2. elevation of the part
        3. incision and drainage
        4. hot wet packs

18. A white blood count will help to determine, but will not give a diagnosis of, inflammation. A high W.B.C. will tell the doctor that

    a. the prognosis is poor
    b. the resistance of the patient is good
    c. the inflammation is severe
    d. the body has the situation under control

        1. all of the above
        2. a and c
        3. b or c
        4. c and d

19. The dilatation of the capillaries in an inflamed part is responsible for the symptom of

        1. pain   3. redness
        2. heat   4. swelling

20. The increased flow of blood to the inflamed part will produce the symptom of

        1. pain   3. redness
        2. heat   4. swelling

21. Rest of an inflamed part is usually prescribed as treatment because

        1. lessened metabolism allows more rapid healing
        2. less fluid accumulates in a part at rest
        3. continuous hot applications will be necessary to increase the blood supply to the part
        4. the heart can bring more blood and nourishing foods to the part during rest

22. An inflammation that is <u>caused by irritation</u> of body cells can be overcome without the help of

        1. exudate   3. phagocytosis
        2. rest   4. hyperemia

23. An effective treatment of an inflammation that the practical nurse can carry out <u>without</u> a doctor's order is

        1. rest of the part
        2. the application of heat
        3. the application of cold compresses
        4. an injection of penicillin

24. The process by which the white blood cells surround and destroy bacteria is known as

   1. metabolism   3. leukocytes
   2. phagocytosis   4. monocytosis

25. The poisonous substances produced by bacteria are known as

   1. exogenous substances
   2. toxins
   3. endogenous substances
   4. lethal

26. An example of a systemic symptom would be

   1. eye strain
   2. a backache
   3. malaise
   4. soreness in the big toe

27. Septicemia, or "blood poisoning", is caused by

   1. pus in the urine
   2. the poisons of the bacteria cir-culating in the blood stream
   3. bacterial invasion
   4. bacteria and their toxins in the blood stream

28. The local heat at the site of an inflammation is the result of

   1. bacteria circulating in the blood
   2. inflammatory exudate
   3. the combination of the swelling and the pain
   4. the increased blood supply to the part

29. Healing cannot begin in an open wound so long as

   1. the skin edges do not come together
   2. healthy cells must reproduce them-selves rapidly
   3. any infection is present
   4. the dietary intake is inadequate

30. The word suppuration refers to

   1. the death of cells
   2. the formation of pus
   3. cleaning out an infected area
   4. the death of cells due to pressure

31. If the bacteria and their toxins from a wound infection circulate throughout the circulatory system, the condition is described as

   1. bacteremia
   2. toxemia
   3. septicemia
   4. pyemia

32. The type of wound that will heal most rapidly because of the kind of cells damaged is

   1. the incision
   2. the puncture wound
   3. the open wound
   4. the abrasion

33. A clean incised wound will heal more rapidly than a lacerated wound because

   1. less tissue is torn
   2. it is always a sterile wound
   3. the wound edges come together in an even line
   4. it is an open wound

34. A bruise would be described as

   1. an abrasion   3. a closed wound
   2. an incision   4. a laceration

35. A surgical incision will become infected only if

   1. some organ has been removed
   2. body fluids are draining through the incision
   3. bacteria invade the tissues
   4. contaminated materials are left in the incision

36. A puncture wound is dangerous if the object that penetrates the tissue carries

   1. dirt
   2. anaerobic germs
   3. rust
   4. infected materials

37. A sprain or a dislocation is classified as a closed wound because

   1. anaerobic germs have been intro-duced
   2. swelling of tissue occurs
   3. tissue fluid accumulates in the part
   4. the skin surface is not broken

38. To increase the body defenses fighting an infection in the big toe, the doctor would probably ask the nurse

    1. to keep the patient flat on his back
    2. to raise the head of the bed
    3. to raise the leg higher than the head
    4. to keep the patient exercising

39. The cardinal symptoms of an inflammation, in the order of their appearance, are

    a. pain
    b. redness
    c. heat
    d. loss or impairment of function
    e. swelling
       1. b-c-a-e-d
       2. c-e-a-b-d
       3. e-a-d-b-c
       4. b-c-e-a-d

40. When dead cells separate from healthy cells and leave a hole that must be filled in, the process is called

    1. sloughing
    2. necrosis
    3. suppuration
    4. leukocytosis

41. The purpose of scar tissue is

    1. to carry on the function of the part
    2. to plug up a hole in an organ
    3. to give the part time to replace damaged tissue
    4. to replace dead tissue cells

42. A tumor of scar tissue that grows on the surface of a scar is called

    1. a debridement   3. an adhesion
    2. a keloid   4. an abscess

43. If much of the normal tissue of an organ has been replaced with scar tissue following repeated inflammations of the organ, the result will be

    1. prevention of further damage to the part
    2. development of an immunity to the inflammation
    3. a need for surgical removal of the part
    4. interference with the functioning of the part

44. An abrasion is the result of

    1. a hematoma
    2. friction that removes the epidermis
    3. a bullet wound
    4. a laceration

45. For a wound to heal by first or primary intention it will be necessary for

    1. the infection to be cleared up
    2. stitches to pull the wound together
    3. the edges to be brought closely together
    4. all damaged tissue to be removed

46. The larger the area that must be filled in with granulation tissue,

    1. the larger the scar will be
    2. the longer it takes to get rid of the infection
    3. the more antibiotics must be given
    4. the more frequently dressings must be changed

47. An area of dead tissue cells is known as

    1. gangrene   3. infarction
    2. necrosis   4. debridement

48. Nutrients valuable in the healing of wounds are

    1. carbohydrates
    2. fats and some minerals
    3. calcium and protein
    4. vitamin C and protein

49. An excess of any normal substance circulating in the blood stream, such as blood sugar or bile, will

    1. increase scar formation
    2. interfere with the healing of a wound
    3. destroy stitches in a wound
    4. destroy granulation tissues

50. The new cells, formed from the healthy cells at the edge of the wound, which fill in a wound, are called

    1. leukocytes
    2. phagocytes
    3. proud flesh
    4. granulation tissue

51. In most open wounds the nurse must be aware of the dangers of

1. inflammation
2. bacterial invasion
3. hemorrhage and infection
4. thrombus formation

52. A surgical incision that is not infected will heal by

1. first intention
2. second intention
3. primary healing
4. forming a scar

53. If a wound is so large that the edges cannot be brought together and held together, healing will take place by

1. primary healing
2. phagocytes
3. granulation
4. second intention

54. A neoplasm is correctly defined as

1. excessive cell growth
2. a new growth
3. hypertrophy
4. a crablike growth

55. When examination of tumor cells reveals that the tumor is benign, this means that it

1. is cancerous
2. will be fatal if not treated
3. spreads by way of the blood stream
4. is not malignant

56. An untreated, malignant growth is

1. contagious
2. dangerous because of the pressure it exerts
3. successfully treated only by surgical removal
4. always fatal

57. The members of the health professions know that a malignancy may

a. occur in all age groups
b. be found more often in the "over 40" group
c. be completely cured with drugs
d. endanger the life of the nurse who cares for the patient

1. none of the above
2. a only
3. a and b
4. b, c, and d

58. Research has demonstrated that one important cause of cancer is

1. a lump in the breast
2. a sore that does not heal
3. chronic irritation from the sun
4. bacterial invasion

59. The term metastasis, applied to a cancerous growth, means

1. the excessive growth of the cells
2. the spread of cancer cells to another part of the body
3. death of the cells close to the malignancy
4. that there is hope of a medical cure

60. Spread of cancer by extension or infiltration means that the cancer cells have

1. spread to nearby tissues or organs
2. been carried by the blood to other parts of the body
3. destroyed the white blood cells
4. involved the lymphatic system

61. Present-day research has proven that cancer can be cured by early and adequate treatment with

a. X-ray
b. drugs
c. radium
d. surgery

1. all of the above
2. d only
3. a and d
4. a, c, and d

62. Precancerous lesions must be recognized by the nurse as

1. warning symptoms of cancer
2. points of chronic irritation
3. possible areas for cancer development
4. evidence of a positive diagnosis

63. The cell growth in a cancer is correctly described as

1. hyperplasia
2. hypertrophy
3. hypertension
4. hypoactive

64. A characteristic common to <u>all</u> malignant tumors, regardless of location or size, is their

1. rapid spread
2. uncontrolled cell growth
3. cure by surgical removal
4. blood stream metastasis

65. Death due to a benign tumor will occur only if

1. it is untreated
2. surgery allows cells to escape into other tissues
3. it is encapsulated
4. a vital organ is involved

66. The nurse will understand that the doctor recommends removal of a neoplasm because

1. the cell increase has no useful purpose
2. it is malignant or will become so
3. it is the only hope for the life of the victim
4. the patient expects this recommendation

67. A common site for the growth of a cancer would be in an area that is

1. exposed to the sun
2. difficult to heal
3. constantly irritated
4. heavily pigmented

68. The <u>most</u> helpful advice the nurse could give friends, relatives, patients, etc., aimed at preventing deaths due to cancer would be to stress treatment of

1. early cancer
2. precancerous lesions
3. persistent indigestion
4. irregular bleeding

69. Nurses should be able to explain that cancer has become a leading cause of death today because

1. we live at too fast a speed
2. we have too many old people
3. it is inherited
4. many other killing diseases are under control

70. Any chemical irritant that will cause normal cells to become cancerous after prolonged exposure to the substance is called

1. palliative   3. causative
2. an irritant   4. a carcinogen

71. The known number of patients with cancer is higher in this country than in many countries because

1. we are more civilized
2. our methods of diagnosis are better
3. more of our people know the warning signs
4. we are exposed to more dangers

72. Examples of precancerous lesions include

a. pigmented moles
b. sores that do not heal
c. leukoplakia
d. persistent cough

1. all of the above
2. c only
3. a and c
4. none of the above

73. A most important reason why many people do not pay attention to the warning signs of cancer is

1. fear
2. the expense of cancer treatment
3. a false idea of its seriousness
4. embarrassment

74. Cancer is one of the few killers of man which

1. gives no warning
2. follows a remission and exacerbation pattern
3. can be prevented by education
4. has no early pain

75. The early symptoms of cancer are often not seen by a doctor because

1. the symptoms are latent
2. adequate clinic facilities are not available in most cities
3. the same kind of symptoms have been safely ignored before
4. the symptoms go away if they are ignored

76. Recognition of the <u>very early</u> signs of cancer must be the responsibility of

 1. the doctor
 2. the nurse
 3. the entire health team
 4. the affected person

77. Cancer cannot be considered cured unless

 1. the patient is alive 10 years later
 2. all cancer cells have been removed or destroyed
 3. a course of irradiation has been completed
 4. treatment is started before metastasis

78. Cancer can spread by <u>metastasis</u> through

 1. the blood and lymph vessels
 2. the adjoining tissues
 3. the respiratory tract
 4. the reproductive hormones

79. If examination of tumor cells from the hip bone show them to have the pattern formation of breast-tissue cells, it is understood that the cancer of the bone is

 1. primary   3. a complication
 2. more serious   4. secondary

80. The nursing care of the terminal cancer patient requires great skill to keep the patient

 1. cheerful
 2. as comfortable as possible
 3. from becoming a drug addict
 4. useful

81. Informed individuals in the critical cancer-age periods should demand that their annual physical examination include

 1. investigation of the danger areas for the age group and sex
 2. complete X-rays of all body cavities
 3. interpretation by specialists
 4. a smear from vaginal secretions

82. The seven danger signals of cancer should be learned because the presence of any one of them is an indication

 1. that immediate cancer treatment is needed
 2. of some trouble that should have medical attention promptly
 3. that moderation in the activities of daily living must be planned
 4. of precancerous lesions

83. Cancer deaths are most often the result of

 1. surgery
 2. metastasis
 3. ulceration
 4. removal of the affected organ

84. Cancer cells interfere with the functioning of normal body cells because they

 a. poison normal cells
 b. crowd out normal cells
 c. use food intended for the normal cells
 d. cut off blood supply to normal cells

 1. b and c
 2. a only
 3. c and d
 4. all of the above

85. No matter how suspicious looking a sore or a tumor may look or feel, it cannot be positively identified as a cancer until

 1. the entire lesion is removed from the body
 2. X-rays have been taken
 3. the pattern of growth is carefully observed
 4. cells from the part are examined under the microscope

86. A blood clot cannot be considered a thrombus unless it is

 1. moving
 2. plugging an artery
 3. attached to the blood vessel wall
 4. located in a vein

87. The formation of a blood clot in a blood vessel that has been cut can be a life-saving mechanism if it

1. keeps the patient from bleeding to death
2. prevents infection from spreading
3. stimulates the growth of new red blood cells
4. increases the blood supply to the part

88. An inflammation of the innermost membrane wall of a vein produces a roughness that allows

1. platelets to break easily as they flow past
2. swelling to plug the vessel
3. fluids to accumulate in the part
4. ascites to complicate the inflammation

89. The circulation of venous blood may be slowed up enough to permit the formation of a blood clot when

1. the heart beats slowly
2. there is constant pressure on the veins
3. the blood pressure is increased
4. the blood vessels are too relaxed

90. It will be dangerous for the nurse to move carelessly an extremity in which a thrombus has formed because

1. gangrene may set in
2. the clot may break loose
3. the circulatory system will be irritated
4. pressure will increase its size

91. The seriousness of a thrombus will be determined by

1. the size of the clot and the size of the blood vessel
2. the size of the blood vessel in which it becomes lodged
3. the degree of infection in the clot
4. its point of origin

92. A blood clot is no longer called a thrombus but becomes known as an embolus when it

1. hardens
2. moves from the site of formation
3. fills up the lumen of the vessel
4. reaches the heart

93. A knowledge of the dangers of thrombi and emboli should keep the practical nurse ever alert to the seriousness of

1. moving the patient without assistance
2. keeping a postoperative patient in a prone position
3. allowing a postoperative patient to get emotionally upset
4. massaging painful legs without the doctor's permission

94. An embolus does not need to be composed of a blood clot. Other substances that may produce an embolus include

a. air
b. bone marrow
c. pieces of diseased heart tissue
d. tumor cells

1. all of the above
2. a and d
3. d only
4. a, b, and d

95. An embolus will plug a blood vessel only when

1. it reaches some vital organ
2. the flow of blood through the part is forceful
3. it reaches one too small to pass through
4. it is a blood clot

96. The seriousness of an embolus will be determined by

1. the importance of the area cut off from a supply of blood
2. the side of the heart it enters
3. the kind of material that has gone into making up the embolus
4. the size of the blood vessel in the lung that is plugged

97. When a large blood clot breaks loose from a valve flap in the left side of the heart, it may be serious to fatal if it

1. enters the general circulation
2. turns into scar tissue
3. plugs a coronary artery of the heart
4. ruptures a blood vessel

98. An effective collateral circulation can be developed only when

1. the blood supply is cut off gradually
2. the heart muscle is involved
3. the clot is in an artery
4. proper medication is given

99. Collateral circulation is the body's way of providing

1. a method of dissolving the blood clots
2. a new circulatory system to replace an area that has been damaged
3. an independent functioning for the part
4. blood to the part that would otherwise not get any

100. The seriousness of a hemorrhage will be determined by

a. the thickness of the heart muscle
b. the type of blood vessel that is injured
c. the size of the vessel or vessels injured
d. the thickness of the blood

   1. b only
   2. a and b
   3. b and c
   4. all of the above

101. The greatest amount of blood will be lost when there is injury to

1. many capillaries
2. a large artery
3. several veins
4. the nerve endings

102. A greater amount of blood will be lost if blood vessel injury results in the flow of blood

1. in spurts
2. in a steady stream
3. as a continuous oozing
4. from an upper extremity

103. A capillary hemorrhage is most easily controlled by

1. applying a tourniquet
2. using an Ace bandage
3. applying a pressure bandage
4. elevating the part

104. The use of a tourniquet to stop a hemorrhage becomes dangerous when

1. tissues are constricted
2. a thrombus forms
3. the part becomes discolored
4. it is forgotten and left on too long

105. The nurse should suspect the patient is hemorrhaging, even though she cannot see the blood, if the patient sud-denly becomes

1. cyanotic   3. dyspneic
2. restless   4. flushed and hot

106. The heart beat is increased during a hemorrhage because the heart is

1. under greater pressure
2. pumping blood that is thicker
3. trying to provide all the tissue cells with sufficient CO_2
4. trying to make a smaller amount of blood do all the work

107. The increased amount of work the heart must do when the patient hemorrhages will produce a pulse that is

1. irregular
2. slow and forceful
3. dyspneic
4. rapid and thready

108. The hemorrhaging patient will become thirsty because

1. tissue fluid is being used to increase the volume of circulating blood
2. the tissues lack an adequate supply of oxygen
3. fluid accumulates as edema in the tissues
4. the heart does not distribute the blood to all parts of the body

109. A calm attitude and an indication that the nurse knows what to do in the situation will be very helpful in relieving the hemorrhaging patient's feelings of

1. distress   3. restlessness
2. anxiety   4. apprehension

110. The patient in psychic shock has too much blood filling

  1. the heart
  2. the lungs
  3. the capillaries
  4. the abdominal veins

111. Regardless of the cause of shock, the symptoms are produced as a result of

  1. emotional complications
  2. some injury that causes loss of blood
  3. reduced volume of circulating blood
  4. some allergy

112. Shock that follows hemorrhage can be expected after a blood loss of

  1. 1 pint   3. 2 to 3 quarts
  2. 1 to 2 quarts   4. 4 quarts

113. If the patient who had just returned from surgery complains of feelings of uneasiness, the practical nurse should appreciate the need to check the possibility of onset of shock by

  1. taking the patient's temperature rectally
  2. checking the pulse and blood pressure
  3. asking the patient questions to determine his degree of consciousness
  4. asking the patient if he feels thirsty

114. Symptoms of shock can be observed by the nurse by the time the blood pressure reading is

  1. 90 or below, systolic pressure
  2. 90 or below, diastolic pressure
  3. higher for the diastolic than for the systolic pressure
  4. irregular

115. The application of hot water bottles to increase the body temperature of the shock patient can be dangerous because

  1. the electrolyte balance can be greatly upset by even limited perspiration
  2. it will speed up the heart beat
  3. the patient will become drowsy and slip into coma
  4. it dilates the surface blood vessels and draws blood from the vital organs

116. The patient recovers quickly from primary shock if placed in

  1. Sim's position
  2. dorsal recumbent position
  3. Fowler's position
  4. jack-knife position

117. The cold skin of the patient in shock is the result of

  1. an inability of body cells to use food substances and oxygen for the process of metabolism
  2. inactivity
  3. constricted blood vessels that limit the flow of warm blood to the surface
  4. fluid loss by evaporation

118. The volume of circulating blood will be built up and will stay up best if the patient is given an intravenous infusion of

  1. normal saline solution
  2. 5% glucose solution
  3. blood plasma
  4. adrenalin

119. The fluid that collects outside the circulatory system when edema is present is located in

  1. a cavity.
  2. the feet and ankles
  3. the blood vessels of the brain
  4. the tissue spaces

120. Edema is characterized by a swelling that is

  1. painless   3. moist
  2. pitted   4. movable

121. Edematous fluid has come from the blood stream through the

  1. capillaries
  2. lymph vessels
  3. arteriole end of the capillary
  4. venule end of the capillary

122. Right-sided heart failure will produce an edema in

  1. the lungs
  2. the lower extremities
  3. the hands and arms
  4. the abdominal cavity

123. Any protein deficiency over a period of time will result in edema because

1. proteins are needed to hold fluid in the blood vessels
2. minerals cannot be properly used
3. metabolism is out of balance
4. fluid intake is excessive to make up for the protein lack

124. Edema is produced when the venous end of the capillaries fail

1. to give up their oxygen and nourishment load
2. to reabsorb excess tissue fluid
3. to hold the plasma proteins
4. to keep the sodium and potassium in balance

125. A right-sided heart failure may be the cause of edema as a result of

1. the slow return of blood through the veins and vena cava
2. high arterial blood pressure
3. decreased solids in the blood
4. too much residual blood remaining in the left ventricle after each beat

126. The doctor will suspect that edema is the result of a kidney disease if

1. the eyelids are puffy in the early A.M.
2. the legs are swollen at the end of the day
3. voiding is scanty
4. the swelling quickly progresses to the rest of the body

127. When edema is the result of inefficient action of the valve between the right auricle and ventricle, the swelling will appear

1. shortly after meals
2. in the early A.M.
3. mid-afternoon or later
4. after any fluid intake

128. Jaundice frequently begins with a yellowish discoloration of

1. the skin
2. the nail beds
3. the lips
4. the whites of the eyes

129. The typical symptoms of jaundice are produced because of the presence of bile in

1. the lymph system
2. the blood
3. the gastric juices
4. the tissue fluid

130. Preoperative vitamin C should be given the jaundiced patient because

1. of the emotional conflicts
2. bile in the blood interferes with healing
3. the patient cannot tolerate the anesthetic
4. any hemorrhage will be fatal

131. If bile cannot get into the small intestine, a vitamin K deficiency in a surgical patient may cause

1. clot formation
2. a fatal postoperative hemorrhage
3. cyanosis
4. many postoperative complications

132. The jaundiced patient will need surgical treatment if the cause of the jaundice is

1. obstructive   3. hemolytic
2. nonobstructive 4. secondary

133. Jaundice may occur as the result of

a. gallstones plugging the common bile duct
b. acute liver infection
c. increased destruction of red blood cells
d. damage to the red bone marrow

1. all of the above
2. a only
3. c or d
4. a, b, or c

134. Ascites is defined as

1. an abnormal collection of fluid
2. a collection of fluid in the tissues
3. a collection of fluid in the lung cavity
4. an abnormal collection of fluid in the abdominal cavity

135. The fluid that accumulates in a condition of ascites comes from

    1. the spinal column
    2. lymph nodes in the groin
    3. capillary oozing
    4. plasma fluid escaping from abdominal capillaries

136. Pressure will produce an ascites as a result of

    1. increased blood pressure
    2. slowed-up circulation
    3. edema
    4. interference with intestinal peristalsis

137. The substances in the blood stream that protect the body from disease invaders are called

    1. immunity   3. antitoxins
    2. antibodies   4. vaccines

138. Substances in the blood stream that fight against only one type of disease organism are called

    1. unicellular   3. singular
    2. serums   4. specific

139. The baby has a positive "take" following a smallpox vaccination. The presence of the scab is evidence of

    1. natural immunity
    2. passive-acquired immunity
    3. active-acquired immunity
    4. prophylaxis

140. A substance most often used when passive-acquired immunity is needed is

    1. a toxin-antitoxin
    2. a toxoid
    3. a serum
    4. a vaccine

141. A child who has been weakened by rheumatic fever is exposed to whooping cough. He has no active immunity to this disease. He should be given a protective dose of

    1. a booster shot of pertussis vaccine
    2. pertussis vaccine at six-week intervals
    3. antibiotics
    4. gamma globulin at once

142. The body can be protected by active immunity as the result of

    a. recovery from the disease
    b. having an undiagnosed infection
    c. administration of antitoxin or gamma globulin
    d. vaccination

        1. a, b, or c
        2. a, b, or d
        3. c and d
        4. all of the above

143. The type of immunity the child will have if he is given immune substances after he has been exposed to the communicable disease will be

    1. short-lasting passive immunity
    2. permanent active immunity
    3. long-lasting passive immunity
    4. autogenous racial immunity

144. Those substances that produce an active immunity are not able to protect the person who has just been exposed to a communicable disease because

    a. several injections may be required
    b. immunity is built up slowly
    c. the reaction is too severe
    d. the immunity does not last long enough

        1. all of the above
        2. a only
        3. a and b
        4. a and d

145. Specific antibodies in the blood stream protect the body from communicable disease when they

    1. kill the causative organism
    2. neutralize the toxins of the bacteria
    3. keep the organism from invading the tissues
    4. stimulate the action of the white blood cells

146. To stimulate the body's production of antibodies, it is necessary to introduce

    1. antigens
    2. gamma globulin
    3. plasma proteins
    4. the disease-producing organism in some form

147. One of the hardest things for most nurses to <u>put into practice</u> as they care for chronically ill patients is

1. to pretend to enjoy this kind of nursing
2. to continue nursing techniques as they have been taught
3. to insist that the patient do as much as he can for himself
4. to place emphasis on body alignment

148. Many chronically ill patients could return to some degree of usefulness if the early emphasis on treatment and nursing was one of

1. overprotection 3. sympathy
2. therapy   4. rehabilitation

149. Many of the chronic diseases in the "50+" age group are described as

1. degenerative   3. functional
2. psychosomatic 4. syndromes

150. The patient and his family may be discouraged by the term "chronic" because most people think of such an illness as

1. terminal 3. incurable
2. fatal   4. contagious

151. A chronic disease, as the term is used by doctors and nurses, describes any disease or condition that

1. requires long-term nursing care
2. will last for a long time
3. will limit the activity of the person
4. requires daily medication or treatment

152. A paralyzed stroke patient who is not receiving total nursing care may have his period of chronic illness lengthened as a result of

1. decubitus ulcers 3. a thrombus
2. insomnia   4. contractures

153. Most people find that a chronic disease is a financial hardship because they

1. have always expected that such care would be furnished by county or state
2. do not carry Blue Cross and Blue Shield insurance
3. have no insurance that pays for long-term disability
4. have no relatives to care for them

154. Rehabilitation efforts for the patient with a long-term illness place the stress

1. on what the patient can do with what he has left
2. on training the patient to be self-supporting
3. on developing a sensible attitude toward his limitations
4. on ignoring the reactions of normal people

155. The elderly patient with an acute illness often becomes the chronically ill patient because his family and nurses fail

1. to make life interesting
2. to stimulate him to try to get well
3. to encourage him to want to go home
4. to provide the proper physical care

156. Even though rehabilitation is expensive, it is still cheaper than custodial care of the chronically ill patient

1. which is a continuing expense
2. who is not covered by insurance
3. who is in need of more skilled medical and nursing care
4. who is in need of such high-cost physical care

157. A point to stress in encouraging an increase in rehabilitation facilities for the chronically ill could well be

1. emphasis on care of these patients in the home
2. public education to provide state facilities for their care
3. to point out how much tax money goes for their care
4. emphasis on the economic value of returning these patients to a tax-paying status

158. The nurse assigned to give "complete nursing care" must have that quality of

1. sympathy 3. courtesy
2. empathy   4. observation

159. If the patient is worried about his failure to meet job and family responsibilities, the nurse should realize that it will be impossible to achieve

1. rest   3. physical comfort
2. sleep 4. emotional rest

160. A patient is described as in a coma when he

    1. talks out of his head
    2. cannot be aroused
    3. is disoriented
    4. cannot cooperate

161. An unconscious patient must not be given food or fluids by mouth because

    1. the swallowing reflex is lost
    2. food accumulates in the mouth and is swallowed infrequently
    3. he cannot chew them adequately
    4. complications are always fatal

162. If the acutely ill patient makes false and strange charges against his nurse, she might well suspect his behavior is the result of

    1. unconsciousness   3. disorientation
    2. coma   4. delirium

163. If the acutely ill, hospitalized patient insists on going "outside and down the path" to the bathroom, he would be considered

    1. hallucinating   3. disoriented
    2. delirious   4. confused

MEDICAL AND SURGICAL DISEASES AND NURSING
PART I

(Answer sheets pp. 317-318)

The review of medical and surgical conditions includes those diseases commonly discussed as part of pediatrics as well as others encountered more frequently in the senescent group. Throughout this section emphasis is placed on the importance of the emotional outlook of the patient and his family and the responsibility of the nurse to recognize and anticipate these emotional fluctuations. Part II of Anatomy and Physiology could have been incorporated in this section on medical and surgical conditions.

1. Mr. A has been told his symptoms are due to an allergy. This could be interpreted as meaning that he is exceptionally sensitive to

   1. most medicines
   2. high-protein foods
   3. a substance or substances harmless to most people
   4. substances eliminated in an emotionally tense situation

2. An allergen invades the body of an allergic person and his system reacts to the invasion by

   1. producing antibodies
   2. developing a papular rash
   3. becoming resistant
   4. producing an immunity

3. Mother has asthma and father has hay fever. The doctor will be able to predict that unless rigid precautions are taken all their children will

   1. be born with some allergy
   2. develop the allergy carried by the father
   3. become allergic to many substances
   4. display symptoms of some allergy at an early age

4. There is a great chance that Johnny inherited a tendency toward allergic reactions. His parents should be advised to delay giving him foods such as

   a. eggs
   b. Karo syrup
   c. cereal
   d. orange juice

      1. a, c, and d
      2. b and c
      3. a only
      4. all of the above

5. Quack medications and fad treatments for allergic conditions are numerous and sell very well because

   1. a prescription is not needed
   2. temporary relief of symptoms is guaranteed
   3. the patient is looking for a quick cure
   4. it increases the psychological attitude of the patient

6. When a person has a diagnosis of "seasonal" hay fever, his symptoms will be present

   1. with each change in season
   2. only when one substance is present in large amounts
   3. most of the time
   4. only in the fall when weeds are going to seed

7. A serious complication of untreated hay fever is

   1. pneumonia   3. otitis media
   2. sinusitis   4. asthma

8. Mr. X has hay-fever symptoms when the air is loaded with ragweed pollens. The symptoms he will complain of are

   a. sneezing
   b. headache
   c. conjunctivitis
   d. increased nasal secretion

      1. all of the above
      2. a only
      3. a, c, and d
      4. c and d

9. The asthmatic wheeze occurs when the individual

   1. inhales
   2. tries to increase the lung capacity
   3. exhales
   4. exerts

10. An individual suspected of having an allergy may have diagnostic patch or skin tests. These are done to attempt to identify

1. a diagnosis
2. the allergens
3. the seriousness of the symptoms
4. effective methods of treatment

11. Mrs. Z is a farmer's wife. She is allergic to house dust. Effective treatment for this woman must be aimed at

1. desensitization
2. filtering all the air she breathes
3. finding a prophylactic medication
4. finding a climate in which she can be symptom-free

12. The stuffy nose that is so often a distressing symptom of hay fever is due to irritation that causes

1. a blocking of the sinuses
2. a drying of the mucosa
3. edema of nasal mucosa
4. capillary nasoconstriction

13. Hospitalization and skilled nursing care are needed for the patient with status asthmaticus. Without adequate treatment, the patient will die from

1. suffocation   3. anoxia
2. strangulation   4. heart failure

14. Parents should be helped to take a very objective attitude toward a child's asthmatic attacks in an effort to prevent

1. them from becoming a habit to control a situation
2. future mental illness
3. serious physical complications in adult life
4. physical and emotional overexertion

15. If anaphylactic shock is going to kill the patient, death will occur

1. immediately
2. in about 2 days
3. before oxygen can be given
4. in 20 to 30 minutes

16. When the patient has been given a medication that is known to produce anaphylactic shock in hypersensitive people, the nurse must observe him closely. The first symptom of anaphylactic shock will appear

1. almost immediately after the allergen is introduced
2. about 24 hours after exposure
3. during sleep
4. too late to give the patient a chance to notify the doctor

17. When anaphylactic shock kills the patient, the death will have been due to

1. the decreased amount of circulating blood
2. anoxia brought about by panic
3. systemic poisoning
4. negligent medical and nursing care

18. The diabetic man-of-the-house gets regular insulin a.c. He insists on shoveling the snow from the sidewalk and driveway before breakfast. This man can expect that before lunch time he will have symptoms of

1. diabetic coma   3. insulin shock
2. excessive hunger   4. acidosis

19. When the diabetic patient who has had the disease under control begins to have frequent insulin reactions, it is important for him to see his doctor. The doctor will need to decide whether

1. he is ill enough to be in the hospital
2. his diet needs to be increased
3. an adjustment must be made in the insulin or the diet
4. oral medication will be less harmful than the injections

20. The nurse should contribute to the good mental health of the newly diagnosed diabetic. She can do this in her teaching when she

1. urges him to keep his weight slightly above normal
2. stresses the need to consult the doctor often
3. tries to convince him that he can lead a normal, useful life
4. tries to help him to understand his physical restrictions

21. The diabetic patient is male, age 40, married, and the father of three children. The doctor's prescription for diet and insulin to keep the disease under control must consider

1. the food habits of the rest of the family
2. his religion
3. his body structure
4. his occupation

22. A noncaloric beverage that the diabetic can order at the "soda fountain" while the rest of the gang drinks cokes is

1. orange juice
2. lemonade
3. coffee
4. rootbeer

23. If the diabetic patient keeps his urine sugar-free over a period of months by following the doctor's plan of treatment, the doctor may reevaluate his prescription and

a. increase the diet
b. increase the carbohydrate
c. decrease the insulin
d. increase the amount of exercise

    1. a only
    2. a or c
    3. b and d
    4. c only

24. If the nurse knows there is a history of diabetes in a family, she can encourage all family members

a. to have a weekly urine test
b. to take additional insulin
c. to be checked periodically
d. to keep weight within normal limits

    1. all of the above
    2. a only
    3. a and d
    4. c and d

25. While the newly diagnosed diabetic patient is still in the hospital, the nurse can best help him to learn the various principles of self-care by

1. giving him pamphlets to read
2. nurse demonstration and patient-return demonstration
3. teaching and reteaching until the patient has the material memorized
4. spending much of her time with the patient

26. It is often very difficult for the small child with diabetes to make a healthy adjustment to the disease because

1. there are too many things he cannot do
2. too many people feel sorry for him
3. his diet is so rigid
4. he dislikes sticking himself with a needle

27. An early symptom of insulin shock the nurse must learn to recognize is

1. blurred vision
2. numbness of lips or tongue
3. nausea
4. excess perspiration

28. The patient must be taught that the beginning of insulin shock may be recognized by his feelings of

1. vomiting
2. hunger
3. anorexia
4. confusion

29. If the diabetic child is ill with a communicable disease, the mother should expect insulin shock to occur in the presence of a symptom such as

1. dyspnea
2. pruritus
3. vomiting
4. photophobia

30. If a diabetic child has frequent emotional tantrums, his insulin needs will be

1. increased
2. ineffective
3. delayed
4. decreased

31. One of the first things the nurse can do to encourage the diabetic child (age 6) to become responsible for his own care is to allow him

1. to select all his own food
2. to take his bath
3. to select and cleanse the area for insulin injection
4. to examine his own urine

32. Parents and the nurse must understand that it is hard for a diabetic child to resist eating forbidden foods when

1. everyone else does
2. his blood sugar is low
3. they are offered to him
4. his own food is not good

33. An excellent way to produce uncoopera-
    tiveness in the preschool diabetic is to
    insist that he

    1. understand the meaning of his
       disease
    2. try to keep up with other children
    3. eat many disliked foods
    4. gradually learn some responsibility
       for his specialized care

34. A mother may find it almost impossible
    to give her diabetic child the insulin
    he needs if she considers the proce-
    dure a form of

    1. sterile nursing technique
    2. discipline
    3. dull routine
    4. punishment

35. The diabetic is encouraged to walk as
    long as shoes and hose fit well and
    posture is good. Walking helps the
    diabetic because it

    a. stimulates the appetite
    b. helps burn up blood sugar
    c. improves circulation
    d. prevents invalidism

       1. c only
       2. b and c
       3. a and b
       4. all of the above

36. Decreased circulation in the feet of
    the diabetic makes it dangerous for
    the affected person

    a. to wear round garters
    b. to sit with knees crossed
    c. to wear tight shoes
    d. to wear hose that are too tight or
       too big

       1. all of the above
       2. b or c
       3. c and d
       4. d only

37. The efficiency of the thyroid gland can
    be determined by checking

    1. with a Geiger counter
    2. the amount of oxygen the body uses
       while at complete rest
    3. the amount of thyroxin in the blood
       stream before and after meals
    4. the brittleness of the bones

38. The results of a basal metabolism test
    would not give an accurate report of the
    efficiency of the thyroid gland if the

    1. patient ate her breakfast
    2. patient read a magazine
    3. patient carried on a conversation
       with her roommate
    4. nurse awakened the patient before
       the test

39. If the patient is tense and worried about
    what will happen to her during the basal
    metabolism test, it is to be expected
    that the results of the test will be

    1. unaffected
    2. higher than her normal rate
    3. lower than her normal rate
    4. dependent on the skill of the tech-
       nician

40. The thyroid gland would be considered
    hyperactive if the basal metabolism
    rate were

    1. +50
    2. unstable
    3. on the "plus" side of zero
    4. higher than a +20

41. A more accurate determination of the
    basal metabolic rate can be obtained
    from the protein-bound iodine test.
    This test is not influenced by

    a. emotions
    b. activity
    c. food
    d. medications

       1. b or c
       2. a, b, or c
       3. a only
       4. all of the above

42. The increased rate of metabolism in the
    patient with a toxic goiter will be
    responsible for the symptoms of

    a. rapid pulse
    b. apathy
    c. breathlessness
    d. bulging eye balls

       1. all of the above
       2. b only
       3. a and c
       4. b, c, and d

43. If the hyperthyroid patient does not get treatment that will lessen the symptoms, death will be due to

   1. physical exhaustion
   2. heart failure
   3. muscle fatigue
   4. toxemia

44. The hyperthyroid patient will lose weight as the result of

   a. increased perspiration
   b. increased peristalsis
   c. overactivity
   d. exaggerated emotions

      1. a and c
      2. b or c
      3. a and d
      4. all of the above

45. The hand tremor characteristic of the hyperthyroid patient will cause the patient to become irritable when she

   1. knows people are staring at her
   2. drops or spills things
   3. makes mistakes
   4. becomes unable to dress herself

46. The patient with hyperthyroidism has been hospitalized to prepare her for surgery. The nurse has the responsibility of helping the relatives to understand that

   1. the only effective treatment is surgery
   2. the personality changes are symptoms of the disease
   3. only in a hospital can the patient be made ready for surgery
   4. the patient actually needs the great amount of food she eats

47. A simple goiter is produced as the body makes an effort to compensate for

   1. the increased rate of growth during adolescence
   2. the increased thyroxin production
   3. inadequate intake of iodine
   4. a calcium imbalance

48. Hemorrhage is the most common complication of a thyroidectomy. Post-operative care must include

   1. checking the pulse every 30 minutes
   2. keeping the patient in a prone position
   3. giving the patient morphine to keep her quiet
   4. inspecting the sides and the back of dressings often

49. The nurse is assigned to set up the recovery room to receive a thyroidectomy patient. It will be most important to include

   1. the oxygen tent
   2. I.V. fluids
   3. the tracheotomy set
   4. ice bags

50. Surgery for the removal of a simple goiter would be necessary only when

   a. great pressure is placed on the esophagus
   b. an increased amount of thyroxin is produced
   c. its size interfered with the growth of the child
   d. pressure is placed on the trachea

      1. d only
      2. a, b, and d
      3. a and d
      4. all of the above

51. The increased production of thyroxin, which produces the symptoms of hyperthyroidism, is the result of

   1. hypertrophy of the gland
   2. dietary excesses
   3. hyperplasia of the gland
   4. a decrease in colloid

52. If the thyroid deficiency of the cretin is not recognized and treated soon after birth, the result will be

   a. giantism
   b. dwarfism
   c. mental deficiency
   d. bone and muscle deformity

      1. all except a
      2. b and c
      3. a and d
      4. b, c, and d

53. The decreased metabolism of the myxedema patient is responsible for sensitiveness to

1. coffee and tea
2. criticism
3. most medications
4. cold

54. Cancer of the thyroid gland is one of the few forms of malignancy in which there are no

1. typical warning symptoms
2. dangers of metastasis
3. effective methods of treatment
4. adequate diagnostic tests known

55. The practical nurse will understand that good medical and nursing care of upper respiratory infections are necessary to prevent

1. such a high death rate
2. the very rapid spread of the disease
3. serious pulmonary complications
4. the expense of antibiotics

56. Good emotional preparation of the child who must have a tonsillectomy makes the procedure safer because

1. the operation can be done faster
2. he will be less disturbed coming out of the anesthetic
3. the parents will not be so emotionally upset
4. he will sleep longer when he returns to his room

57. The warning symptom of cancer of the larynx is

1. hemorrhage
2. persistent cough with thick sputum
3. persistent hoarseness
4. increasing pain and dyspnea

58. Any patient with a respiratory disease described as chronic and progressive must be taught the importance of avoiding

1. alcoholic drinks
2. milk and eggs
3. recreation
4. upper respiratory diseases

59. A major concern in the nursing care of the acutely ill pneumonia patient is to provide for

1. improved circulation through coughing
2. stir-up exercises
3. rest
4. an increased oxygen supply

60. Efforts to discover cancer in the outer part of the lung in time to effect a cure will require

1. paying careful attention to all warning symptoms
2. an annual physical examination
3. treating every cough as if it were a warning symptom
4. a chest X-ray every 6 months

61. When the diagnosis is essential hypertension, the doctor's advice may include a combination of

a. weight reduction diet
b. limited use of coffee
c. frequent small feedings
d. rest and relaxation before meals

1. all of the above
2. c and d
3. a only
4. a, b, or d

62. The person with hypertension must be reassured that

1. he can continue his previous activities
2. the seriousness is not decided by the height of the pressure
3. complications are seldom serious
4. daily medication will cure the disease

63. Hypertension that accompanies a kidney disease is classified as

1. primary
2. secondary
3. metastatic
4. toxic

64. The presence of hypertension is frequently discovered

1. from the patient's complaints
2. by examining the arteries
3. by use of the electroencephalogram
4. in the process of a routine physical examination

65. A symptom commonly associated with excitement, accompanied by an increase in blood pressure, is

    1. anorexia
    2. dyspnea
    3. headache
    4. tympanites

66. Hypertension does not always develop in the person with an explosive personality. Increased blood pressure is also a danger in the individual with a personality that

    1. depends too much on others
    2. is too aggressive
    3. does more than his share of the work
    4. feels like blowing up but is afraid to do it

67. Hypertension is a condition in which the blood pressure remains high. A blood pressure reading that would mean hypertension is

    1. 110/72
    2. 120/55
    3. 120/140
    4. 150/100

68. The patient with a severe decrease of heart function will need to be taught the importance of

    1. exerting himself as little as possible
    2. eating a high CHO diet
    3. planning life as if he had only a short time to live
    4. exercising regularly after each meal

69. The order for "absolute rest" for the cardiac patient will include

    1. complete inactivity
    2. limited motion in bed
    3. medication to keep the patient drowsy most of the 24 hours
    4. freedom from physical activity and emotional tension

70. If the cardiac patient becomes too tired while the nurse is giving morning care, she will be wise

    1. to give the patient a sedative so that care can be completed
    2. to do partial care and finish when the patient is rested
    3. to omit all care until the following day
    4. to limit visitors the rest of the day

71. "Absolute rest" will be difficult to obtain if the nurse permits

    1. medications to be spaced at 2-hour intervals
    2. the patient to be placed in a 2-bed room
    3. the relatives to stand outside the room door and talk in whispers
    4. the patient to arouse from sedation

72. In the presence of arteriosclerosis, the heart may enlarge and continue to function efficiently within the framework of moderation. The heart action is described as

    1. compensation
    2. decompensation
    3. hyperplasia
    4. infarction

73. The patient with a heart attack will be fearful. This emotion will be increased by

    1. inactivity
    2. boredom
    3. an attitude of panic on the part of the nurse
    4. telling the patient he has nothing to be afraid of and that everything will be O.K.

74. The cardiac patient must not become constipated because

    1. death may result from the accumulation of toxic substances
    2. special medications will be habit forming
    3. straining at the stool will increase the work of the heart
    4. heart stimulants cannot be so effective as planned

75. When the cardiac patient is allowed only limited fluid intake, the nurse can keep the patient most comfortable by

    1. removing the water pitcher from the room
    2. giving him an injection of atropine
    3. providing for fluids to be given throughout the 24 hours
    4. eliminating all between-meal fluids

76. The cardiac patient with severe dyspnea is usually most comfortable

   1. lying on his side with his heat flat
   2. lying prone with the head of the bed elevated
   3. dorsal recumbent with a pillow under his head
   4. sitting up, resting his arms and head on the over-the-bed table

77. Following a heart attack, the patient will be placed on "complete bed rest" to enable collateral circulation to develop effectively. The nurse understands that such an order means

   1. she must do everything for the patient
   2. it is all right to permit bathroom privileges
   3. his family must not be allowed to upset him
   4. heavy doses of morphine will be necessary

78. The major change the angina pectoris patient must make in his daily activities is

   1. to lose weight
   2. to increase his daily exercise
   3. to slow down
   4. to stay on a salt-free diet

79. The nurse must appreciate that the ordered rest for the patient with a coronary thrombosis is to help establish collateral circulation. Unless the nurse knows the value of such rest, she may be tempted

   1. to permit visitors to stay too long
   2. to give too much nursing care
   3. to feel it is necessary to keep up his spirits by keeping him busy with a passive sport such as chess
   4. to encourage the patient to do things for himself because he says he feels fine

80. The patient with Buerger's disease can always expect the doctor to insist that he discontinue the use of

   1. alcohol
   2. hot water bottles
   3. tobacco
   4. bandages

81. Symptoms of Raynaud's disease are spasmodic and not continuous because

   1. medication temporarily reduces them
   2. the blood vessels are affected by the position of the patient
   3. circulation decreases as the day advances
   4. they are affected by external temperatures

82. The subjective symptom that is most distressing to the patient with Buerger's disease is

   1. vertigo
   2. tingling and numbness
   3. muscle aching
   4. severe pain

83. Nicotine increases the symptoms of Buerger's disease because it

   1. increases the spasms of the muscles of the blood-vessel walls
   2. poisons the whole system
   3. slows up the circulation to a point of danger
   4. interferes with the amount of oxygen the red blood cells carry

84. The person with varicose veins will wear elastic stockings or bandages for the purpose of

   1. increasing the efficiency of the valves in the veins
   2. relieving pressure and lessening the pain
   3. slowing down the flow of venous blood
   4. stimulating and speeding up circulation

85. The patient with varicose veins should be instructed to apply elastic bandages when

   1. standing   3. lying down
   2. sitting   4. in motion

86. Whether treatment of varicose veins is medical or surgical, the result of the treatment is

   1. stimulation of the affected veins
   2. destruction of the affected veins
   3. dilatation of the affected veins
   4. seldom satisfactory

87. Following the removal of varicose veins, the patient must be impressed with the dangers of

   a. using circular garters
   b. injuring the leg
   c. prolonged standing
   d. sitting with the legs crossed

      1. all of the above
      2. a and d
      3. b only
      4. a and b

88. A blood clot may form on the wall of an infected vein. Such a clot would be especially dangerous as an embolus because

   1. it always results in sudden death
   2. it increases in size as it travels
   3. a secondary infection is set up where it stops
   4. the symptoms are so mild that the patient refuses to follow the doctor's orders

89. The nurse is instructed never to massage the cramping legs of a surgical patient without specific medical orders. Such massage could be dangerous because

   1. spasms in the veins are increased
   2. a thrombus may become an embolus
   3. pain spreads upward and downward
   4. administration of narcotics is necessary to relieve the pain caused by the increased circulation

90. Symptoms suspicious of thrombophlebitis should be called to the doctor's attention immediately. Such symptoms would include

   1. increased blood pressure and headache
   2. dyspnea and dizziness
   3. redness and tenderness along a vein
   4. large, irregular bumps or knots along the course of a vein

91. The prognosis in pernicious anemia is good as long as the patient appreciates the need for

   1. continuing his medicine
   2. weekly blood counts
   3. periodic care in the hospital
   4. the services of a specialist

92. Thrombophlebitis can probably be prevented as a postoperative complication if the nurse will encourage the patient

   1. to keep his knees elevated
   2. to keep pillows under both knees for support
   3. to move about in bed
   4. to take deep breaths

93. Further attacks of Raynaud's disease may be prevented if the patient is careful

   1. to control situations leading to emotional stress
   2. to plan all activities to avoid fatigue
   3. to apply continuous ice packs faithfully
   4. to concentrate on a rigid, high-protein, high-vitamin diet ·

94. The prognosis of other types of anemia will depend on

   1. treatment with the right kind of medicine
   2. finding and correcting the cause
   3. skilled nursing care
   4. the patient's ability to stay on his diet

95. If the greatest degree of rehabilitation is to be obtained for the pernicious anemia patient, teaching must stress the need for

   1. retirement and complete rest
   2. continued liver-extract therapy
   3. emotional calm
   4. life in a warm climate

96. Recreational therapy for the anemic patient should be aimed at

   1. lessening feelings of depression
   2. stimulating the appetite
   3. developing a hobby at home
   4. improving the general metabolism

97. The most satisfactory type of mouth care for the anemic patient would be

   1. vigorous massage with a stiff brush
   2. use of a strong mouthwash
   3. gentle cleansing with cotton swabs
   4. usual mouth care with a toothbrush

98. The decreased efficiency of the circulation makes the anemia patient
very susceptible to

1. pneumonia   3. pressure sores
2. black outs   4. drafts

99. Because the nourishment supply to
the nerves is decreased, the nurse
can expect the anemic patient to be

1. helpless   3. in great pain
2. complaining 4. irritable

100. Because the nurse recognizes the
problems of circulation in the
anemic patient, she will be very
careful in her application of

1. external medications
2. heat
3. hematinics
4. cold compresses

101. The anemic condition of the leukemia patient causes symptoms
of

1. anorexia
2. dyspnea and fatigue
3. depression
4. diarrhea and constipation

102. The average leukemia patient often
causes a problem for the community
because

1. he cannot be taken care of in
many hospitals
2. he needs help with his family
responsibilities
3. the cost of medications is too
high to be covered by insurance
4. he lives so long and requires so
much care

103. The palliative nursing care of the
patient with leukemia is aimed at

1. keeping the patient alive as
long as possible
2. treating the symptoms to keep the
patient comfortable
3. providing sufficient recreational
therapy
4. keeping up an adequate nutritional
level

104. An important nursing responsibility
in the care of the patient with leukemia
is

1. force feeding an adequate diet
2. to give medication even if the
patient must be awakened
3. gentle and frequent mouth care
4. to check the pulse often

105. Death in leukemia is often the result
of

1. hemorrhage or intercurrent
infection
2. exhaustion
3. malnutrition
4. loss of the will to live

106. The prognosis in leukemia is discouraging because

1. the patient cannot remain on the
severe treatment
2. the family interferes with the
necessary discipline
3. treatment is available in only a
few medical centers
4. the cause of the disease is not
known

107. Usually the first symptom of Hodgkin's
disease is

1. painless swelling of the lymph
nodes of the neck
2. pallor due to anemia
3. sore, red, "beefy" tongue
4. painful swelling of the spleen

108. The kind of symptoms that give the
patient with Hodgkin's disease the
most trouble will depend on

1. the stage of the disease
2. his reaction to treatment
3. the form of radiation used
4. which glands are swollen

109. X-ray treatments in Hodgkin's disease
are intended

1. to cure the condition
2. to relive pressure symptoms for
a while
3. to give the patient hope
4. to give the patient a mental boost

MEDICAL AND SURGICAL DISEASES AND NURSING

110. One of the hardest things about caring for a young man with Hodgkin's disease is

   1. trying to overcome his feelings of hopelessness
   2. trying to limit visitors
   3. overcoming a desire to spoil him
   4. overcoming your own feelings of disgust at the sight of him

111. The first attack of rheumatic fever can best be avoided by

   1. giving the child oral penicillin every day
   2. staying out of all crowded places
   3. keeping the child away from persons with upper respiratory infections
   4. keeping the child home from school during the winter

112. Parents often fail to recognize early symptoms of rheumatic fever. Such failure is based on the false belief that

   1. the child should not miss school
   2. growing pains are normal between 5 and 10 years of age
   3. the child really does not feel too sick
   4. treatment of the disease is too severe

113. The joint pains characteristic of rheumatic fever are located in

   1. all the weight-bearing joints
   2. first one joint and then another
   3. the elbows first
   4. the fingers and toes

114. During the acute stage of rheumatic fever a daily sponge bath is essential because

   1. it will stimulate circulation
   2. there is a sour odor to the perspiration
   3. the heat relieves the joint pains
   4. health habits must not be discontinued

115. The child hospitalized with rheumatic fever can be expected to show regression in the form of

   1. apathy
   2. aggression
   3. refusing medications
   4. thumb sucking

116. The hospital that specializes in the care of rheumatic fever will be the best place for the child during

   1. the acute stage
   2. the subacute stage
   3. the convalescent stage
   4. the chronic stage

117. Rheumatic fever affects the nervous system. Parents should be taught to be more patient with the symptom of

   1. repeated convulsions
   2. bed wetting
   3. blurred vision
   4. emotional irritability

118. The patient and his family must understand that once the attack of rheumatic fever has subsided, the great stress will be on the need for

   1. a hot climate
   2. frequent medical check-ups
   3. a complete, high-caloric diet to offset the fever
   4. always being a spectator in any sport or game

119. Rheumatic fever is different from most communicable diseases of childhood because

   1. an immunity to streptococcus infections is produced
   2. the child becomes more susceptible to further attacks of the disease
   3. positive diagnosis cannot be made until complications begin
   4. the variety of causative organisms changes the symptom pattern

120. Parents are encouraged to prevent rheumatic fever in their children. One method of doing this is

   1. to keep the child out of all crowds during the winter
   2. to insist on hospitalization whenever the child has an upper respiratory infection
   3. to get medical advice for upper respiratory symptoms
   4. to keep each child in a single room

121. The child who has recovered from rheumatic fever must be taught the importance of bed rest at the first sign of an infection. This is done to prevent

    1. recurrence of the deformity
    2. increased resistance to other contagious diseases
    3. valvular hypertrophy
    4. progressive damage to the heart

122. During the <u>acute</u> stage of rheumatic fever the child's interest in his surroundings should be <u>limited</u> to an activity such as

    1. television programs of football, wrestling, etc.
    2. watching a bowl of goldfish
    3. cutting out paper dolls
    4. a radio story of the Lone Ranger

123. The rheumatic fever patient convalescing at home might feel more like a <u>useful member</u> of the family if he is assigned the task of

    1. running the vacuum cleaner
    2. dusting
    3. folding tea towels
    4. pulling weeds

124. The school teacher will need to make special plans for the child with heart damage due to rheumatic fever. During recess play activities the teacher could safely assign the child the task of

    1. playing baseball
    2. watching baseball as a spectator
    3. scorekeeper
    4. umpire

125. Bacterial endocarditis, a complication of rheumatic fever, can be dangerous because

    1. emboli containing bacteria may spread throughout the body
    2. the resistance of the lining membrane of the heart is low
    3. heart murmurs result from the inflammation of the valves
    4. we do not know how to treat and cure it

126. When an inflamed eye is sensitive to light, the symptom is known as

    1. photophobia   3. mystagmus
    2. strabismus   4. vertigo

127. The rheumatic fever patient should be protected from bacterial endocarditis because

    1. the symptoms last so long
    2. it is too often fatal
    3. any heart damage produced will be permanent
    4. all activities will be restricted even during convalescence

128. Diplopia is defined as

    1. extreme thirst
    2. spots before the eyes
    3. farsightedness
    4. double vision

129. Because of the intraocular pressure in glaucoma, a patient with this condition would be advised

    1. to wear dark glasses in the sun
    2. to avoid worry, fear, anger, and excitement
    3. to eat foods high in vitamin A
    4. to use Murine eye drops several times a day

130. Every person over 40 should be encouraged to have an annual check-up for symptoms of glaucoma by

    1. a specialist
    2. an optometrist
    3. an ophthalmologist
    4. an otolaryngologist

131. "Pink eye" is one form of

    1. iritis   3. conjunctivitis
    2. trachoma   4. cataract

132. Cataracts may be the result of

    a. acquired infection
    b. injury at time of birth
    c. nutritional deficiency
    d. degeneration

        1. d only
        2. a and b
        3. c and d
        4. all of the above

133. All aspects of postoperative care following cataract surgery are aimed at preventing

1. excitement or worry
2. any increase of intraocular pressure
3. detaching the retina
4. a corneal infection

134. A person recently blinded is often made an invalid when cared for at home because

1. he is overprotected
2. the darkness frightens him
3. he enjoys the attention
4. the home is not arranged to be safe for the blind

135. All sighted members of the family of a blind person who lives at home must be alert to the need

1. for a simple daily routine
2. for keeping up a steady flow of conversation to keep the patient's mind active
3. for leaving furniture in the same place
4. for using their voices to guide the patient

136. If the nurse can put herself in the place of the person who cannot see, she will never fail

1. to keep the patient informed of what is going to happen to him
2. to understand why he is so fearful
3. to tell him what is on his tray and where it is placed
4. to get his attention before she starts to talk

137. The nurse will increase the security of the hospital patient who cannot see if she will remember to

1. introduce herself each time she speaks to the patient
2. arrange his food for his convenience
3. keep the call bell where the patient can get it
4. bring visitors into the room quietly

138. When the nurse hears a hissing sound with each inspiration, she knows the tracheotomy patient

1. is breathing normally
2. is practicing speech exercises
3. is trying to get her attention
4. needs the suction used at once

139. The adult tracheotomy patient should be provided with

1. recreational materials
2. pencil and paper
3. special nurses
4. a high-vitamin, high-protein diet

140. The safest way to attempt the removal of a foreign object of vegetable origin from the external auditory canal is to shrink it with

1. soda bicarbonate solution
2. boric acid solution
3. sweet oil
4. alcohol

141. A large per cent of the deafness in adults can be traced to

1. inadequate high school vocational guidance
2. failure to take enough cod liver oil
3. failure to do periodic urinalysis
4. inadequate care during childhood diseases

142. The reason many people cannot get maximum return of hearing ability either by surgery or a hearing aid is

1. the personality block to adequate treatment
2. failure to recognize any decrease in hearing until almost 75% is lost
3. the result of inadequate testing equipment
4. the type of nerve damage that has been done

143. You would suspect that an infant had an earache when his behavior included

1. running an elevated temperature
2. having a convulsion
3. rolling the head from side to side
4. refusing to eat, vomiting

144. Deafness may be produced by a chronic middle-ear infection. Hearing loss results from

1. perforation of the inner eardrum
2. adhesions that limit movement of the ossicles
3. interference with the vibration of the perilymph
4. damage to the auditory nerve

145. If a cotton plug is packed so tightly in the external auditory canal that drainage from the middle ear is prevented, the complication resulting will be

1. extension of the infection to the Eustachian tube
2. perforated round window
3. stabilization of the stirrup
4. mastoiditis

146. Pus in the middle ear is best drained by a myringotomy. The advantage of this procedure is

1. the ability to schedule the drainage at the patient's convenience
2. the opportunity to remove all the pus quickly
3. healing with minimal scar tissue
4. prevention of all known complications

147. Surgery to restore hearing may be as simple as

1. a mastoidectomy
2. a tympanotomy
3. a D. and C. of the Eustachian tubes
4. an adenoidectomy

148. The seriousness of the prognosis, when symptoms indicate some involvement of the facial nerve following a mastoidectomy, depends on whether these symptoms are observed

1. immediately after surgery or hours later
2. during the surgery and treatment begun stat
3. before the patient leaves the unit
4. before or after the first change of packing

149. Immediately after cleft-lip repair it will not be safe to place the baby

1. in a supine position
2. on its abdomen
3. in a dorsal recumbent position
4. in a Fowler's position

150. The patient can be helped to relax during a gynecological examination if the nurse will tell and show her how

1. to hold her breath
2. to put her feet into the examining-table stirrups
3. to breathe through her mouth
4. to keep covered with the gown and sheet

151. Immediate rinsing in cold water of the rubber gloves worn during a vaginal examination will

1. kill only venereal disease germs
2. prepare them for use on the next patient
3. get them ready for boiling later
4. remove the protein material of body secretions

152. The patient will be more comfortable and the doctor will be better able to do a pelvic examination, if the nurse has prepared the patient for examination by encouraging her

1. to rest
2. to empty the bladder
3. to tell the doctor all her symptoms
4. to answer only the questions the doctor asks

153. Spotting of blood between menstrual periods should be viewed with alarm as a possible warning sign of

1. menopause
2. gonorrhea
3. carcinoma
4. menorrhagia

154. Dysmenorrhea is more often a problem in the adolescent girl who

1. begins menstruating early
2. has been poorly prepared for this event
3. does not start her menstrual cycle until 16
4. is not athletic

155. Cervicitis may be a predisposing cause of cancer of the cervix, since

    1. inflamed tissue is readily infected
    2. the leukorrhea acts as a constant irritant
    3. scar tissue takes the place of normal tissue
    4. it is always due to tears produced during childbirth

156. An early symptom, and often the only warning symptom of cancer of the cervix, is

    1. menorrhagia   3. leukorrhea
    2. metrorrhagia   4. vaginitis

MRS. X HAS JUST HAD SIX RADIUM NEEDLES INSERTED INTO A CANCER ON HER CERVIX.

THE NEXT FOUR QUESTIONS TEST THE STUDENT'S KNOWLEDGE OF THE NURSING CARE AND RESPONSIBILITIES FOR SUCH A PATIENT:

157. An indwelling catheter was inserted into the bladder in the operating room. The chief reason for this catheter is

    1. to prevent any contamination of the gauze packed in the vagina
    2. to prevent a distended bladder getting in the way of the radium rays
    3. to prevent cystitis from frequent catheterizations
    4. to keep the bladder collapsed and the patient comfortable

158. The nurse will be responsible for seeing that the radium is not lost while the patient is in the ward unit. She will do this by

    1. keeping all soiled linen in a special hamper until the radium is removed and accounted for
    2. staying with the patient at all times until the radium is removed
    3. keeping the patient in one position until the radium is removed
    4. allowing nothing to be taken from the room until the radium has been returned to the safe

159. Since the treatment might be stopped if the doctor knew the patient had symptoms of radiation sickness, it is important for the nurse to recognize the early symptoms as

    1. vaginal hemorrhage
    2. itching of the vulva
    3. burning on the perineum
    4. elevated temperature, nausea, and vomiting

160. The safety of the patient requires the nurse to assume responsibility for notifying the surgeon when the ordered time for removal of the needles is approaching. The nurse is aware that

    1. the doctor will get busy and forget
    2. overdosage may result in a burn
    3. the treatment is too expensive for the patient to be charged overtime
    4. the patient is anxious to move about more freely

161. Chronic cervicitis is most often due to infection that follows

    1. exposure to the gonococcus
    2. routine daily douching
    3. pelvic surgery
    4. cervical tears during childbirth

162. A woman of 40 expresses her fears of the approaching menopausal period. The informed nurse can reassure her by advising

    1. "People won't expect you to do anything when you reach that age"
    2. "You won't have any trouble if you limit your physical and social activities"
    3. "A long period of bed rest will prevent any serious physical symptoms"
    4. "It is a natural physiological process which bothers only a few women"

163. Gonorrhea is so often the cause of sterility because the inflammation

    1. dilates the hymen
    2. prevents ovulation
    3. obstructs Bartholin's glands
    4. blocks the Fallopian tubes

164. Johnny's mother apologizes to the nurse for being so critical of her son's care. "I'm just not myself. I have the most distressing vaginal discharge that has me worried." The nurse would be correct to suggest

1. "Most women have a vaginal discharge sometimes"
2. "All vaginal secretions are normal"
3. "Most discharges are annoying but harmless. You should let your doctor find the cause"
4. "When you get home, try a strong antiseptic solution daily as a douche"

165. Many of the emotional problems upsetting patients hospitalized for surgery of the female reproductive organs have their foundation in

1. superstitions and misinformation
2. the knowledge that menopause will occur earlier
3. the seriousness of the disease requiring such surgery
4. unreasonable modesty

166. The nurse has a friend, age 60, who complains of occasional vaginal bleeding. The nurse will be most concerned with impressing on her friend the need to determine

1. the time the bleeding occurs
2. the amount of the bleeding
3. the reason for the bleeding
4. her red blood count and hemoglobin level

167. Elaborate sterilization of linens and equipment used by the gonorrheal patient is not necessary because

1. after the third month she is not infectious
2. the germs do not live long outside the human body
3. the discharge is usually confined to a pad or a dressing
4. all gonorrheal patients are taken care of in the same ward unit

168. The nurse can adequately protect herself from infection with gonorrhea from the patient with genital discharge by

1. soaking her hands in Lysol solution
2. wearing a gown and a mask
3. carrying out full isolation technique
4. washing her hands thoroughly

169. In an institution in which a group of young patients is being cared for nursing personnel could be responsible for an epidemic of gonorrhea by

1. placing two patients in one crib
2. failing to isolate suspected cases
3. using contaminated rectal thermometers
4. failing to use prophylactic eye drops

170. Gonorrhea and syphilis are both

1. the same disease
2. different stages of the same disease
3. highly contagious
4. more common in men

171. The only positive way to avoid infection with syphilis is

1. to keep the blood stream full of long-acting penicillin
2. to avoid exposure to the infection
3. to enter a monastery
4. to maintain an optimum level of health

172. It is more difficult to make an early diagnosis of syphilis in women than in men because

1. women refuse to seek medical advice
2. the chancre is less painful in the women
3. the chancre is hidden in the vagina
4. the symptoms are milder

173. Inadequate treatment of syphilis is as dangerous to the person affected as no treatment at all because

1. it will lead to insanity
2. he will infect his whole family
3. he will soon be unable to work
4. in time, complications will disable him

174. The best way to kill the germs causing gonorrhea is to use

1. adequate soap, water, and a brush
2. a 5% Lysol solution
3. a strong Listerine solution
4. boiling water

175. Nursing service personnel are most likely to get a gonorrheal infection from patients through

1. sexual intercourse
2. discharges getting in the eyes
3. soiled surgical instruments
4. food contamination

176. The most distressing symptoms of early gonorrhea are

1. abdominal pains
2. itching and burning on urination
3. the open sores
4. fever, headache, and nausea

177. Gonorrhea is not like many infectious diseases because

1. aseptic precautions are not necessary
2. there is no immunity after one attack
3. more men are affected than women
4. there is no specific treatment

178. Syphilis is becoming an increasing community problem because of the greater number infected

1. in the female sex
2. in the teen-age group
3. in the wage-earning class
4. who are filling our mental institutions

179. The most dangerous and infectious stage of syphilis is

1. the incubation period
2. the chancre stage
3. the rash stage
4. the latent period

180. The most distressing symptoms of cystitis are

1. the frequency and urgency of urination
2. severe abdominal cramping
3. high blood pressure and headache
4. retention of urine and distention of the bladder

181. The toxins of the hemolytic streptococcus are responsible for the kidney damage that produces

1. pyelitis   3. nephritis
2. cystitis   4. nephrosis

182. Bacteria are not present in the urine of the patient with nephritis. This means that the symptoms are produced as a result of

1. obstruction due to stones
2. action of the leukocytes against the infection
3. inflammation
4. ureteral peristalsis

183. Regardless of the amount of kidney damage, by the time the diagnosis of chronic nephritis has been made the disease will be correctly classified as

1. chronic and progressive
2. terminal
3. acute and fulminating
4. metastatic

184. A common upper respiratory infection which may precede the onset of acute nephritis is

1. pleurisy   3. bronchiectasis
2. bronchitis   4. pharyngitis

185. A common symptom of bladder tumors is

1. nocturia   3. hematuria
2. dysuria   4. oliguria

186. Health teaching of the patient with nephritis must include stress on the importance of preventing future attacks by

1. prophylactic doses of penicillin
2. prevention or prompt treatment of upper respiratory infections
3. a high-protein, high-vitamin diet
4. limited activity and a change of climate

187. The negligent nurse may be responsible for the production of kidney stones in the chronically ill patient following care that permits

a. an inadequate fluid intake
b. a diet high in CHO
c. an emotional outlook in the patient
d. a prolonged supine position

    1. all of the above
    2. a, b, and c
    3. a and d only
    4. c and d

188. A diagnosis of kidney stones or suspected kidney stones will require the nurse to strain all urine through a sieve and fine gauze to make it possible

1. to determine when all stones have been passed
2. to reassure the patient that surgery will not be necessary
3. to plan the necessary nursing care
4. to recover stones no larger than grains of sand

189. Any disease of the urinary system that makes it necessary to restrict fluid intake will require the nurse to provide frequent mouth care in an effort to help

1. ease the pain of fever sores
2. lower the body temperature
3. make the restricted intake easier to accept
4. prevent serious dehydration

190. An early symptom of prostatic hypertrophy which is commonly ignored in the man over 40 is

1. hematuria   3. anuria
2. dysuria   4. nocturia

191. The immediate postoperative care of the prostatectomy patient which will detect complications early will include

1. sedatives to keep the patient from getting out of bed
2. frequent check of pulse and blood pressure
3. attachment of the catheter to the suction bottle
4. nasal oxygen

192. The nursing care following a perineal prostatectomy requires special caution to prevent

1. rupture of the incision
2. drainage of urine through the incision
3. contamination of the incision
4. retention of urine

193. When the prostatectomy has been done through a perineal incision, it will not be safe for the nurse

1. to get the patient up in a chair without help
2. to take a rectal temperature
3. to insist the patient force fluids
4. to leave the patient alone

194. Circumcision would be an emergency operation in an older male child or adult if

1. a tight foreskin produced pain
2. the foreskin became tight enough to interfere with circulation and voiding
3. an inflammation caused the penis to swell
4. an accumulation of sebaceous secretions was a predisposing cause of cancer

195. The incidence of cancer of the breast is higher in women during the

1. child-bearing period
2. menstrual period
3. geriatric period
4. menopausal period

196. Metastasis of breast cancer is more frequent and rapid by way of the

1. bone   3. pectoral muscle
2. lymphatic system 4. veins

197. The most frequent location for breast cancer is in

1. the breast
2. the upper outer quadrant
3. the inner upper quadrant
4. the apex

198. The dimpling of the skin over the breast cancer is described as

1. orange peel in appearance
2. exanthema
3. hyperemia
4. hyperplasia

199. Symptoms of breast cancer that are referred to the nipple include

a. mastitis
b. bleeding
c. retraction
d. sharp, boring pain

    1. all of the above
    2. all but d
    3. b only
    4. b or c

200. The rate of cure for cancer of the breast is higher when the cancer is diagnosed and treated while

1. the general health will stand the shock
2. treatment for menopausal symptoms is in progress
3. the cancer is localized in the breast
4. the woman is still in the age group 40 to 50

201. A positive diagnosis of cancer in the breast requires examination of

1. all the female reproductive organs
2. the tumor cells through biopsy
3. the chest wall by X-ray
4. the breast tissue with cell dyes

202. The prompt removal of benign tumors of the breast is recommended in order

1. to prevent cell change to cancer
2. to relieve the patient's fears
3. to make the patient cancer conscious
4. to remove all causes of breast cancer

203. If breast cancer cannot be removed by surgery, its growth may be controlled by use of

1. antibiotics   3. radium
2. physiotherapy 4. chemotherapy

204. In an effort to kill any cancer cells in the breast that may not be removed by surgery, the doctor may prescribe

1. Mustargen
2. X-ray before and after surgery
3. heat treatments postoperatively
4. wound irrigation with chlorine solution

205. If metastasis of breast cancer is suspected, the doctor will be sure to remove

1. the axillary lymph nodes
2. the uterus
3. the other breast
4. the breast bone on the affected side

206. Following a radical mastectomy, the nurse would check for hemorrhage by examining

1. the pulse
2. skin color and texture
3. suture line
4. dressings under the axilla

207. Postoperative lymphedema is often prevented by

1. hyperextending the affected area
2. supporting the affected area on a pillow
3. keeping the patient on the affected side
4. a high Fowler's position

208. Most physicians prescribe exercise of the affected area the day after surgery. Such exercise would be described as

1. active   3. resistive
2. passive   4. individual

209. Contracture will be the result if the patient with a mastectomy is not encouraged to practice exercises that will

    1. maintain the function of the ball and socket joints
    2. daily increase her ability to raise the arm above the head
    3. keep her responsible for self-care
    4. increase the muscle strength

210. One of the best ways to help a patient accept the scheduled mastectomy is

    1. to give her complete information about the surgery to be done
    2. to give her a clear picture of the distress ahead of her if surgery is not done
    3. to prepare her husband for the results
    4. to have a successfully operated patient visit her

211. Monthly examination of the breast, done correctly, will enable the woman to feel the presence of a lump when

    1. it has only been growing for 2 months
    2. the breasts enlarge at her menstrual period
    3. it reaches the size of a golf ball
    4. visual examination is done

212. Breast self-examination includes the techniques of

    a. auscultation
    b. inspection
    c. palpation
    d. percussion

        1. all of the above
        2. b only
        3. b and c
        4. b and d

213. Successful removal of a breast cancer that results in a cure will depend on

    a. early diagnosis
    b. emotional outlook
    c. the degree of immunity built up
    d. adequate treatment

        1. b or d
        2. d only
        3. a and d
        4. a only

214. Cancer of the breast is more serious if it develops during pregnancy or lactation because it will

    1. grow and metastasize more rapidly
    2. be passed on to the fetus
    3. be malignant
    4. interfere with the development of the fetus

215. If the patient with a breast cancer, either before or after surgical removal, complains of back pain, metastasis is suspected to

    1. the kidney   3. the pelvic bones
    2. the vertebrae   4. the ribs

216. The recommended time for monthly examination of the breast in the premenopausal woman is

    1. just before the menstrual period
    2. on a set date each month
    3. just after the menstrual period
    4. every other month

217. Fear of breast cancer is aided because information stresses

    1. the number who die rather than the number saved
    2. the hereditary aspects of this type of cancer
    3. the danger of all lumps in the breast
    4. difficulties in emotional adjustments before and after surgery

218. The emotion most often noticed in the postoperative mastectomy patient is that of

    1. irritability   3. rejection
    2. panic   4. depression

219. No patient should go to surgery for biopsy of a breast tumor without understanding that

    1. a cancer is suspected
    2. mutilating surgery will be done only as a last hope
    3. breast removal will be done if cancer cells are present
    4. the postoperative period will be a most uncomfortable one

220. As a first aid measure, the pain of a severe burn can be lessened just by

1. covering to prevent exposure of the nerve endings to air
2. leaving it alone
3. covering it with sterile cotton
4. tea-soaked packs

221. A large or a deep burn should never be covered with a grease such as lard or butter because

1. evaporation is prevented
2. the absorption of fat interferes with healing
3. it prevents the formation of a crust
4. it is difficult and painful to remove

222. Clothing that has burned onto the skin should not be removed by a first aider because

1. the epidermis will be killed
2. this forms a sterile dressing
3. too much plasma will be lost
4. the needed antiseptic solution must be prescribed

223. A burn is most serious when it

1. is deep
2. crusts over
3. covers a large skin area
4. is caused by a match

224. Shock may complicate a severe burn that covers a large body area because of the loss of

1. blood   3. sweat glands
2. skin   4. plasma

225. Hospitalization is recommended for any burn patient if the area involved covers

1. 1% of the skin surface
2. 5% of the skin surface
3. 10% of the skin surface
4. part of an extremity

226. The badly burned patient will not lose so much body fluid if the doctor applies

1. a pressure dressing
2. moist heat
3. cold applications
4. potassium permanganate

227. The severely burned patient can be cared for with the least amount of pain and discomfort if he is placed on

1. sterile sheets
2. a rubber mattress
3. a Gatch bed
4. a Stryker frame

228. It would be important to check the blood pressure of a severely burned patient every hour for

1. 24 hours   3. 7 days
2. 48 hours   4. 2 weeks

229. The severely burned patient is in great danger of infection in the burned tissues from

1. contamination
2. environmental dusts
3. the staphylococci
4. upper respiratory discharges of the doctor and nurses

230. A record of urinary output would be important in the care of the burned patient because loss of body fluid through the burn would normally result in

1. polyuria   3. oliguria
2. anuria   4. glycosuria

231. If the burned patient is in shock for several hours, the decreased blood pressure would cause

1. anuria   3. pyuria
2. albuminuria   4. polyuria

232. The nurse should recognize that the patient's emotional reaction to the burn is based on the fact that

1. his job is insecure
2. the burn is the result of an accident
3. lengthy hospitalization is expensive
4. he fears deformity

233. Extensive burns on the face and the neck should be avoided if this is possible because

1. burns in these areas will be fatal
2. skin grafting cannot be done here
3. scars will be disfiguring
4. brain damage results from toxins absorbed

234. Skin from a healthy person may be used as a graft for a burned area because it

1. stimulates the tissue cells to reproduce skin cells
2. acts as a protective dressing to lessen serum and protein loss
3. contains antibodies that protect the patient
4. protects against infection

235. I.V. fluids given shortly after a severe burn must attempt to replace

1. plasma proteins   3. salts
2. blood sugar   4. tissue fluid

236. Deformity following a massive burn will usually consist of

a. psychosis
b. scar tissue
c. asthenia
d. contracture

     1. any of the above
     2. a and d
     3. b only
     4. b or d

237. Death shortly after a severe burn is usually the result of

1. exposure   3. hemorrhage
2. shock   4. infection

238. Research has shown that most migraine or "sick" headaches are the result of

1. cancer   3. neuroses
2. mental illness   4. emotional strain

239. The patient with a migraine headache will most often complain of a pain that is

1. spasmodic and intense
2. one-sided and throbbing
3. general and stabbing
4. constant and increased by postural changes

240. The headache of the migraine patient is an expression of the mental mechanism known as

1. projection   3. conversion
2. compensation   4. regression

241. It is often difficult for the informed migraine patient to pin point the cause of any particular headache because

1. it is the end result of several emotional pressures
2. any looking back into past experiences is too painful
3. there is amnesia for the attack
4. thinking ability is affected

242. Do-it-yourself treatment of headaches that occur frequently can be dangerous because

1. the frequency of the pain will result in overdose of medicine
2. the headache may be a symptom of a serious condition
3. the symptoms will become latent
4. this involves practicing medicine without a license

243. The prodromal symptom of a typical migraine syndrome is

1. nausea
2. numbness
3. thick tongue
4. visual disturbance

244. Several of the nervous-system diseases are characterized by diplopia, which means

1. spots before the eyes
2. double vision
3. dizziness
4. disturbances in gait

245. A neighbor's child has had a convulsion. This is the first one he has ever had. The practical nurse must know enough about epilepsy and convulsions to reassure the parents that

1. medications can control future convulsions
2. epilepsy is not the only cause
3. the convulsions will disappear at puberty
4. the public understands and accepts convulsions

246. The epileptic patient requiring the most careful nursing care is the one who has

1. grand mal seizures
2. petit mal seizures
3. Jacksonian seizures
4. status epilepticus

247. The practical nurse must know the progress of a grand mal seizure to safeguard the patient. The mouth wedge must be placed between the teeth

1. before the aura
2. before the tonic stage begins
3. during the tonic stage
4. during the clonic stage

248. A symptom that cannot be controlled, yet one that the epileptic will find most embarrassing as he regains consciousness following a convulsion, is

1. disorientation   3. a sore tongue
2. confusion   4. incontinence

249. An epileptic employee has just had a grand mal convulsion. He is not trying to get out of his assignments when he complains of

1. feeling irritable
2. mental confusion
3. nausea and vomiting
4. headache and sleepiness

250. The nurse suspects the patient's convulsion is on a hysterical basis. One of the quickest ways to check the patient's level of consciousness is to test for the presence or absence of

1. incontinence
2. the corneal reflex
3. the toe reflex
4. a knee jerk

251. The cry the epileptic gives as he falls in a grand mal convulsion is the result of

1. extreme fear of the convulsion
2. forceful contraction of the respiratory muscles
3. the aura
4. extreme muscle pain preceding the convulsion

252. The immediate nursing care of the patient who is just beginning a grand mal convulsion includes

a. placing him flat on the floor
b. protecting the tongue with a mouth wedge
c. controlling the muscle twitchings
d. protecting him from environmental dangers

1. b and d
2. a and b
3. b, c, and d
4. all of the above

253. Before the nurse assigns any job to an epileptic patient, it is essential that she consider all the possibilities of

1. overexcitement
2. his physical and mental ability
3. upsetting the medication routine
4. danger to the patient and others in the environment

254. Part of the teaching responsibility of the nurse caring for epileptic patients is stressing that the number of seizures will be increased as the result of

1. overeating   3. excesses
2. overactivity 4. excitement

255. The nurse on night duty will need to watch epileptic patients very closely as she makes her rounds during the night because during a seizure

1. the patient will wet the bed
2. the patient can bite his tongue severely
3. it is possible for the patient to smother in his pillow
4. the patient can become confused and get out of bed

256. Nurses who are regularly assigned to work with epileptic patients should be prepared to care for the convulsing ones. This would include keeping readily available

1. some anticonvulsant medication
2. a metal airway
3. a first aid kit
4. a padded mouth wedge

257. Messages that put the skeletal muscles of the nurse in action when she sees a patient fall in a grand mal seizure are carried by

1. the motor nerves
2. the sensory nerves
3. the cranial nerves
4. the peripheral nerves

258. The bedfast stroke patient will have poor circulation. To keep the skin from breaking down, the nurse must

1. force fluids
2. massage the back and bony prominences each time the patient is turned
3. exercise the patient at least 45 minutes a day by means of passive therapy
4. encourage the patient to move about in bed with the aid of a trapeze

259. It will be easier for the paralyzed patient to eat comfortably if the person feeding him will remember

1. to keep up a constant stream of conversation
2. to allow him to rest an hour before meals
3. to place food in the unaffected side of the mouth
4. to let the patient hold the spoon

260. Huntington's chorea is correctly described as an inherited disease. This means that

1. both parents suffered from the disease
2. the disease was present from the time the egg and sperm united
3. the symptoms of the disease are present at birth
4. all the children born of these parents will develop symptoms of this disease

261. Sydenham's chorea, or St. Vitus's dance, is considered a complication of

1. measles
2. nephritis
3. rheumatic fever
4. bacterial endocarditis

262. The greatest emotional adjustment to an amputation occurs when the surgery is necessitated by

1. deformity
2. circulatory disturbance
3. diabetes
4. injury

263. The patient who is least disturbed emotionally by the need for an amputation is the patient who is

1. emotionally mature
2. financially independent
3. in severe pain
4. psychiatrically prepared

264. Many amputee patients hesitate to leave the hospital environment because of a dread of

1. being pitied
2. having to work for a living
3. becoming too independent
4. having to take care of himself

265. Following an amputation, the immediate postoperative complication that is most serious is

1. gas gangrene   3. infection
2. hemorrhage   4. contractures

266. In an attempt to prevent a contracture of the thigh or the knee joint after a lower leg amputation, the patient must be regularly encouraged

1. to exercise daily, from the first day
2. to lie on his abdomen, twice daily
3. to massage the stump daily
4. to begin using his prosthesis at once

267. The stump will be elevated on a pillow for the first 24 hours postoperatively. At the end of that time the pillow must be removed to prevent

1. infection
2. pressure sores
3. continuous serous oozing
4. muscle contractures

268. It will not be possible to fit a workable prosthesis in the presence of

a. stump infection
b. muscle contractures
c. tight bandages
d. scar tissue

    1. a only
    2. a and b
    3. a, b, and d
    4. all of the above

269. A prosthesis can be used most efficiently if the entire body is in good physical condition. To keep in good condition, the bedfast amputee must be encouraged

    1. to put all joints through range-of-motion activities
    2. to keep his body in perfect alignment
    3. to remain in a prone position
    4. to help himself

270. Complications resulting from the cast can be prevented if the nursing care is guided by the philosophy that

    1. constant observation will prevent deformities
    2. all cast patients will be uncomfortable and complaining
    3. the first day in the cast requires the most complete care
    4. no pain is too slight to investigate

271. The presence or absence of circulatory irregularities in the extremity in the cast can be determined by observation of

    1. the pulse and respiration
    2. the fingers or toes
    3. the blood pressure
    4. the skin temperature

272. Unless the nurse investigates even minor complaints of pain, it is possible for a pressure area to develop under a cast

    1. without other warning signs
    2. over night
    3. which will require amputation
    4. at points of contact with the bed

273. The nurse is instructed in the need for careful handling of a wet cast to prevent

    1. indentations that will cause pressure points when dry
    2. changing the alignment of the wet plaster
    3. the cast from remaining wet and rubbery
    4. cracks in the plaster that will later pinch the skin

274. The wet cast has been molded to the shape of the part it is encasing. To preserve this contour, the part in the cast should be placed on

    1. a fracture board
    2. a foam rubber mattress
    3. complete bed rest
    4. correctly arranged pillows

275. A wet cast will dry more rapidly if the following conditions exist:

a. high humidity
b. good circulation of air
c. frequent turning of the patient
d. fan turned directly on the cast

    1. all of the above
    2. a and b
    3. c only
    4. b and c

276. If a blower at high heat is turned directly on the wet cast, the cast will

    1. dry more rapidly
    2. dry on the outside, remain wet on the inside
    3. become firm and shiny
    4. be more comfortable for the chilled patient

277. It will be most important to report to the doctor if the patient in a cast shows any indication of

a. a cold extremity under the cast
b. an elevated temperature
c. inability to wiggle fingers or toes
d. numbness or tingling

    1. all of the above
    2. a and d
    3. a, c, and d
    4. b, c, and d

278. The principle of body mechanics which should be practiced by the nurse who helps to move a patient in a <u>full body cast</u> is that of

1. bending at the hips
2. balancing the weight on both feet
3. bending from the waist
4. flexing the hips and knees

279. The patient with a broken bone must be moved very carefully from the scene of the accident to the hospital or the doctor's office to prevent

1. shock
2. turning a simple fracture into a compound fracture
3. pain
4. complicating the symptoms and the diagnosis

280. It will not be so hard to reduce a fracture if it is done soon after the bone is broken because

1. the muscles have not yet gone into spasm
2. the patient has had medication for relief of pain
3. the patient will already be in shock
4. the healing process has not yet begun

281. Emotional problems will always accompany a fracture, since the broken bone is the result of

1. carelessness
2. an occupational hazard
3. an accident
4. reckless driving

282. The broken bone described as a green stick fracture is one in which the bone is

1. cracked in several places
2. difficult to heal
3. compounded
4. broken only on one side

283. The nurse can expect that even after the broken bone is set and immobilized, the patient will complain of

1. coldness of the part
2. pressure of the cast
3. fatigue from one position
4. pain

284. Unless the uninjured leg is kept in good body alignment, the patient with a fracture of the right femur will find, when he tries to walk again, that he has complications of

a. external hip rotation
b. foot drop
c. sciatic nerve paralysis
d. crutch paralysis

1. all of the above
2. b only
3. a, b, or c
4. a or b

285. The broken bone begins to heal just as soon as

1. reduction is done
2. a clot forms
3. the part is put at rest
4. the calcium goes into solution

286. Treatment and nursing care of the fracture patient should be directed toward

1. complete rehabilitation
2. a permanent cure
3. return to normal activity as soon as possible
4. prevention of muscle weakness

287. The purpose of the CALLUS that forms in the process of healing a fracture is to act as

1. a splint around the broken bone ends
2. a supply of calcium
3. a source of new bone cells for repair
4. the first step in the healing

288. Unless the fracture patient in traction is moved so that body alignment is maintained, the result will be

1. extreme pain
2. delayed repair of the fracture
3. disturbance of the bone setting
4. increased tendency to develop pressure sores

289. The most important SUBJECTIVE symptoms the fracture patient will complain of are

1. pain
2. redness and elevation of temperature
3. loss of function and pain
4. headache and mental confusion

MEDICAL AND SURGICAL DISEASES AND NURSING

290. Osteoarthritis is a degenerative disease of advancing age. On this basis, it is to be expected that the affected joints will be those that are

1. weight bearing
2. most often exposed
3. seldom used
4. engaged in pleasurable activities

291. Personality characteristics seem to be a positive predisposing factor in the development of

1. osteomyelitis
2. rheumatoid arthritis
3. osteoarthritis
4. bursitis

292. The doctor suspects that the patient's right arm has been fractured. To enable the doctor to examine it closer, the nurse would remove the man's coat and shirt by

1. removing the right sleeve first
2. removing the left sleeve first
3. cutting out the right sleeve, being careful to follow the seam
4. cutting the garment down the middle of the back to make removal easy

293. The pattern of rheumatoid arthritis is characterized by

1. its chronicity
2. remissions and exacerbations
3. little relief from aches and pains
4. periods of ambulation alternating with periods of helplessness

294. The location of the pains, and the type of pains, associated with rheumatoid arthritis in the young woman are responsible for confusing the diagnosis with

1. strep. sore throat
2. rheumatic fever
3. rheumatism
4. "housemaid's knee"

295. The remission that follows the first attack of rheumatoid arthritis can be prolonged if the patient can practice

1. daily exercises as prescribed
2. adequate dietary habits
3. discontinuance of all pain relieving medicines
4. moderation in attitudes and in activities

296. The principles of good body alignment that are so important in preventing deformities in the orthopedic patients have equal value in the care of

1. patients with bone disorders
2. patients with nervous system diseases
3. arthritis
4. any patient with a long-term illness

297. In congenital dislocation of the hip the head of the femur does not fit securely into the pelvic socket because the acetabulum is

1. too small   3. absent
2. too shallow   4. deteriorated

298. The most perfect results of treatment of congenital dislocation of the hip occur when treatment is begun

1. before 3 months of age
2. at the age of 1 year
3. before the child starts to walk
4. after the muscles have been strengthened by walking

299. If the abduction ability is limited, the nurse could expect that hip joint movement would be decreased when an effort was made

1. to rotate the hip inward
2. to rotate the hip outward
3. to flex the hip
4. to place weight on the pelvic girdle

300. The crippling effects of arthritis are to be feared by the patient with a diagnosis of

1. rheumatism
2. bursitis
3. rheumatoid arthritis
4. osteoarthritis

MEDICAL AND SURGICAL DISEASES AND NURSING
PART II

(Answer sheets pp. 319-320)

1. If the walk of the child with dislocation of the hip could accurately be described as a "duck waddle," the nurse would know the involvement was

   1. unilateral
   2. bilateral
   3. associated with club foot
   4. beyond surgical repair

2. The baby with a corrective pillow splint may be cared for at home. It will be most important for the mother to have instruction and supervised practice in the application of this splint because

   1. it is a time-consuming task
   2. the baby will be uncomfortable in a poorly positioned splint
   3. this procedure is difficult and complicated
   4. it must be removed and reapplied each time the diaper is changed

3. If a small baby is placed in a corrective cast, the most difficult nursing tasks will include

   1. steps to insure normal emotional growth
   2. keeping the baby happily occupied
   3. keeping the cast dry and clean
   4. maintenance of correct body alignment

4. Several members of one family have club foot. The suspected <u>cause</u> would be

   1. poor prenatal care
   2. faulty nutrition habits
   3. defective germ plasm
   4. a hereditary tendency

5. The Achilles tendon is shortened if club foot is not corrected. Such shortening will not allow

   1. the heel to touch the ground
   2. the foot to be fitted with a shoe
   3. the child to walk
   4. for normal growth and development

6. The club foot has been recognized at the time of delivery. It would be best to begin treatment on this baby

   1. at about 6 months of age
   2. before the child is ready to walk
   3. after the body has reached its maximum growth
   4. before the newborn leaves the hospital

7. If it becomes the responsibility of the nurse to do the corrective manipulation of a club foot, it is most important for her to have

   1. a course in physiotherapy
   2. instruction and supervision by the doctor
   3. a knowledge of the bones and muscles of the foot
   4. an understanding of the principles of physics

8. Once a club foot has been corrected, the parents must be completely convinced of the need for

   1. surgical correction
   2. correction under hospital supervision
   3. medical supervision until the child is full grown
   4. providing special recreation and activity during the growing stage

9. The small baby is wearing corrective casts for club feet. Both the nurse and the mother must recognize that special care and observation are needed to prevent

   1. an unstable emotional personality
   2. circulatory complications
   3. an attitude of invalidism
   4. deterioration of the cast

10. An <u>excoriation</u> is defined as

    1. a fissure
    2. a break in the continuity of the skin
    3. an emergency lesion
    4. a sloughing away of tissue

11. A pustule occurs as the result of

    1. a systemic infection
    2. a secondary infection in a vesicle
    3. cross infection
    4. careless personal hygiene habits

12. A wheal is best described as

    1. an oversized papule
    2. an allergy
    3. an inflammatory lesion
    4. a raised, edematous welt

13. Athlete's foot most often begins

    1. on the sole of the foot
    2. under the toe nails
    3. between the fourth and fifth toes
    4. on only one foot

14. Athlete's foot can be prevented by

    a. wearing a <u>foot covering</u> in wet, damp areas
    b. keeping the area between the toes clean and dry
    c. wearing summer shoes that allow for sweat evaporation
    d. wearing wool socks to absorb the perspiration

        1. all except d
        2. b only
        3. a and d
        4. all of the above

15. The most frequent complication of untreated athlete's foot is

    1. gangrene, necessitating amputation
    2. joint mice
    3. secondary infection that gains entrance to tissues through fissured epidermis
    4. a slow, progressive extension to the rest of the body

16. Nits are difficult to remove from the hair shaft because

    1. they look like dandruff
    2. a gluelike substance holds them to the hairs
    3. they fasten themselves into the hair shaft
    4. they are nourished from the same source

17. Following the prescribed treatment for head lice, the hair is fine-combed to remove nits and lice. The hair combings are destroyed by

    1. wrapping them in newspaper
    2. soaking in hot, soapy water
    3. burning
    4. flushing them down the hopper

18. The nurse on a pediatric ward should suspect that the newly admitted child has head lice when she observes

    a. blood
    b. him frequently scratching his head
    c. scratch marks at the nape of the neck
    d. an excess loss of hair when it is combed

        1. any of the above
        2. c only
        3. all except a
        4. b and c

19. Once the nits have been loosened from the hair shafts by treatment, they are removed from the hair by

    1. shampooing
    2. brushing with nylon bristles
    3. combing with a fine comb
    4. a vinegar rinse

20. The admitting nurse would expect to check new patients for the presence of lice. She would find evidence of body lice by examining the

    1. seams of clothing
    2. eyebrows
    3. inner hatband
    4. hair on the chest

21. The characteristic skin evidence of the presence of body lice includes

    a. a pin-point-size lesion
    b. redness
    c. scratch marks on the chest and back
    d. swelling around the bite

        1. all of the above
        2. a and c
        3. c only
        4. all except b

22. D.D.T. powder is effective in ridding a person of

1. the nits of scabies
2. nits and lice
3. only the male itch mite
4. all parasites

23. Itching is a frequent symptom of louse infestation. The itching may occur day or night because it is produced by

1. movement of the lice
2. hatching of the nits
3. deposits of excreta on the skin or hair
4. the bite of the louse as it feeds

24. It would be possible for one person to pass along the itch mite of scabies to a second person during an activity such as

1. swimming   3. card playing
2. square dancing   4. bowling

25. The deposit of excreta by the itch mite as she burrows into the epidermis is responsible for producing

1. itching
2. an inflammatory reaction out of proportion to the number of mites
3. a vesicle
4. a discoloration which may be mistaken for a sliver

26. The activity of the itch mite increases when it is warm. On this basis, the itching would be increased

1. during a bath
2. after the victim had gone to bed
3. on a hot, humid day
4. following a high-fat, high-CHO meal

27. Pediculosis and scabies are considered predisposing causes of impetigo. The causative organism of impetigo gains entrance to the body as a result of

1. toxic absorption
2. respiratory invasion
3. the weakened condition of the body
4. scratching

28. The transfer of erysipelas from one hospitalized patient to another is extremely dangerous because one of the characteristics of the causative organism is its ability to

1. be air borne
2. increase in virulence while outside the body
3. increase in virulence on transfer
4. reproduce rapidly

29. A common cosmetic habit that should be discouraged because it is known to be a predisposing cause of erysipelas is

1. squeezing pimples
2. pulling hairs out of the nostril
3. daily use of vanishing and cleansing creams
4. continued use of detergent-type soaps

30. A nurse who cares for a patient with a third-degree burn must be alert to prevent secondary erysipelas. One of her responsibilities is

1. to keep the patient's environment sterile
2. to isolate the burn patient
3. to apply sterile dressings frequently
4. to cover her nose and mouth with a mask

31. Mr. Jones has a varicose ulcer and secondary erysipelas. The nurse in charge of changing dressings on a surgical ward would know that it is important

1. to change Mr. Jones's dressing last
2. to clean the dressing cart before caring for Mr. Jones
3. to use recently sterilized instruments and dressings
4. to have assistance from another nurse

32. The prodromal symptoms of erysipelas could best be described as

1. local   3. circulatory
2. systemic   4. diagnostic

33. Because of the method of extension of erysipelas, the topical application of any medication would be done by

1. using an atomizer or spray can
2. continuous irrigation
3. starting at the periphery of the lesion and applying toward the center
4. first removing all medications remaining from the last treatment

34. In addition to the pain of erysipelas, other symptoms distressing to the patient include

a. burning
b. hyperemia
c. itching
d. eupnea

1. b, c, and d
2. a only
3. a and c
4. all of the above

35. The absorption of the toxins from the Streptococcus causing erysipelas is responsible for the symptoms of

a. tachycardia
b. hyperpnea
c. hyperpyrexia
d. edema

1. all of the above
2. c only
3. all except b
4. a, b, and c

36. The patient with erysipelas should receive 3000 c.c. to 4000 c.c. of fluid per day because

1. he will quickly become dehydrated
2. the absorbed toxins of the streptococcus may damage the kidneys
3. the systemic symptoms will improve more rapidly
4. the causative organism will thus be flushed out of the body

37. The local heat and edema accompanying erysipelas can best be relieved by

1. antipyretic medication
2. aspirin and other salycilates
3. alcohol sponge baths
4. cold, moist compresses

38. The typical lesions of psoriasis that cause so much emotional distress to the patient would be described as

1. red and weeping
2. deeply ulcerated and circumscribed
3. definitely outlined, shiny, frosty scales
4. symmetrical

39. Psoriasis of the scalp will not be confused with ringworm of the scalp because in psoriasis

1. there are definite patches of baldness
2. the scalp looks "moth eaten."
3. the scales look like dandruff
4. hair growth is not affected

40. The patient with psoriasis is not distressed by one symptom that is common to most skin conditions. The absent symptom is

1. itching   3. erythema
2. scaling   4. local fever

41. Psoriasis can best be described as a chronic disease characterized by

1. skin lesions that are always present
2. extreme emotional involvement
3. remissions and exacerbations
4. intense pain, relieved only by narcotics

42. Psoriasis improves on exposure to ultraviolet rays. Therefore, the lesions could be expected to improve

1. in Arizona
2. during the summer
3. with hydrotherapy treatments
4. under a home-type "sun lamp"

43. The patient with psoriasis is seldom hospitalized because of this disease. The office nurse should explain to the patient that stained bed linens could be prevented by

1. covering the ointment-treated parts with wax paper
2. applying the ointment only in the morning
3. sleeping in long underwear
4. using sheets that are already stained

44. Herpes zoster is usually preceded by 3 or 4 days of

1. anorexia
2. gastric upsets
3. general malaise
4. systemic symptoms

45. The location of the pain associated with herpes zoster will depend on

   1. the physical resistance of the patient
   2. the nerve involved
   3. which organ is the weakest of the body
   4. the presence or absence of referred pain

46. The lesions of herpes zoster go away without treatment. In spite of treatment, the patient may continue to have

   1. persistent neuralgic pain for months
   2. small vesicles and crusts
   3. general malaise
   4. loss of function

47. The nurse could reassure the adolescent with eczema that the skin lesions will not leave a scar unless

   1. the treatment is discontinued too quickly
   2. they become hemorrhagic
   3. they are overtreated
   4. a secondary infection follows scratching

48. It would be expected that the eczema classified as contact dermatitis could be cured if

   1. the allergen could be identified and eliminated
   2. a change of occupation could be arranged
   3. an elimination diet was followed
   4. desensitizing injections were given

49. If both parents have a past history of allergies, it would be wise to try to prevent the appearance of infantile eczema in the newborn by

   1. placing it in a foster home for the first year
   2. omitting or delaying its exposure to known allergens
   3. restricting the diet to milk until the danger period is past
   4. prophylactic visits to the dermatologist

50. The nurse must recognize that the distress of infantile eczema includes

   a. deep neuralgic pain
   b. shame and resentment by the parents
   c. malnutrition and stunted growth
   d. extreme itching of the lesions

      1. all of the above
      2. d only
      3. b and d
      4. all except a

51. All nurses should recognize the warning signs of skin cancer which include

   a. leukoplakia
   b. any sore that does not heal within three weeks
   c. increase in the size of a mole
   d. increase in pigment coloring of a mole

      1. all of the above
      2. a only
      3. b and c
      4. b, c, or d

52. A general predisposing cause of cancer which is also true of skin cancer, is the presence of

   1. abnormal cells
   2. cell irritation
   3. a systemic virus
   4. leukoplakia

53. Most skin cancers, other than malignant moles, are known to grow

   1. sporadically   3. slowly
   2. rapidly   4. peripherally

54. Some skin cancers metastasize rapidly, others slowly, and others not at all. This variation is due to

   1. the different type of cells involved
   2. the original cause of the cancer
   3. the presence or absence of precancerous lesions
   4. the stage of the cancer at the time of the diagnosis

55. With the exception of the malignant moles, most skin cancers metastasize by

   1. way of the blood stream
   2. development of an embolus
   3. extension to the bone
   4. way of the lymphatic system

56. It should be encouraging to know that regardless of the type of skin cancer diagnosed

    1. it is seldom fatal
    2. complete removal is always possible
    3. early treatment could insure a 100% cure
    4. there is never any danger of spread

57. Tuberculosis must be considered a dangerous disease today because

    1. so many people have it
    2. not much is known about the cause
    3. it is not possible to get rid of the predisposing causes
    4. about one third of the active cases are not getting treatment

58. One reason for stressing regular chest X-rays is to help

    1. everyone to stay on the job
    2. diagnose persons with no symptoms of the disease
    3. to keep the lead as the healthiest country in the world
    4. to protect the next generation

59. Since the causes and the method of spread are known, tuberculosis is a disease that can be classified as

    1. preventable   3. congenital
    2. acute   4. functional

60. If the chest X-ray discovers active tuberculosis in one member of a family, an effective safeguard of the public health would require

    1. a survey of all the people who worked for the same company
    2. sterilization of all public transportation used by the person
    3. X ray of members of the immediate family
    4. quarantine of the whole family

61. When an infant develops tuberculosis, the assumption is usually correct that contact with the germs came

    1. through the birth canal
    2. from the baby's home
    3. from the newborn nursery
    4. from the germ plasm

62. A positive reaction to a tuberculin skin test tells the doctor that the patient

    1. has good resistance to tuberculosis
    2. is, or has been, attacked by the tubercle bacilli
    3. has tuberculosis and should have a chest X-ray
    4. is cured of tuberculosis and never needs to worry again

63. A positive reaction to a tuberculin test is not enough to make a diagnosis of tuberculosis. An accurate diagnosis can be made only if

    1. a chest specialist reads the skin reaction
    2. the person is hospitalized at once
    3. a chest X-ray is also done
    4. a sputum examination is done

64. The best way to get tuberculosis under control and stop the increase in the number of persons with the disease is

    1. to reassure the patient and his family
    2. to find the unknown cases
    3. to keep young children from being exposed
    4. to increase the facilities for the care of active cases

65. Nursing measures to kill the tubercle bacilli are stricter than for most other diseases of the respiratory system because

    1. the tubercle bacilli can live for months in dust
    2. the patient is seldom interested in cooperating
    3. specific techniques to kill them are not known
    4. the longer it stays outside the human body, the more dangerous it becomes

66. Tuberculosis is never considered cured because even though the bacilli have been sealed up by the body it is possible

  1. for them to keep the patient in ill health
  2. to pass them on to other people
  3. for the bacilli to fight their way through the walls of the tubercles
  4. for the germs to again become active if body resistance gets low

67. All persons who are around a newly diagnosed tuberculosis patient should understand the value of using rehabilitation principles as soon as he

  1. is able to meet with other patients for group therapy
  2. feels at home in the sanatorium
  3. is given the diagnosis
  4. accepts the need for changing his whole life

68. One of the reasons we try so hard to help the patient to understand his disease is the knowledge that the more he understands about the cause and the spread of tuberculosis

  1. the more frightened he will become
  2. the easier it will be to talk about his fears
  3. the easier it will be to follow the rules of care
  4. the more he will realize that there is little he can do except remain in the hospital

69. When the wage earner of the family has tuberculosis and he tells you he is worried about the financial needs of his family, you can reassure him by saying,

  1. "They will be all right. They have their health"
  2. "Don't worry. They are taken care of"
  3. "I can understand your concern, I will ask the social worker to tell you what help is available"
  4. "It will take several agencies to meet all their needs, but among them, they will do a good job"

70. It is important to tell the tuberculosis patient that a good way to help rid himself of this disease is to

  1. become a doctor
  2. buy Christmas seals
  3. follow precautions that will prevent the spread of germs to others
  4. remain in the sanatorium and help to care for patients more ill than he

71. One of the first things a hospitalized patient with tuberculosis is taught for the protection of employees and visitors is

  1. to be happy doing nothing
  2. to dispose of his sputum to avoid spreading germs
  3. to avoid close contact with all people
  4. to keep up a good nutritional state by eating all the food on his tray

72. If it were possible, every tuberculosis patient should be urged to ensure his peace of mind while he is in the hospital by

  1. insisting on going home every week-end
  2. keeping busy all the time with occupational therapy projects
  3. putting his personal affairs in order before entering the sanitorium
  4. making arrangements for his wife to work and asking the bank for an extended loan

73. When the newly diagnosed tuberculosis patient feels there is nothing more he can do with his life, the nurse might try to raise his spirits by encouraging him

  1. to snap out of it
  2. to join a church
  3. to read one of the books written by an ex-T.B. patient
  4. to look around at the patients who are worse off than he is

74. The bedfast tuberculosis patient needs to work on some occupational therapy project to stimulate a feeling of

  1. recovery   3. being wanted
  2. accomplishment 4. importance

75. The tubercle bacillus trapped in the tubercle is considered to be <u>dormant</u>. This means that the germ is

1. dead
2. weakened
3. very actively reproducing itself
4. sleeping

76. The tuberculosis patient who has been released from a sanitorium is safe to work with because

1. he is now immune
2. he prefers to work alone
3. he has frequent, regular check-ups and chest X-rays
4. he understands that his associates will be afraid of him

77. One of the hardest things for the inactive tuberculosis patient to accept after he has been released from the sanitorium is

1. the fear that his friends and business associates show toward him
2. the need to get back to work
3. the fact that his family got along all right when he was away
4. admitting he has been ill with tuberculosis

78. Tuberculosis is most serious in those age groups from

a. birth to 3 years
b. school age to adolescence
c. 16 to 35
d. 50 to 60, if male

1. all of the above
2. c only
3. a, c, and d
4. all except d

79. The death rate from tuberculosis in the United States has decreased 90% in 60 years. Much of this achievement is based on

1. increased public education and improved health policies
2. free treatment
3. occupational and recreational therapy
4. increasing supplies of surplus foods

80. The practical nurse could make it easier for the inactive T.B. patient to return to his home and job if

1. she arranged for someone to do all his heavy jobs
2. she helped him find a job where he could work alone
3. she warned him constantly that a relapse could send him back to the hospital
4. she helped the community to understand what hospitalization did for the patient and his disease

81. In this country the death rate from tuberculosis is higher among negroes than white persons. The informed individual knows this is because the nego group is

a. more susceptible to the disease
b. less resistant
c. exposed at an earlier age
d. reluctant to accept treatment

1. all of the above
2. a only
3. b and c
4. a and d

82. The incidence of tuberculosis is higher among people who are employed in

1. strenuous jobs
2. confined areas
3. inside occupations
4. dusty trades

83. There are fewer undiagnosed cases of tuberculosis in our communities. There are also fewer people with a positive reaction to the tuberculin test because

1. more people get only a chest X-ray
2. people have physical examinations annually or semiannually
3. school children are vaccinated against tuberculosis
4. fewer people are exposed to the germs

84. The persons responsible for the greatest spread of tuberculosis are those who

1. are ambulatory
2. prefer to stay at home
3. will not wear a mask
4. are undiagnosed

85. Development of active tuberculosis by exposure to a diseased person will depend on

   a. the length of time exposed
   b. the virulence of the bacilli
   c. the age of the T.B. patient
   d. the resistance of the exposed individual

      1. all of the above
      2. b only
      3. b and d
      4. a, b, and d

86. One of the characteristics of primary tuberculosis is

   1. a negative sensitivity test
   2. absence of specific symptoms
   3. increased susceptibility
   4. susceptibility to secondary lung infections

87. The presence or absence of tuberculosis at this specific moment cannot be told from a positive reaction to the sensitivity test. The individual with such a reaction must still have

   1. a complete physical examination
   2. a bronchoscopy
   3. a large chest X-ray
   4. blood and urine tests

88. When the tubercle bacilli enter the lungs, the body defenses are called into action. The initial body reaction is called

   1. necrosis   3. petechia
   2. calcification   4. inflammation

89. Adults with negative reaction to the sensitivity test should be given skin tests twice a year. This can be an important way

   1. to check the stability of the immunity
   2. to determine the value of the X-ray
   3. to diagnose tuberculosis early
   4. to discover primary tuberculosis

90. The outside temperature is 20° above zero. The tubercle bacilli in expectorated sputum will characteristically

   1. die
   2. be unaffected
   3. form a protective spore
   4. live but will not multiply

91. The tubercle bacilli will be walled off by calcification in the body with good resistance. The possessor of the tubercles should clearly understand that it is still possible

   1. to have all the symptoms of tuberculosis
   2. to run an elevated temperature
   3. for the patient to be sick enough to require sanatorium care
   4. for the bacilli to break through and reactivate the disease

92. Many persons have been exposed to the tubercle bacilli, have had primary tuberculosis, and have been unaware of the invasion. One objective sign of such tuberculosis would be

   1. calcifications
   2. the X-rays
   3. a negative tuberculin test
   4. a positive sputum

93. The chest X-ray is most effective in locating early tuberculosis in apparently healthy people because

   1. even minimal lesions are seen
   2. the location of cavities can be seen
   3. the activity of the bacilli can be visualized
   4. the bacilli are very sensitive to X-rays

94. We know the body has been exposed to the tubercle bacilli when the reaction to the tuberculin test is positive because

   1. the reaction of cell proteins indicates previous contact with the bacterial proteins
   2. the immune substances in the body easily defeat the invading bacilli
   3. most people have a positive reaction
   4. injection starts up the old lesion

95. The tubercle bacilli of the human variety are spread to others only from

   1. articles contaminated with bacilli
   2. tubercle laden dust
   3. sputum containing active bacilli
   4. bacilli leaving the body of the person with active tuberculosis

96. All newly diagnosed patients with tuberculosis should be hospitalized. This is important

    a. to teach him about the disease
    b. to help him adjust to the diagnosis
    c. to teach him to protect those around him
    d. to teach him how to rest

        1. all of the above
        2. a only
        3. a and d
        4. b, c, and d

97. Most tubercle bacilli enter the human body through the process of

    1. ingestion
    2. inhalation
    3. absorption
    4. assimilation

98. Spread of the tubercle bacilli from the lung to other parts of the body is accomplished by

    a. contaminated food
    b. the lymph vessels
    c. the tissue fluid
    d. the blood stream

        1. any of the above
        2. d only
        3. b and d
        4. a, b, and c

99. The tubercle bacilli present in moist sputum can be most effectively killed by

    1. burning
    2. disinfection
    3. soaking with 5% Lysol solution
    4. covering with chloride of lime

100. The tuberculosis patient is taught to protect other people by caring for his nose and throat discharges correctly. Such teaching is based on the fact that

    1. coughing with productive sputum nauseates other people
    2. the blood produced is bright and frothy
    3. the tubercle bacillus lives outside the body in the sputum
    4. there is great danger of reinfecting himself

101. People are more susceptible to invasion by the tubercle bacilli if their diets have long been lacking in adequate

    1. calcium   3. protein
    2. iron   4. fats

102. Tuberculosis of the bone is most often the result of

    1. extension from the lungs
    2. drinking milk containing tubercle bacilli
    3. earlier bone infection
    4. careless child management

103. Tuberculosis of the bone produces deformities in children because the disease destroys

    1. nerve stimulation to the bone
    2. the ability of muscles to contract
    3. the ends of the bones
    4. body resistance to disease

104. The usual treatment of tuberculosis of a long bone results in

    1. elimination of the adjoining joint
    2. injection of penicillin into the joint
    3. decreased production of red blood cells
    4. increased sensitivity to heat and cold

105. Tuberculosis of the spine most frequently affects those in the age group from

    1. birth to 3 years   3. 12 to 15
    2. 2 to 10   4. 45 to 50

106. An early symptom of tuberculosis of the bone that may not be recognized as serious by parents is

    1. an elevated temperature
    2. easy fatigue
    3. night cries
    4. pain in the vertebrae

107. If the spine is not maintained in good body alignment the patient will complain of pain caused by

    1. joint inflammation
    2. muscle spasm
    3. pressure of pus on the cord
    4. nerve tension

108. Good body alignment in tuberculosis of the spine is best maintained by

1. generous use of sandbags
2. application of a body cast
3. pillows placed in all body curvatures
4. using two nurses to turn the patient

109. Tuberculosis of the bone most often leads to

1. pulmonary complications
2. emotional depression
3. limited function of the part
4. spread of the disease to other organs

110. A beginning symptom of tuberculosis of the hip is

1. a scissors gait
2. night sweating
3. muscle spasm
4. a limp of increasing severity

111. T.B. meningitis in children is usually the result of

1. a spinal injury
2. spread from a pulmonary lesion
3. a run down physical condition
4. spinal fluid infection

112. Because T.B. meningitis is an inflammation of the meninges covering the brain, a constant symptom of the disease is

1. heat   3. headache
2. edema   4. convulsions

113. If the T.B. process in the meninges blocks the free flow of spinal fluid, the symptoms will be those of

1. a tumor in the brain
2. inflammation in the brain
3. an internal hydrocephalus
4. increased pressure in the spine

114. The formation and healing of T.B. ulcers on the intestinal lining is often complicated by

1. obstruction
2. hemorrhage
3. shock
4. extension to the liver

115. When the tubercle bacilli invade the kidney, the symptoms may occur only when

1. both kidneys are involved
2. ulcers are formed in the bladder
3. urine formation is decreased
4. the ureters become involved

116. A urine examination is often delayed until the patient with tuberculosis of the urinary tract complains of

1. backache
2. pain in the groin
3. pus in the urine
4. blood in the urine

117. When the kidney is infected with tuberculosis, the nurse must take special precautions in her care of

1. bony prominences
2. all body discharges
3. the urine
4. all bath equipment

118. The only successful treatment of tuberculosis of the kidney is

1. complete removal of the organ
2. use of mercurial diuretics
3. medication which changes the concentration of urine
4. ureteral catheterization

119. If tuberculosis affects the one remaining kidney, the outcome will be

1. toxemia
2. alkalosis
3. increased waste output by other organs
4. death due to uremia

120. The informed practical nurse will understand how important it is to recognize leukoplakia as

1. an early stage of cancer
2. a medical emergency
3. the normal deterioration of old age
4. a precancerous lesion

121. An examination for leukoplakia in the upper digestive tract would include inspection of

    a. the lower lip
    b. the tonsils
    c. the cheeks
    d. the tongue

        1. all of the above
        2. a only
        3. a and b
        4. a, c, and d

122. Leukoplakia would be recognized as a mucous membrane patch that

    a. forms a crust
    b. is thin and white
    c. is dark brown in color
    d. is not easily removed

        1. all except c
        2. d only
        3. b and d
        4. a and c

123. Leukoplakia is best treated by

    1. giving up all habits that would stimulate its growth
    2. removal of false teeth
    3. routine use of an alkaline mouth wash
    4. surgical removal

124. Chronic irritation of the lip can be caused by

    a. whistling
    b. a hot pipestem
    c. sun and wind
    d. lipstick

        1. b only
        2. b, c, and d
        3. b and c
        4. c and d

125. Cancer of the mouth can often be traced to the effects of

    1. continued irritation
    2. tobacco
    3. rays of the sun
    4. irritation of teeth

126. A person who wears false teeth should protect himself from a chance of developing an oral cancer by

    1. cleaning them several times a day
    2. being sure that they fit correctly
    3. soaking them in Polident daily
    4. using mouthwashes often

127. A friend or relative should be encouraged to see a doctor if an ulcerated area on his lip

    1. is infected
    2. needs treatment with an antibiotic
    3. has been present more than two weeks
    4. is not a healthy color

128. We would be more suspicious that a lesion on the lip was cancer if we knew the person who had the lesion was

    a. a man
    b. a pipe smoker
    c. red-haired
    d. past 40

        1. b only
        2. a and b
        3. a, b, and d
        4. all of the above

129. We would not suspect that a recent lesion on the lip or in the mouth was a cancer if it

    1. bled easily
    2. was painful
    3. rapidly increased in size
    4. looked like a wart

130. The mucous membranes of the mouth may be continually irritated by

    1. the daily use of a strong mouthwash or gargle
    2. chewing gum
    3. rough, coarse foods
    4. the daily use of very hot foods and fluids

131. Most people have a lesion in the mouth once in a while. The degree of seriousness of a lesion can often be judged by

    1. the length of time it lasts
    2. the production of pus
    3. the symptoms of inflammation
    4. the response to antiseptics

132. An open lesion may not be present in cancer of the mouth. Early cancer should also be suspected if

   1. the tissues are sore
   2. bleeding occurs
   3. a painless lump can be felt
   4. food and drink irritate the tissues

133. Factors that increase the chances of cancer of the mouth in older men are

   a. they have used tobacco over a period of years
   b. oral hygiene is often poor
   c. the teeth are more likely to be rough
   d. a vitamin B deficiency is more apt to be present

      1. a and c
      2. a, b, and d
      3. b, c, and d
      4. all of the above

134. Since surgery to remove a cancer of the mouth or the lip will disfigure the patient, the nurse must always remember the importance of

   1. respecting the patient's desire to be left alone
   2. controlling her expression when she changes dressings
   3. sympathy toward his discomforts
   4. assuring the patient everything will be all right

135. The patient should be told that for a while after the surgical removal of an oral cancer he will be fed

   1. through a straw
   2. through a gastrostomy opening
   3. through a tube from the nose into the stomach
   4. by intravenous injection

136. The prognosis is more serious because metastasis is more rapid when the oral cancer is located

   1. on the tongue
   2. on the cheek
   3. on the lip
   4. in the corner of the mouth

137. A child who has swallowed lye must not be encouraged to vomit because

   1. the esophagus will rupture
   2. stomach tissues will be damaged
   3. tissue destruction will increase as the chemical comes up the esophagus
   4. once the gastric juices are lost by vomiting, it will be difficult to replace them

138. After a caustic substance has been swallowed, it must be recognized that in immediate first aid treatment the safety of the patient will require

   1. removal of the substance from the body
   2. neutralization of the substance
   3. a stomach washing
   4. use of a laxative

139. A chemical burn of the esophagus will eventually narrow the esophagus because

   1. the scar tissue will constrict
   2. edema is produced
   3. of the inflammatory process
   4. scabs fill in the burned area

140. The victims of cancer of the esophagus often admit an early symptom that they overlooked was

   1. a hacking cough after eating
   2. dyspnea
   3. dysphagia
   4. slight difficulty swallowing dry foods

141. Most patients hospitalized with cancer of the esophagus will need the kind of nursing care described as

   1. group nursing   3. careful nursing
   2. hourly nursing   4. terminal nursing

142. The term "indigestion" does not accurately describe the patient's complaint of a stomach upset because

   1. it is a diagnosis
   2. it has a different meaning to different individuals
   3. he is tempted to take baking soda to relieve it
   4. most people think of this as a serious condition

143. The greatest harm comes to the person with repeated attacks of indigestion as a result of

    1. self-medication
    2. heartburn
    3. reverse peristalsis
    4. overeating

144. An ulcer is most often found in a person who has no acceptable outlet for his frequent

    1. indifference
    2. hypermotility
    3. insomnia
    4. emotional tenseness

145. A peptic ulcer often has its beginning when tense, nervous behavior is carried over into the individual's

    1. eating habits
    2. sleep habits
    3. business activities
    4. habits of personal hygiene

146. The peptic ulcer is a lesion best described as

    1. organic   3. psychosomatic
    2. functional   4. hypertrophy

147. The ulcer patient is often not able to admit he enjoys being waited on. The mental mechanism, overcompensation, may cause him to react to such nursing care

    1. in an indifferent manner
    2. as a semi-invalid
    3. in an embarrassed way when care is given
    4. in a sharp, overcritical way

148. The nurse can best reassure the hospitalized ulcer patient, already nervous and scared, by

    1. moving quietly about his room
    2. keeping the room darkened
    3. advising visitors to stay only a few minutes
    4. preparing the patient carefully for each examination and treatment

149. The nurse's notes on the patient's chart would help the doctor to make a diagnosis of peptic ulcer if the observations and notations included

    1. the patient's complaints of constipation
    2. the onset of pain in relation to the time of eating
    3. the patient's reaction to gas-forming foods
    4. the presence or absence of flatus

150. Relief from the pain of a stomach ulcer can be expected

    1. as soon as the chyme becomes alkaline
    2. as soon as the gastric juice is diluted or neutralized
    3. when the food substances pass into the duodenum
    4. only after an antacid medication is given

151. The mental mechanism of overcompensation allows the ulcer patient with an unconscious wish to be dependent to behave instead as

    1. a meek, mild, fearful individual
    2. a tactless, irritable individual
    3. an aggressive, go-getter type
    4. a persecuted individual

152. A second ulcer may develop following the surgical removal of the first lesion if no effort has been made

    1. to help the patient modify his personality problems
    2. to remove all the ulcer cells
    3. to remove the adjoining lymph glands
    4. to regulate the postoperative diet

153. An ulcer will perforate as a result of

    1. hemorrhage
    2. digestion of the three muscle coats in the area of the ulcer
    3. coarse, fibrous foods in the diet
    4. pressures from overeating

154. The symptoms accompanying perforation of an ulcer are

    a. hematemesis
    b. apnea
    c. abdominal rigidity
    d. sudden, sharp abdominal pains

        1. all of the above
        2. a, b, and c
        3. a and d
        4. c and d

155. If the patient shows no improvement after several weeks of treating a suspected ulcer, surgery will be advised in order

    1. to cure the patient
    2. to rule out the possibility of cancer
    3. to provide an opening for feeding the patient
    4. to repair the ulcer

156. Bleeding slowly, but steadily, from a stomach ulcer or cancer, should be suspected in the presence of

    1. bright red, frothy emesis
    2. black, tarry stools
    3. continuous abdominal cramping
    4. low blood pressure

157. If a man had always been healthy and usually symptom-free, stomach cancer, in its early stage, might be diagnosed if he sought medical advice at the first signs of

    1. digestive distress
    2. abdominal pain
    3. heartburn
    4. vomiting

158. The onset of pain in relation to the time of eating is important to the diagnosis of cancer or ulcer of the stomach. The pain of cancer tends to appear

    1. before meals
    2. only at bedtime
    3. after the food leaves the stomach
    4. immediately after meals

159. The nurse can help the patient with a partial gastrectomy to prevent regurgitation of food by advising him

    1. to eat a liquid diet
    2. to eat less and more slowly
    3. to eat a high-fat diet
    4. to concentrate on protein foods

160. Malnourishment and vitamin deficiencies will follow prolonged periods of diarrhea because

    1. passage of intestinal contents through the large intestines is too fast
    2. digested materials are incompletely absorbed by the villi
    3. the person does not have strength enough to eat well
    4. there will be a shortage of digestive juices

161. Rectal bleeding is most serious when "self-diagnosis" concludes that the cause must be

    1. capillary fragility
    2. chronic hemorrhoids
    3. roughage in the diet
    4. inactivity

162. An inguinal hernia is more common in boys than in girls because of

    1. too strenuous play
    2. the restrictive type of clothing worn
    3. the usual weight differences between sexes
    4. a muscle weakness present at birth

163. A cure for chronic ulcerative colitis most often requires a combination of

    a. medicines
    b. surgery
    c. psychotherapy
    d. physical therapy

        1. all of the above
        2. b and c
        3. b, a, and d
        4. c and a or b

164. Undiagnosed rectal bleeding may be caused by

a. hemorrhoids
b. peptic ulcers
c. colitis
d. cancer of the rectum

    1. all of the above
    2. d only
    3. a and d
    4. a, c, or d

165. Following a hemorrhoidectomy, the first bowel movement is made easier by

a. an oil-retention enema
b. a high-cellulose diet
c. a cleansing enema
d. a laxative

    1. d, a, then c
    2. all of the above
    3. a only
    4. b, d, then c

166. The patient who has had a hernia repair will not be allowed to do any heavy lifting or straining

1. for an indefinite period, to avoid a recurrence
2. unless a truss is worn
3. until a strong scar tissue has developed
4. for at least a year or two

167. An infection in an abdominal incision should be prevented because it might be a predisposing cause of

1. hemorrhoids   3. hernia
2. shock   4. adhesions

168. The nurse who is successful in teaching a colostomy patient to care for his own irrigations is one who

1. avoids any expression that indicates she finds the care unpleasant
2. spends time explaining how lucky he is to be alive
3. allows other patients to observe her care of the colostomy
4. makes him assume full responsibility for its care soon after surgery

169. The patient is discouraged from buying a colostomy bag to collect feces because

1. the bag is unsanitary
2. the patient refuses to learn how to empty the bag
3. other members of the family are disturbed by the constant odor
4. the patient becomes dependent on the bag and does not try to become regulated

170. When the pyloric sphincter muscle hypertrophies, symptoms are produced because

1. the nerve supply of the sphincter is interfered with
2. the tumor collapses the pyloric opening
3. the gastric contents pass into the duodenum too rapidly
4. thickened muscle narrows the sphincter opening

171. Pylorospasm implies that the symptoms are produced when

1. pyloric sphincter muscles go into spasm
2. peristalsis is decreased
3. gastric juices do not prepare food for intestinal digestion
4. production of bile is affected

172. When the infant's feedings have been accumulating in the stomach, the nurse can expect the emesis to be

1. stimulated by excitement
2. thin and watery
3. projectile
4. coffee-ground in appearance

173. The nurse's observations and recordings will be most important if pyloric stenosis is suspected. It is especially important that the nurse's notes give information about

1. the color of the vomitus
2. the odor of the vomitus
3. the symptoms displayed by the baby at the time of the emesis
4. the time of the emesis in relation to feeding

174. The behavior of the infant with pyloro-spasm will be characterized by

1. stupor
2. lethargy
3. indifference
4. tension

175. If the nurse is to function effectively in the preparation of a baby for stomach X-ray to diagnose pyloric stenosis, she cannot allow her sympathy

1. to convince her the baby should be fed if it is hungry
2. to interfere with the procedure of the technician
3. to upset the emotions of the baby
4. to interfere with her understanding of the problems of the X-ray

176. The surgical treatment of hypertrophy of the pyloric sphincter does not upset the baby's feeding schedule for more than 8 to 12 hours because

1. surgery takes place through a bronchoscope
2. the incision is not made through the mucous-membrane layer
3. the ability to nurse is instinctive
4. tissue repair is rapid in the infant

177. The job of the nurse assisting the doctor who is doing a paracentesis is to observe the cardinal symptoms closely and to report at once any symptoms indicating

1. shock
2. hemorrhage
3. anemia
4. nervous irritability

178. Predisposing causes of gallbladder diseases will include

a. marital status
b. presence of chronic disease
c. age 40 or over
d. obesity

   1. b and c
   2. c and d
   3. all except a
   4. none of the above

179. The patient with cholecystitis usually gives a history of symptoms of

1. gallstones
2. long-standing indigestion
3. a constant urge to eat
4. persistent diarrhea

180. Cholecystitis may be caused by

1. irritation from gallstones
2. irritation of concentrated bile
3. extension of respiratory infections
4. obstruction to the flow of bile

181. Since gallbladder surgery requires an incision near the diaphragm, post-operatively, the patient with such surgery will need extra encouragement

1. to get up to the bathroom the day of surgery
2. to cough and breathe deeply
3. to take sufficient fluids
4. to check nausea and vomiting

182. If a drain into the gallbladder is pulled out postoperatively, the result of the escape of bile from the gall-bladder will be

1. hemorrhage
2. peritonitis
3. suppuration
4. hypertrophy

183. Food substances stored preoperatively that will protect the liver during the postoperative period of limited food intake include

1. vitamins A and C
2. CHO and starch
3. protein and glucose
4. thiamine and niacin

184. The patient with liver disease would probably not be given a narcotic medication for the relief of pain as long as he complained of

a. headache
b. nausea
c. tenesmus
d. dizziness

   1. all but c
   2. c and d
   3. b and c
   4. all of the above

222

185. A liver abscess can be relieved surgically by

1. removal
2. drainage
3. section
4. plastic surgery

186. Liver abscess is one of the few diseases in which treatment is more effective

1. after complications develop
2. after jaundice develops
3. when palliative measures are used
4. with oral medications than with needle injections

187. The patient with cirrhosis of the liver usually does not seek medical aid until the disease is well advanced because

1. none of the symptoms is distressing
2. symptoms are not present until much of the liver is destroyed
3. the symptoms are considered the result of aging
4. the beginning symptoms are common and come and go

188. Regardless of the predisposing cause, the primary cause of cirrhosis of the liver is believed to be

1. alcohol
2. malnourished liver cells
3. carcinoma
4. irritation from bile

189. Statistics concerning cases of infectious hepatitis admit the number given is not a true picture of the incidence. They are not accurate because

1. the disease is not reportable
2. most cases are misdiagnosed as mononucleosis
3. many children are anicteric and thus undiagnosed
4. there is no positive way of making a diagnosis

190. Many persons most probably are exposed to virus A as the result of contact with

1. contaminated household linens
2. contaminated blood or plasma
3. unpasteurized milk
4. a subclinical case

191. It is known that virus A, which causes infectious hepatitis, can be found in the feces of the patient or a carrier. Predisposing factors that would tend to increase the spread by the "anus-to-mouth" route include

a. use of an outdoor toilet
b. life along a large body of water, such as Lake Michigan
c. crowded living conditions
d. poor sanitary facilities

1. all except b
2. c only
3. c and d
4. all of the above

192. Epidemics of infectious hepatitis are often present in institutions responsible for the custodial care of individuals. A common source of contamination is

1. the drinking bubbler
2. the rectal thermometer
3. the community roller towel
4. the floor in the shower room

193. If there is a virus A carrier employed in a restaurant, one health habit that would probably prevent an epidemic outbreak is

1. thorough handwashing after each use of the toilet
2. routine covering of all coughs and sneezes
3. thorough evacuation of the bowel contents daily
4. complete cap, gown and mask technique

194. On the basis of the predisposing causes of infectious hepatitis, it is to be expected that the highest incidence would be among those

1. in low-income areas
2. working in communicable disease units
3. living in the northern states
4. with a hereditary predisposition

195. One symptom of infectious hepatitis that is most common in adults and seldom present in children is

1. fever
2. irritability
3. upper respiratory signs
4. anorexia

196. If it is given before the onset of symptoms, gamma globulin or immune globulin serum may be effective prophylaxis against

1. infectious hepatitis
2. serum hepatitis
3. mononucleosis
4. viral hepatitis

197. It is known that the incidence of hepatitis, A and B, is high among hospital personnel. One source of contamination that should be recognized and respected accordingly is

1. the needle used for any type of skin puncture
2. tissues soiled with nasal discharges
3. the rectal thermometer
4. the soiled bed pan or urinal

198. Serum hepatitis, or infection with virus B, can be transmitted only following

1. close person-to-person contact
2. the injection of the virus through puncture of the skin
3. contact with contaminated feces
4. a break in the nursing technique when a patient has infectious hepatitis

199. The death rate is higher following serum hepatitis than after an attack of infectious hepatitis. This is probably because

1. more young people have the disease
2. the symptoms make it almost impossible to supply the body nutrient needs
3. the disease is secondary to some illness requiring some type of injection
4. the virus is more toxic

200. Abdominal distress due to the inflammatory process in the liver may be present in

a. the epigastric region
b. the pyloric area
c. the perineal region
d. the upper right quadrant

1. any of the above
2. d only
3. a or d
4. all except c

201. Mrs. B. has a diagnosed case of hepatitis B. In an effort to determine the possible source of infection, the nurse or the doctor would question her in regard to any

a. solutions or blood received by I.V. in the last 6 months
b. medications received by hypo or I.M.
c. withdrawal of blood for examination purposes
d. recent tatooing

1. a only
2. all of the above
3. all except d
4. a or b

202. If we were to compare infectious hepatitis with serum hepatitis on the basis of onset, we would say that

1. serum hepatitis comes on more rapidly
2. the onset of infectious hepatitis is insidious
3. the onset of infectious hepatitis is more abrupt than the onset of serum hepatitis
4. the onset of both infectious hepatitis and serum hepatitis is characterized by jaundice

203. The jaundice that often accompanies viral hepatitis is caused by

1. viral irritation of liver cells
2. necrosis of liver cells
3. replacement of liver cells with scar tissue
4. pressure from the edema on the bile ducts

204. One symptom disappears or is greatly lessened once the jaundice appears. This symptom is

1. anorexia   3. fever
2. nausea   4. pain

205. The severer the jaundice, the more likely the patient will be greatly distressed by

1. clay-colored stools
2. pruritis
3. dark-colored urine
4. diarrhea

206. If one of the outstanding symptoms of hepatitis is swelling of the cervical lymph nodes, a common misdiagnosis is

1. mumps
2. Hodgkin's disease
3. tonsillitis
4. mononucleosis

207. If the patient with viral hepatitis cannot be kept from overactivity during the acute stage and for several weeks thereafter, the greatest danger will be

1. a relapse
2. a carrier condition
3. irreversible jaundice
4. cirrhosis of the liver

208. Death from viral hepatitis may be the result of

a. chronic hepatitis with progressive liver damage
b. intercurrent infection
c. suicide
d. infection with a very virulent strain of the virus

1. any of the above
2. all except c
3. d only
4. a, or b, or d

209. Maintenance of the blood sugar level above the point of hypoglycemia is the responsibility of the healthy liver. When the liver is busy trying to overcome hepatitis, it is essential that the food intake be more than adequate in

1. protein
2. vitamin C
3. carbohydrates
4. vitamin K

210. If the protein intake is not high enough to allow the liver cells to regenerate, recovery may be complicated by

1. formation of a liver abscess
2. achlorhydria
3. a complete failure to digest fats
4. the replacement of necrotic tissue with scar tissue

211. A symptom that can be expected to accompany prolonged nausea, vomiting, and anorexia is

1. diplopia
2. weight loss
3. hypotension
4. tenesmus

212. To be sure that the causative viruses of hepatitis are no longer capable of causing the disease, all contaminated articles must be

a. boiled at least 30 minutes
b. burned
c. autoclaved
d. destroyed and discarded

1. any of the above methods
2. c only
3. only b or c
4. b, or c, or d

213. Attempts to transfer mononucleosis from the infected person to volunteer humans or to animals have not been successful. Because this is true, it is very difficult to justify nursing care that insists on

1. disinfection of urine and feces
2. complete and absolute isolation technique
3. careful collection and burning of tissues contaminated with nose and throat secretions
4. isolation of the patient in a single room

214. The suspected method of passing on mononucleosis seems to coincide with the age group most often affected. These seem to be the years when one could expect increased

1. excesses
2. nutritional deficiencies
3. effect of daily tensions
4. close oral contact

215. The presence of petechiae may be the confirming factor of the diagnosis mononucleosis. The nurse would expect the doctor to look for this symptom

1. at the junction of the hard and soft palate
2. in the area of the spleen
3. on the extremities
4. along the conjunctiva

216. Immune serum globulin will be used

1. to prevent mononucleosis
2. to protect all contacts
3. to treat the symptoms of mononucleosis
4. to produce an immunity to mononucleosis

217. Most of the diseases accompanied by swollen cervical lymph glands would be ruled out because the swelling lasts 2 weeks or longer. It would be possible, however, for a sporadic case of mononucleosis to be mis-diagnosed as

1. pharyngitis
2. peritonsillar abscess
3. Hodgkin's disease
4. parotitis

218. A symptom that is always present in mononucleosis, if the doctor does enough examinations to find it, is

1. jaundice
2. enlargement of the spleen
3. pruritis
4. nausea, vomiting, and diarrhea

219. The symptoms of a ruptured spleen closely resemble those that accompany

1. chronic appendicitis
2. a perforated peptic ulcer
3. ulcerative colitis
4. bowel obstruction

220. Laboratory examinations that give information of value in the diagnosis of mononucleosis include

a. complete blood count (C.B.C.)
b. total white blood count
c. specific gravity tests
d. differential blood count

   1. b and d
   2. a only
   3. all except d
   4. all of the above

221. The severity of mononucleosis cannot be determined on the basis of

1. the objective symptoms
2. the subjective symptoms
3. the laboratory reports on the W.B.C.
4. the response to gamma globulin

222. Swelling of the spleen and rupture of the spleen in mononucleosis can be understood when it is remembered that the spleen is responsible for

1. screening all toxic substances
2. our reserve blood supply
3. manufacture and storage of lymphocytes
4. production of antibodies

PHARMACOLOGY AND DRUGS AND SOLUTIONS

(Answer sheets pp. 321–322)

Basic information on the understanding of various symbols and abbreviations needed to interpret written medical orders correctly is treated first, along with the metric and apothecary systems. General information concerning groups of drugs and specific drugs follows. Only those drugs in popular use are included, and no attempt is made to test the students' knowledge of the many variations of the basic drugs.

1. The convalescent patient will usually not need his temperature taken any oftener than B.I.D. You would expect to take his temperature

    1. at 8:00 A.M. and 8:00 P.M.
    2. after meals
    3. twice a day
    4. at bedtime

2. A teaspoon of medicine given in the home would be ordered in the hospital as ʒi. This would be measured as

    1. 1 c.c.
    2. 5 c.c.
    3. 15 c.c.
    4. 1 ounce

3. A bad-tasting medicine is often ordered c̄ aq. This directs the nurse

    1. to give as needed
    2. to give with meals
    3. to give the medicine in milk
    4. to give with water

4. A laxative ordered for H.S. is intended to be given

    1. after meals
    2. once only
    3. at bedtime
    4. 3 times a day

5. Before most surgical patients are discharged as recovered, the doctor will have written an order "Out of bed, ad. lib." The nurse would expect the patient

    1. to get out of bed whenever he wished
    2. to sit up in a chair for meals
    3. to get up for a tub bath
    4. to stay up all day

6. A T.I.D., a.c. medicine to stimulate the appetite should be given

    1. 30 minutes after each meal
    2. 30 minutes before each meal
    3. at mealtime, with the food
    4. before meals

7. An S.O.S. medication can be given

    1. whenever the patient's symptoms indicate a need for it
    2. if the patient requests it
    3. once only, if the nurse feels the patient needs it
    4. at bedtime, for relief of pain

8. A stat. medication is ordered to be given

    1. immediately
    2. only if the nurse can justify its need
    3. whenever the patient's symptoms are serious
    4. after first consulting the R.N. or the M.D.

9. A medicine ordered Q.I.D. will be given

    1. after meals
    2. well diluted with water
    3. at 8, 12, and 4
    4. at 8, 12, 4, and 8

10. A medicine ordered for q.6.h. will be be given

    1. at 8, 2, 8, and 2
    2. after meals and at bedtime
    3. only while the patient is awake
    4. at 2 and 8 A.M. and 2 P.M.

11. If the doctor orders soda bicarbonate gr. XV, and the strength on hand is 0.5 Gm., the nurse will find she needs to give the patient

    1. 1 tablet
    2. 2 tablets
    3. 3 tablets
    4. 5 tablets

12. An order for penicillin, 250,000 units, q.d., will be given

    1. every hour, starting with the time the order was noted
    2. by injection, deep into the muscle
    3. at bedtime
    4. once only, every day

13. A P.R.N. order for morphine gr. 1/4 (H) that has been given at 4:00 P.M. cannot, without special medical permission, be given again until

    1. 5:00 P.M.   3. 7:00 P.M.
    2. 6:00 P.M.   4. 8:00 P.M.

14. A medication ordered given q.4.h. must be given

    1. a.c.
    2. p.c.
    3. when it will do the patient the most good
    4. even if the patient must be awakened

15. If an average adult dose of a medicine is gr. i, the nurse could expect the child's dose to be about gr. ss, or

    1. 0.5 gram   3. 1/2 grain
    2. 1 c.c.   4. 3 minims

16. A pain-relieving medication is ordered P.R.N. when the doctor decides that the nurse is able

    1. to prepare and give hypodermic medicines
    2. to supervise the patient as he takes the medicine
    3. to determine when the patient needs the medicine
    4. to give the patient supportive nursing care

17. If the patient has stopped breathing, a stat. order for a stimulant will be given

    1. hypodermically
    2. immediately
    3. by the doctor
    4. at once and every 2 hours

18. Irritating oral medicines will be ordered given p.c. in order

    1. to increase the appetite
    2. to stimulate digestion
    3. to increase absorption from the stomach before food dilutes it
    4. to mix them with food in the stomach

19. A relaxing drug that is ordered as a T.I.D. and H.S. medication will be given

    1. at 8, 12, 4, and 8
    2. 3 times a day and at bedtime
    3. 30 minutes after meals and at 9:00 P.M.
    4. whenever the patient complains of feeling tense

20. The ʒ symbol means

    1. 1 dram   3. 1 c.c.
    2. 1 ounce   4. 1 gram

21. The meaning of the symbol s̄s̄ is

    1. take   3. one half
    2. one of each 4. at once

22. If the doctor wanted to give a patient 15 grains of medication, but wrote it in the metric system, it would read

    1. 0.5 Gm.   3. gram. 1.0
    2. 1 gram   4. 1.0 Gm.

23. If a fraction of a grain of morphine were ordered in the apothecary system, the order would be written

    1. gr. 1/4   3. 0.25 gr.
    2. Gm. 0.25   4. 1/4 Gm.

24. Seven and one half grains in the apothecary system is written in the metric system as

    1. gr. v̄īīs̄   3. 0.5 Gm.
    2. 1.0 Gm.   4. m. xv

25. When the doctor wants the patient to have a full ounce of medicine, the symbol he will use is

    1. ʒ̄   3. s̄s̄
    2. ʒ   4. m.

26. The symbol for the dram stands for

    1. a larger dose than the ounce symbol
    2. the same dose as the ounce symbol
    3. pouring drugs that are solid sub-
       stances
    4. a smaller dose than the ounce symbol

27. Fifteen grains of medication will equal
    the metric measurement of

    1. 1 ounce   3. 8 drams
    2. 1 gram   4. 1 minim

28. The liquid measure in the metric sys-
    tem is 1 c.c. The equivalent weight
    measure in this system is

    1. 5 minims   3. 1 gram
    2. 1 pint   4. 1 ounce

29. One milligram in the metric system
    has the same value in the apothecary
    measurement of

    1. 3 minims   3. gr. 1/60
    2. one c.c.   4. 0.064 gram

30. The ℥ symbol means

    1. 1 dram   3. 1 c.c.
    2. 1 ounce   4. 1 gram

31. The apothecary equivalent of 0.064
    Gm. is

    1. 1 grain   3. 1 dram
    2. 1 c.c.   4. 1 milligram

32. 0.5 Gm. is equal to

    1. 15 minims   3. 2 ounces
    2. 15 grains   4. gr. v̄īīss

33. Thirty c.c. poured into a medicine
    glass will equal

    1. 5 minims   3. 3 grams
    2. 1 dram   4. 1 ounce

34. A 1-quart measuring pitcher will hold

    1. 2000 c.c.   3. 1500 c.c.
    2. 4000 c.c.   4. 1000 c.c.

35. The liquid measurement equal to one
    grain of weight is

    1. 1 gram   3. 1 dram
    2. 1 c.c.   4. 1 minim

36. How many grains of medicine can be
    contained in one gram?

    1. 5   3. 15
    2. 10   4. 30

37. A pill containing 1 gram of medicine has
    the same value as the liquid measure of

    1. 1 minim   3. 1 pint
    2. 1 c.c.   4. 1 ounce

38. The apothecary equivalent of 1 c.c. of
    liquid is

    1. 4 to 5 minims   3. 10 minims
    2. 8 minims   4. 15 minims

39. One quart of solution is the same as

    1. 10 ounces   3. 1 gallon
    2. 2 pints   4. 15 minims

40. One pint of solution equals

    1. 2 quarts   3. 250 c.c.
    2. 4 ounces   4. 500 c.c.

41. If we figure 5 c.c. to a dram, there will be,
    in 1 ounce, an equivalent of

    1. 2 drams   3. 6 drams
    2. 4 drams   4. 8 drams

42. A 1-ounce measurement can be changed to
    the apothecary equal of

    1. 30 minims   3. 450 to 480 minims
    2. 150 minims   4. 1000 minims

43. The weight measure that is equal to the
    liquid minim is

    1. 1 grain
    2. 1 gram
    3. 1 c.c.
    4. 1 dram

44. A measuring pitcher filled to the 1000 c.c. mark will hold

1. 1 pint
2. 1 quart
3. 1 gallon
4. 1 dram

45. When an H.S. medication is ordered to provide rest and sleep for the patient, it should be given

1. before visiting hours
2. at 8:00 P.M.
3. following P.M. care
4. when the patient is ready to sleep

46. If the nurse gives a P.R.N. medication for the relief of pain, her charting responsibility will include

1. recording the name of the doctor writing the order
2. some notation on the narcotic record
3. some observation of the effects of the drug
4. a complete description of her method of preparation

47. A new medication considered a specific in treatment of thrush is

1. tr. myrrh
2. Tr. Merthiolate
3. Mycostatin
4. sulfacetamide

48. Medication must be applied very carefully to the lesions of thrush to prevent

1. toxic symptoms from too much medicine
2. upsetting baby's appetite
3. spreading the lesions
4. injury to the mucous membranes

49. Griseofulvin is a new medication that is taken orally yet it is effective in the treatment of ringworm. The fungus is killed when

1. the medication reaches the fungus by way of the blood stream
2. it invades the lymph vessels
3. it eats the cells of the epidermis that previously had absorbed the medicine
4. the medication leaves the body through the sweat glands

50. The application of medication to the lesions in the mouth is correctly described as

1. topical
2. parenteral
3. specific
4. systemic

51. Most of the patent-medicine ointments are not effective in the treatment of athlete's foot. The fungus is not destroyed because

1. it burrows into the epidermis and the medicine does not reach it
2. any medicine strong enough to kill the fungus will destroy the tissue
3. it is too difficult to keep the fungus in contact with the medicine constantly
4. it is anaerobic

52. Kwell or benzyl benzoate lotion may be applied to kill the itch mite. Directions for use will include

a. taking a hot, cleansing bath
b. covering surfaces of the body
c. keeping the medication away from the eyes
d. not bathing or changing clothes until the treatment is concluded

1. all of the above
2. a, c, and d
3. b and d
4. all except c

53. D.D.T. powder is effective in ridding a person of

1. the nits of scabies
2. nits and lice
3. only the male itch mite
4. all parasites

54. In the acute stage of erysipelas the patient would be given penicillin. The nurse could expect orders for

a. procaine penicillin, daily
b. aqueous penicillin G, q.3.h.
c. oral penicillin, tablets ii, T.I.D.
d. penicillin ointment, q.h.

1. b only
2. a and b
3. c and d
4. all of the above

55. A 3% vinegar solution is needed to loosen the nits of head lice. This will be prepared by

1. diluting household vinegar on a 1 to 3 ratio
2. measuring 30 c.c. vinegar and adding enough water to make 1000 c.c.
3. measuring 150 c.c. vinegar and adding it to 350 c.c. water
4. measuring 3 parts of vinegar for every 10 parts of water

56. If respiration is depressed, the burned patient would not be given

1. phenobarbital for sleep
2. morphine to relieve pain
3. codeine to relieve cough
4. oxygen by nasal catheter

57. When both orders are available, it is often up to the nurse to decide whether the medication needed by the burned patient is

1. a pain reliever
2. a narcotic or a sedative
3. a tranquilizer
4. a deodorant or a hyperemic

58. Adrenalin would be given in the emergency treatment of anaphylactic shock. This drug is valuable because of its rapid action as

1. a respiratory relaxant
2. a vasoconstrictor
3. a cardiac stimulant
4. a diuretic

59. An asthmatic attack would be treated with an antispasmodic medication. Such a medicine could be expected

1. to reduce nasal edema
2. to relax the smooth muscles of the bronchi and bronchioles
3. to produce mucus or to liquify thick mucus
4. to reduce emotional tensions and help the patient to relax

60. Elixer of terpin hydrate with codeine might be given during an asthmatic attack. It would act

1. to increase mucus production
2. to help the patient sleep
3. to relax the bronchioles and stop the wheeze
4. to control the cough reflex in the brain

61. Benadryl cannot be used as a daily medication to keep allergic symptoms under control. An unpleasant side effect of this drug which would make continuous administration undesirable is that of

1. dry mouth   3. drowsiness
2. diplopia   4. anorexia

62. A vasoconstrictor drug such as ephedrine is placed in the nose to relieve symptoms of sinusitis because

1. drainage is increased when the mucous membrane of the nose shrinks
2. less blood flowing to the head will lessen symptoms of pressure
3. the secretions are liquified and drain more easily
4. the heart does not pump so much blood to that area

63. Codeine is given to the patient with a continuous, unproductive cough for the purpose of

1. loosening the cough
2. allowing the patient to get some rest
3. putting the patient to sleep
4. relieving chest pains

64. The doctor will expect the pneumonia patient to receive ordered sulfa drugs

1. q.4.h. while the patient is awake
2. with a high fluid intake
3. q.4.h. day and night
4. and a diet restricted in salt

65. A medication often used for its expectorant effects is

1. codeine   3. ammonium chloride
2. chloroform   4. ephedrine

66. An <u>acutely ill</u> pneumonia patient needs to be given the kind of pencillin that is

1. absorbed rapidly in a 3-hour period
2. effective for 8 hours
3. absorbed slowly over 24 hours
4. effective when given with sulfa drugs

67. Codeine is effective in the relief of a cough because it acts on

1. the cough reflex in the brain
2. the swallowing reflex in the larynx
3. the mucous membrane of the bronchi
4. the alveoli directly

68. One purpose of an <u>expectorant</u> cough medicine is

1. to lower the cough reflex
2. to stop the symptoms
3. to reduce the swelling of the mucous membranes
4. to liquify the bronchial mucus

69. A cough medicine that is used to loosen mucus and stop tickling in the throat cannot be effective if it is given

1. with water
2. every time the patient coughs
3. when there is food in the stomach
4. while the patient is at rest

70. If you are ready to give a pneumonia patient a "stat." order of streptomycin and the patient says, "I hope that isn't streptomycin, I'm allergic to it", the practical nurse should recognize the need

1. to give the shot and report the comment of the patient to the head nurse
2. to do a sensitivity test and then give the medicine
3. to notify the doctor
4. to omit the dose until the doctor sees the patient

71. Lipoid pneumonia may follow the aspiration of

1. sputum   3. blood
2. fruit juices   4. oily nose drops

72. It will be easier to get the tonsillectomy patient to eat if the throat pains are relieved by

1. gargles before meals
2. the application of heat
3. Aspergum, chewed 1/2 hour before meals
4. preparatory intake of citrus-fruit juices

73. Morphine is used with great caution in the treatment of an elderly patient with a respiratory disease because this drug

1. decreases the cough
2. is addicting
3. causes mental confusion
4. decreases the expansion of lung tissue

74. An anticonvulsant medication taken to control <u>nocturnal</u> seizures would be given

1. after meals
2. with several glasses of fluid
3. dissolved in warm milk
4. at bedtime

75. Tridione has proven most effective in controlling the petit mal seizures of

1. mentally retarded children
2. adult males
3. adults with nocturnal seizures
4. children

76. Mysoline is widely used in the control of epileptic seizures because it

1. produces no toxic effects
2. is effective in all types of seizures
3. is easy to give parenterally
4. stops status epilepticus

77. The reason for urging the migraine patient to take her medicine as soon as the first warning of a headache appears is to give the medicine a chance

1. to test the cause of the headache
2. to prevent or shorten the attack
3. to lower the blood pressure
4. to take effect before nausea begins

78. Oral Cafergot is of value only during the early stages of the attack. Once the person becomes nauseated, he must take the Cafergot by

    1. hypodermic   3. I.V.
    2. I.M.   4. suppository

79. When patients with Parkinson's disease are placed on the newer medications such as Artane and Rabellon, the doctor must depend upon the nurse to know and recognize the toxic symptoms of these drugs because

    1. an overdose may prove fatal
    2. the dosage is gradually increased until toxic symptoms appear
    3. the symptoms increase if the patient gets too much medicine
    4. the nurse is responsible for regulating the dose

80. An unpleasant side effect of the administration of belladonna preparations, such as atropine, in the control of symptoms of Parkinson's disease is

    1. dizziness
    2. ringing in the ears
    3. dry mouth
    4. bleeding gums

81. Drugs such as Tolserol and Artane are effective in some patients with Parkinson's disease because they

    1. control all of the undesirable symptoms
    2. act as mental stimulants
    3. lessen muscle rigidity
    4. improve the emotional outlook

82. An anticonvulsant drug like Dilantin is better than phenobarbital for most mentally normal epileptics because it

    1. will cure the epilepsy
    2. limits the seizures to the sleep period
    3. does not make the patient drowsy
    4. is easier to swallow in capsule form

83. Control of seizures in a newly diagnosed epileptic may be a matter of trial and error. The nurse will need to reassure such a patient that he will

    1. soon get complete relief from his seizures
    2. probably have to try several drugs in various dosages
    3. probably get only the newer medications
    4. have more severe reactions to the medicine until he develops a tolerance

84. The nurse would report symptoms indicating a toxic reaction to Dilantin. The most common of these symptoms would be

    1. headache and blurred vision
    2. hypertrophy and bleeding of the gums
    3. constant drowsiness and confusion
    4. acnelike rash and hematuria

85. When the epileptic develops toxic symptoms from Dilantin, the doctor will usually decrease the drug and add small amounts of

    1. bromide   3. phenobarbital
    2. Nembutal   4. Tridione

86. To lessen the irritation of the stomach when the patient is on regular doses of Dilantin, the nurse should be sure to give the medicine with

    1. large amounts of cream
    2. sodium bicarbonate
    3. at least 1/2 glass water
    4. fruit juices

87. The patient who has had almost any type of orthopedic surgery has pain great enough to require use of

    1. morphine or Demerol
    2. aspirin compound
    3. an antispasmodic
    4. tranquilizers

88. Early symptoms of toxic effects from high dosages of aspirin include

    1. change of voice and growth of facial hair
    2. gastritis and flatulence
    3. psychotic behavior
    4. ringing in the ears and deafness

89. In the combination of aspirin and sodium bicarbonate given to the arthritic the aspirin is given

   1. to reduce the pain
   2. increase the benefits of the sodium bicarbonate
   3. quiet the nerves
   4. control the fever

90. The many patent medicines available at a great variety of prices to treat arthritis are chiefly

   1. ineffective
   2. unsafe
   3. only an unreasonably priced form of salicylate
   4. considered valuable by those who have been cured by them

91. Chronic osteomyelitis with its multiple abscesses could be prevented by treating the acute stage with

   1. an anesthetic injected into the bone shaft
   2. skin traction on the part
   3. enough activity to keep the blood circulation stimulated
   4. large doses of penicillin

92. The antipyretic action of sodium salicylate makes the patient in an acute attack of arthritis more comfortable by

   1. fighting the infection
   2. absorbing the inflammation
   3. reducing the fever
   4. changing the acid-base balance

93. The arthritic patient who gets relief of symptoms from cortisone must also have information that will prepare her to expect

   1. her menstrual periods to become irregular
   2. symptoms of overdose that are worse than the arthritic symptoms
   3. return of symptoms shortly after discontinuing the drug
   4. the effects of the drug to decrease gradually

94. Meticortone has the benefits of Cortone but has the advantage of

   1. being easier to take
   2. decreased cost
   3. producing no toxic effects
   4. fewer side effects

95. The patient with rheumatoid arthritis should understand that cortisone or ACTH will probably relieve the painful symptoms

   1. with no deformity
   2. within 48 hours
   3. for only a brief period
   4. and lead to a cure after a few months

96. Cortisone is given in dosages of 100 milligrams per day until the symptoms are relieved. The patient is then placed on

   1. a week of medication, 10 days rest, then repeat
   2. a maintenance dose
   3. slowly absorbing preparation once a month
   4. the maximum amount the patient can tolerate without toxic symptoms

97. During an acute attack of arthritis the nurse on the morning shift could expect to give the patient aspirin in an amount totaling

   1. 10 milligrams   3. 45 grains
   2. 500 milligrams   4. 3.0 grams

98. A diuretic medication increases the output of urine because of its ability

   a. to draw tissue fluid into the blood stream
   b. constrict the capillaries in the glomeruli
   c. prevent the reabsorption of a greater amount of water
   d. increase the glomerular filtrate

   1. all of the above
   2. d only
   3. a, c, or d
   4. a or d

99. Before moleskin is used on the patient in skin traction, tincture of benzoin painted on the skin is useful in

  1. lessening skin irritation
  2. removing tiny body hairs
  3. slowing up the hair growth
  4. sterilization of the skin

100. The patient who has just been put in a full body cast because of multiple fractures will need an injection of morphine gr. 1/4. Tablets on hand are of a strength gr. 1/6. The nurse will prepare and give the hypodermic in the following way:

  1. Dissolve one tablet morphine gr. 1/6 in m. 15 sterile distilled water. Discard m. 5. Give the patient m. 10 to equal the ordered gr. 1/4.
  2. Dissolve 2 tablets morphine gr. 1/6 in m. 20 sterile distilled water. Discard m. 5. Give the patient m. 15 to equal the ordered gr. 1/4.
  3. Dissolve one tablet morphine gr. 1/4 in 60 c.c. sterile distilled water. Give the patient 2 1/2 c.c. to equal the ordered gr. 1/6.
  4. Dissolve two tablets morphine gr. 1/6 in m. 12 sterile distilled water. Give the patient m. 12 to equal the ordered gr. 1/4.

101. Whenever a medication is ordered for its diuretic effect, the nurse should understand, without a doctor's written order, the importance of

  1. forcing fluids
  2. placing the patient on bed rest
  3. measuring all fluid output
  4. sending a daily urine specimen

102. Regardless of the cause of the cystitis, sodium bicarbonate may be given for the purpose of

  1. applying an antiseptic to the bladder walls
  2. making the urine alkaline to relieve burning on voiding
  3. stimulating the production of body defenses
  4. increasing the urinary output and thus diluting the urine

103. The nurse must know the special characteristics of each sulfa drug she gives in the treatment of urinary diseases so that she will understand

  1. why the prescribed dose is ordered
  2. the importance of asking the patient frequently to describe his symptoms
  3. what medication changes she can recommend to bring symptomatic relief
  4. the need to increase, or decrease, fluid intake or hold it at normal level

104. The patient with severe uremia will be given epsom salts B.I.D. to allow

  1. the elimination of accumulated wastes through the feces
  2. an increased fluid intake to prevent dehydration
  3. the reaction of the blood to remain acid
  4. fluid to be drawn from brain tissue and prevent confusion and delirium

105. Ammonium chloride is given to the patient receiving methenamine (Urotropin) because it provides

  1. increased permeability of the tubules
  2. a dissolving agent necessary to make the Urotropin effective
  3. an acid urine, necessary for the medicine to be effective
  4. a neutralizing agent that prevents toxic reactions

106. The ready solubility of Gantrisin makes it quite safe to use in the treatment of urinary infections with fear of

  1. severe toxic reaction
  2. crystalluria starting stone formation
  3. changing the color of the urine
  4. eliminating it through perspiration

107. Gantrisin does not have to be given in combination with other medication because it is effective

  1. only in the production of urine
  2. in an acid or an alkaline urine
  3. as a urinary antiseptic
  4. only when it can coat the mucous membrane

108. A daily blood count should be done on a patient receiving Gantrisin over a long period of time in order to determine when the drug begins to

    1. cause a leukocytosis
    2. stimulate the production of an excess of blood cells
    3. affect the blood-producing organs
    4. destroy the hemoglobin content of the red blood cells

109. Sodium bicarbonate is effective in controlling the multiplication of the colon bacillus in the bladder because

    1. the organisms die when the sodium coagulates their protoplasm
    2. they are anaerobic germs
    3. the organisms grow only in an acid urine
    4. the increased urine output keeps pushing the germs from the bladder

110. Diuril is an effective diuretic in nephrosis because the tubules are able

    1. to work more rapidly when stimulated by the drug
    2. to eliminate more salt and therefore more water
    3. to be more selective in the substances filtered from the blood
    4. to keep the output in balance with the fluid intake

111. The caffeine group of diuretics are considered stimulant diuretics because they act by

    1. stimulating the tubule cells
    2. increasing peristalsis of the ureters
    3. stimulating the nerve supply to the bladder
    4. increasing the supply of blood through the glomeruli

112. Women with menstrual difficulties are often given a medication known as testosterone. This medicine is

    1. one of the female sex hormones
    2. the male sex hormone
    3. a pituitary extract
    4. a product of the gonads

113. Gastric distress is lessened when ammonium chloride is given

    a. with enough water for good dilution
    b. along with sodium bicarbonate
    c. by using an enteric-coated tablet
    d. at mealtime

        1. all of the above
        2. c only
        3. a, b, and d
        4. a, c, and d

114. Mercurial diuretics cannot be used when the glomeruli are inflamed because

    1. they increase the acid reaction of the urine
    2. an overdose produces poisonous effects
    3. the irritating effects of the mercury increase the kidney damage
    4. they remove too many solids from the blood stream, thus concentrating the urine

115. Diamox is an effective oral diuretic. It produces its effect by lessening the activity of the kidney tubules which results in

    1. a decrease in fluids reabsorbed from the tubule
    2. a retention of sodium and potassium in the blood stream
    3. an increase in the sugar content of the urine
    4. failure of the glomeruli to filter out as much water from the blood

116. The ordered dose of Theelin 1.0 milligram is equal to

    1. 1.0 c.c.   3. 1/1000 gram
    2. 1.0 gram   4. 1/500 grain

117. Most estrogenic substances are ordered in milligram dosages because

    1. the substances are poisonous
    2. it is so expensive to prepare them
    3. the toxic symptoms may be fatal
    4. the substances are so potent only a small amount is needed

118. The estrogenic substances given to the senile patient with vaginitis are effective because they

1. kill the causative organisms
2. restore the normal pH to vaginal secretions
3. stimulate hormone production
4. stop the pruritis

119. If dysmenorrhea is due to spasms of the muscles of the uterus, a most effective medication would be a form of

1. analgesic   3. emetic
2. antacid   4. antispasmodic

120. The undesirable reactions that accompany treatment of menopausal symptoms with stilbestrol affect

1. the gastrointestinal tract
2. the nervous system
3. the circulatory system
4. the endocrine system

121. Most patent medicines for the relief of dysmenorrhea are effective because they contain

1. narcotics
2. sedatives
3. aspirin preparations
4. male or female sex hormones

122. Medications to treat senile vaginitis would be most effectively administered by

1. mouth   3. intramuscularly
2. hypodermic   4. suppository

123. Undesirable effects of continued treatment of menstrual disorders with testosterone include

1. the appearance of masculine characteristics
2. nausea, vomiting, headache
3. dermatitis
4. an increase of menstrual flow

124. Pyrodoxine may be given the patient receiving deep X-ray therapy because of its value in

1. building up a tolerance to the X-ray
2. making the X-ray more effective
3. stimulating the appetite
4. relieving or preventing nausea

125. An estrogenic substance that is mixed with oil would be given

1. I.M.   3. I.V.
2. orally   4. by suppository

126. If the doctor wanted to prevent a patient from having a bowel movement for several days following repair of a cystocele and rectocele, he might effectively order

1. emetine   3. paregoric
2. Pro-Banthine   4. Furadantin

127. Mycostatin is considered specific in the treatment of

1. trichomonas vaginitis
2. senile vaginitis
3. moniliasis
4. cervicitis

128. Administration of the male sex hormone testosterone is intended to affect the breast cancer in the female by

1. causing it to atrophy
2. preventing metastasis
3. localizing the cancer cells so that complete removal is possible
4. neutralizing the female sex hormone that stimulates the cancer-cell growth

129. The nurse must appreciate that any hormone-type drug must be prescribed

1. for the rest of the person's life
2. according to the physiological needs of the individual
3. for only brief periods of time, with rest periods between courses
4. in gradually increasing doses

130. An iodine solution should be given in milk or fruit juice because

1. the taste of the drug is unpleasant
2. it irritates the lining of the stomach
3. the effects of the drug are increased
4. it destroys the teeth

131. Thyroid preparations given to the patient with myxedema will begin to be effective within

1. 24 hours
2. 5 to 7 days
3. 2 weeks
4. 3 months

132. Antithyroid medications are usually taken for several months before any results are apparent. This is because they are not effective until

1. the body builds up a tolerance to it
2. the blood stream is saturated
3. all the stored thyroxin has been used
4. the drug is absorbed into the lymphatic system

133. It is most important that the nurse follow an injection of insulin by

1. checking the insulin order
2. charting the injection in red ink
3. checking the time the last dose was given
4. charting the location of the injection

134. Oral medications, such as Orinase, cannot correctly be called

1. effective
2. oral insulin
3. synthetic preparations
4. safe for older diabetics

135. The doctor has ordered 60 units of insulin. You have on hand 80 units of insulin and a 2-c.c. hypodermic syringe with which to give it. It will be correct to give

1. 1/2 c.c. of U. 80 insulin
2. 3/4 c.c. of U. 80 insulin
3. 1-1/2 c.c. of U. 80 insulin
4. 12 minims of U. 80 insulin

136. The reason many diabetics get a prebreakfast dose of crystalline or regular insulin plus the protamine zinc insulin is to allow

1. the dosage of protamine insulin to be reduced
2. a lessened expense to the patient
3. some insulin to be quickly available to act on the CHO of the breakfast
4. a slower absorption rate of the protamine insulin

137. When the nurse is assigned to clean out the ward refrigerator containing medications, it is most important to check the insulin boxes for

1. the amount of insulin left in each bottle
2. the color of the insulin
3. the expiration date
4. the odor of the insulin

138. If two types of insulin are being mixed in one syringe, the first type of insulin to be drawn into the syringe should be

1. the long-acting insulin
2. figured for the individual patient
3. the regular insulin
4. the larger dose

139. Ordered - insulin U 25. Strength on hand - U. 40. Syringe available - insulin U 40. It will be correct to measure

1. 10 minims   3. 0.6 c.c.
2. 25 units   4. 50 units

140. The nurse has a 40-80 insulin syringe. Insulin strength on hand is 80 units. Ordered dosage 20 units. If the nurse fills the syringe to the U-20 mark on the 40-unit side of the syringe her mistake will be in giving the patient

1. twice as much as is ordered
2. half as much as is ordered
3. an overdose
4. an incorrect amount

141. Insulin given by I.V. in an emergency must be

   1. rapid acting
   2. regular, aqueous insulin
   3. fortified with zinc crystals
   4. long lasting in its effects

142. Dosage ordered — U 70. Strength on hand — U 80. Syringe available — 2-c.c. hypodermic syringe. It will be correct to measure

   1. 1/2 c.c. of U 80 insulin
   2. 1-1/2 c.c. of U 80 insulin
   3. 3/4 c.c. of U 80 insulin
   4. 14 minims of U 80 insulin

143. Dosage ordered — U 42. Insulin on hand — U 80. Syringe available — insulin syringe U 40 calibration. It will be correct to measure

   1. U 21   3. 22.5 units
   2. U 25   4. U 20

144. Information on the label of a bottle of insulin will tell the nurse

   a. the kind of insulin in the bottle
   b. the peak of effects
   c. the number of units per cubic centimeter
   d. an expiration date
      1. all of the above
      2. a and c
      3. b, c, or d
      4. all except b

145. The dosage range safest for the patient receiving insulin is

   1. 4 to 12 minims 3. 32 minims
   2. 8 to 20 minims 4. 40 to 80 units

146. Protamine zinc insulin is kept in the refrigerator. Its desired effectiveness will depend on the nurse's knowledge of the need

   1. to shake the bottle before drawing out the dose
   2. to warm the bottle under the hot water faucet before removing the insulin
   3. to distribute evenly the particles of the suspension before withdrawing the dosage
   4. to prepare the dosage quickly before the insulin has a chance to warm up

147. The diabetic who receives insulin will have a late evening snack prescribed if

   1. he feels hungry at bedtime
   2. his diet is high in CHO
   3. a slow-acting insulin, such as protamine, is used
   4. he frequently goes into coma

148. One characteristic of protamine zinc insulin that will influence the preparation of the dosage is its ability

   1. to become cloudy
   2. to separate into layers
   3. to bubble
   4. to clog the needle

149. Regular or crystalline insulin will be circulating in the bloodstream and ready to begin action in about

   1. 5 to 10 minutes   3. 30 to 45 minutes
   2. 15 to 20 minutes   4. 2 hours

150. Special precautions are stressed when a long-acting and a short-acting insulin are combined in one syringe to avoid the need for two separate injections. The greatest concern is to prevent

   1. precipitation of the insulin
   2. mixing the insulins in the stock bottle
   3. contaminating the needle
   4. injuring the tissue at the site of injection

151. Diabetes has responded best to Orinase in patients

   1. under 10 years of age
   2. 15 to 40 years old
   3. of the male sex
   4. over 40 years of age

152. Insulin is effective in the control of diabetes because it

   1. prevents accumulation of carbohydrates
   2. neutralizes carbohydrate
   3. lowers blood sugar by aiding metabolism of carbohydrates
   4. prevents fats from being changed to glucose

153. When the nurse teaches the patient how to prepare and give his own insulin injections, she must stress the importance of

1. rotating the insulin bottle
2. figuring the dosage in minims
3. keeping the needle and syringe sterile
4. always taking the insulin as soon as he gets up

154. The patient should be advised to wear dark glasses to protect his eyes from photophobia when eye drops are used that are classified as

1. mydriatics
2. miotics
3. atropines
4. antiseptics

155. Before the tonometer is used, eye drops will be placed in the eye that will

1. dilate the pupil
2. contract the pupil
3. relax the muscles
4. anesthetize the cornea

156. Since eye medications can produce a serious effect if not properly given, the nurse would need to check carefully

1. the appearance of the solution
2. her equipment
3. the patient's blood pressure
4. the corneal reflexes

157. If a blind person had to be responsible for taking his own oral medications at home, the only safe way to avoid a mix-up would be

1. to have each medicine in a bottle of different size and shape
2. to package the medicines in individual doses
3. to have the visiting nurse supervise him
4. to order harmless drugs

158. It would be most dangerous to the glaucoma patient to have the nurse mistakenly use eye drops that would

1. contract the pupil
2. dilate the pupil
3. change the shape of the iris
4. irritate the sclera

159. The control of glaucoma in its early stages can often be done by the use of

1. exercises to speed up the absorption of aqueous humor
2. surgery to provide a greater area for the outflow of aqueous humor
3. eye drops to dilate the pupil
4. Diamox to slow down the inflow of aqueous humor

160. Since glaucoma is a chronic condition, Diamox is considered useful in treatment because it can be applied

1. safely by the lay person
2. over a period of years with only unpleasant rather than toxic symptoms
3. without a doctor's prescription
4. in a wide variety of disease conditions with a high degree of success

161. Dizziness and nausea will follow the fenestration operation. This can be relieved by use of

1. gingerale
2. penicillin
3. Dramamine
4. Terramycin

162. Excoriation of the skin covering the auricle of the ear can be prevented when purulent drainage is excessive. Preparations best able to protect the skin are

1. aluminum paste and Gelusil
2. Merthiolate or mercurochrome
3. petrolatum and zinc oxide
4. rubbing alcohol or body lotion

163. Mastoiditis could probably be prevented if at the beginning of an upper respiratory disease the child is given prophylactic doses of

1. sulfa drugs
2. penicillin
3. Neo-Synephrine
4. salicylates

164. A sedative drug that would be safe to give an infant 8 to 10 weeks old following repair of a cleft lip is

1. syrup of codeine
2. paregoric
3. aspirin compound
4. elixir of phenobarbital

165. Following a tracheotomy it would not be safe to attempt to ease the patient's discomfort with injections of

1. morphine or codeine
2. sodium phenobarbital
3. an analgesic
4. a hypnotic

166. Wax in the ear may be softened and removed by

a. cotton applicators
b. hydrogen peroxide drops
c. Cerumenex or Kerid
d. soda bicarbonate solution irrigation
   1. a and d
   2. b or c and d
   3. a, b, and d
   4. b only

167. Diseases of the middle ear and the inner ear must, because of their anatomical structure, be treated with medications that

1. produce direct effects
2. circulate in the blood stream
3. affect the nerve endings in the ear
4. can be placed in the external auditory canal

168. Drugs that do not produce toxic effects when used to treat the digestive tract are those that

1. are given with plenty of water
2. are not absorbed from the stomach or intestines
3. are absorbed only in an alkaline environment
4. are eliminated from the body too rapidly

169. A medication classed as an antacid is given in conditions that produce

1. increased peristalsis
2. irritation of the intestinal mucous membrane
3. excessive flatus
4. gastric juices of a high acidity

170. In the presence of an ulcer or a cancer in the stomach irritation is decreased if the nurse will remember

1. to place all tablets in a smooth capsule
2. to crush tablets before administration
3. to accompany all medicines with sodium bicarbonate
4. to give medicines only when there is food in the stomach

171. Dramamine or Bonamine are medications that can be obtained without a prescription for the relief of

1. motion sickness   3. diarrhea
2. constipation   4. flatulence

172. Some of the distress of a peptic ulcer is relieved by Banthine or Pro-Banthine because of their ability to decrease

1. secretion of bile
2. nausea and vomiting
3. stomach peristalsis
4. the raw surface of the ulcer

173. Banthine is an example of a drug classified as

1. an antacid   3. an emetic
2. a digestant   4. an antispasmodic

174. Emotional tension would be lessened if one of the medications prescribed for the ulcer patient contained

1. a stimulant   3. a cathartic
2. a sedative   4. an appetizer

175. The temporary relief of stomach pains provided by baking soda or a commercial preparation such as Tums comes from their ability

1. to coat the ulcer
2. to put something in the stomach so the lining walls do not rub together
3. to act on the pain center in the brain
4. to neutralize the gastric juices

176. The patient with cancer of the stomach may die as a result of his self-medication. This most often occurs because the cancer victim

1. takes an overdose
2. gets enough relief to keep him from seeing a doctor
3. speeds the metastasis of the cancer
4. is unable to digest his food

177. A medication from the group classified as antacids will be given in disease conditions that produce

1. increased peristalsis
2. irritation of the intestinal mucous membrane
3. excessive flatus
4. gastric juices of a high acidity

178. Medications cannot relieve the pain and stomach distress of an ulcer unless the nurse is always careful

1. to explain the action of the drug
2. to hide the fact that a medicine is being given
3. to give the medicine promptly at the stated time intervals
4. to hold the medication until the stomach is empty

179. Aluminum hydroxide gel (Amphojel) is used in the medical treatment of a gastric ulcer because it

1. stimulates healing
2. forms a protective coating over a raw surface
3. constipates the patient
4. produces a vasoconstriction

180. Aluminum hydroxide gel (Amphojel), used to neutralize hydrochloric acid in the stomach, must be given

1. a.c.   3. q.i.d.
2. p.c.   4. q.h.

181. Even though the doctor orders dilute hydrochloric acid, the nurse must still give it to the patient

1. through a gavage tube
2. with false teeth or no teeth
3. in one-half glass of water
4. daily, before breakfast

182. The group of medications given because they stimulate vomiting is known as

1. anthelmintics
2. analgesics
3. enterics
4. emetics

183. Atropine will be given the baby with pylorospasm for the purpose of

1. relieving nausea and vomiting
2. contracting the cardiac sphincter of the stomach
3. relaxing the muscle spasm
4. stimulating gastric secretions

184. The earliest sign of atropine toxicity is

1. dilated pupils   3. jaundice
2. diarrhea   4. flushed skin

185. Phenobarbital is often given the baby suffering with pylorospasm for its

1. stimulating effects
2. sedative effects
3. healing properties
4. antiemetic effects

186. The person who takes mineral oil regularly over a considerable period of time will be annoyed by its tendency to

1. lose its effect
2. produce indigestion
3. leak from the anus
4. produce a diarrhea

187. Epsom salts is an example of a saline cathartic that acts by

1. irritating the lower bowel
2. increasing peristalsis
3. lubricating the content of the bowel
4. drawing water from the tissues into the bowel

188. A candylike cathartic that may produce severe results in children if they get an overdose is

1. castor oil
2. Ex-Lax
3. Petrogalar
4. cascara

189. Castor oil should be kept on ice because it

1. changes color
2. loses its strength
3. becomes rancid
4. becomes more concentrated

190. A good way to hide the unpleasant taste of castor oil is

1. to put ice chips in the glass
2. to put it between layers of orange juice
3. to give it per rectum
4. to enteric-coat it

191. Sulfa drugs used before surgery on the intestines are considered antiseptic because they

1. sterilize the operative area
2. build up the resistance of the patient to infection
3. reduce the number of bacteria in the intestine
4. flush out the entire bowel

192. Sulfasuxidine and Sulfathaladine can be effective without forcing fluids because their action is dependent on their

1. stimulation of peristalsis
2. coating of a lesion
3. diluting the gastric juice
4. high concentration in the intestine

193. Daily use of a harsh laxative will

1. cause hemorrhoids
2. cause a loss of appetite
3. be irritating to the entire body
4. lower the ability of the bowel to act for itself

194. Nupercaine ointment, applied to hemorrhoids for the relief of pain, would be classified as

1. an antipyretic   3. an antiseptic
2. a hypnotic   4. an analgesic

195. An antidiarrheic that acts by slowing up intestinal peristalsis is

1. paregoric   3. charcoal
2. Kaolin   4. hexylresorcinal

196. A jaundiced patient would be given vitamin K before and after surgery because this vitamin will supply

1. the antiseptic needed to prevent infection
2. the material needed to return the skin to its normal color
3. the material that is necessary for the blood to clot
4. the stimulus for the gallbladder to contract and free the bile

197. The nurse should be sure to explain to the patient who is receiving Priodax in preparation for gallbladder X-ray that he may feel

1. dizzy
2. constipated
3. weak and lethargic
4. nauseated

198. Vitamin K must be given to the jaundice patient by I.M. because

1. vomiting results from the gastric distress produced by the oral route
2. it is never effective by any other route
3. the process of digestion changes its structure
4. it is not absorbed from the intestine in the absence of bile

199. If vitamin K is not available to the liver, any disease will be further complicated by the danger of

1. generalized ecchymosis
2. the increased clotting time
3. avitaminosis
4. disturbance of the electrolyte balance

200. Since morphine increases the contraction of the gallbladder, its use in gallbladder colic must be accompanied by

1. atropine to relax the muscles
2. an antidiarrheic
3. vitamin K to control hemorrhage
4. phenobarbital to produce a sedative effect

201. The patient with ascites may be given a diuretic medication in an attempt

 1. to stop the infection
 2. to increase fluid output through the urinary system
 3. to prevent the escape of fluids
 4. to produce a diarrhea

202. If the nurse gave Synkamine, a vitamin K preparation, but forgot to give the bile salts ordered, the result would be

 1. extreme discomfort
 2. toxic reaction
 3. an emergency situation requiring a transfusion
 4. failure of vitamin K to absorb from the intestines

203. Dilute HCl will be given to the patient through a drinking tube to prevent

 1. staining the teeth
 2. aspiration
 3. refusal because of the bad taste
 4. formation of ulcers in the mouth

204. Dilute HCl, a.c., is given to the anemic patient for the purpose of

 1. aiding the absorption of vitamins from the stomach
 2. making the liver extract more effective
 3. lessening gastric symptoms
 4. stimulating the action of the liver

205. Liver extract is not the only medication useful in treating pernicious anemia. Another medication that is just as effective is

 1. folic acid
 2. vitamin B_{12}
 3. glutamic acid
 4. protamine zinc insulin

206. Ascorbic acid is often given with ferrous sulfate in the treatment of one type of anemia because it

 1. prevents gastric distress
 2. stimulates the reproduction of cells
 3. increases the absorption of iron
 4. increases the appetite

207. After daily doses of liver extract have built up the blood, the doctor will order

 1. all medications stopped
 2. daily liver in the diet to prevent further symptoms
 3. a maintenance dose
 4. hospitalization for liver extract twice a year to keep the patient well

208. The patient who receives ferrous sulfate should expect to find a change in

 1. the color of the feces
 2. emotional outlook
 3. skin texture
 4. the color of the whites of the eyes

209. The dosage of vitamin B_{12} is higher if it is given

 1. by rectum   3. intramuscularly
 2. orally   4. subcutaneously

210. More benefit is received from liver extract when it is given

 1. by mouth   3. intramuscularly
 2. sublingually   4. by rectum

211. The label on the bottle of liver extract will inform the nurse of

 a. the number of cubic centimeters to give
 b. the need to keep it refrigerated
 c. the expiration date of effectiveness
 d. the grams of medication per cubic centimeter

  1. all of the above
  2. b and c
  3. b only
  4. a, b, and d

212. The patient with pernicious anemia must fully recognize that neither iron, B_{12}, nor liver extract will

 1. relieve the major symptoms
 2. increase the hemoglobin level
 3. relieve the anorexia
 4. cure the disease

213. If the patient with pernicious anemia fails to continue with medication as prescribed, the result of a relapse is

1. prolonged hospitalization and delirium
2. coma, convulsions, and death
3. central nervous sytem damage that cannot be repaired
4. extreme pain relieved only by narcotics

214. The patient may rightly prefer injections of vitamin B_{12} rather than liver injections because B_{12} is

1. painless
2. cheap
3. not affected by lack of refrigeration
4. easily administered by the nurse

215. An extract from the liver of animals contains the antianemia factor. The body needs this factor for the purpose of

1. stimulating the reuse of hemoglobin from worn out cells
2. adequately manufacturing R.B.C. in the bone marrow
3. keeping a balance between R.B.C. and W.B.C.
4. increasing the absorption of essential nutrients from the intestines

216. The missing intrinsic factor may be replaced orally by giving the patient

1. dried hog stomach
2. iron preparations such as Feosol
3. dilute HCl
4. an extract of pancreatic juice

217. The medication given to supply the extrinsic factor that is normally supplied by the diet is

1. dessicated hog stomach
2. Blaud's pills
3. vitamin B_{12}
4. hydrochloric acid

218. Once the blood picture and the symptoms of pernicious anemia have improved with liver injections, the maintenance dose would probably be

1. 1 c.c. I.M. daily
2. 1 c.c. at weekly intervals
3. 10 c.c. I.M. every 2 weeks
4. 1 to 2 c.c., I.M., per month

219. The dosage of liver injection is not standard. The nurse may need to reassure patients that variations in dosage occur according to

a. the age of the patient
b. the extent of the symptoms
c. socioeconomic status
d. blood levels

    1. all of the above
    2. d only
    3. b and c
    4. a or b

220. Some improvement of the symptoms of pernicious anemia can be expected as soon as

1. the blood stream absorbs the medication
2. the patient learns the value of moderation
3. 48 hours after I.M. injection of liver
4. the appetite increases

221. Intramuscular injections of liver must be given

1. deep in the gluteal muscle
2. in the anterior aspect of the thighs
3. into the subcutaneous fat
4. into the deltoid muscle group

222. The patient may object to semimonthly or monthly I.M. injections of liver because of

1. the inconvenience
2. the local pain and tenderness
3. the embarrassment of exposure
4. the added cost of nursing services

223. Oral iron preparations should be given

1. a.c.
2. p.c.
3. with meals
4. between meals

224. If the symptoms of pernicious anemia are well advanced before treatment is started, the patient and his family must understand that no amount of medication will bring about the disappearance of

1. the red, raw tongue
2. achlorhydria
3. respiratory and circulatory symptoms
4. the neurological symptoms

225. If the patient complains of gastric distress in spite of the time the iron preparation is given, it may be necessary for the doctor to change the form of the medication to one that

1. is enteric-coated
2. can be given parenterally
3. is easily dissolved in gastric juices
4. can be hidden in food

226. The patient receiving iron medications should be instructed to expect gastro-intestinal changes such as

a. flatulence
b. diarrhea
c. constipation
d. black, tarry stools

1. all of the above
2. b and c and d
3. a and c
4. d and b or c

227. Iron preparations, used alone, are of value only in the treatment of

1. iron deficiency anemias
2. posthemorrhage deficiency
3. pernicious anemia
4. nutritional deficiencies

228. The patient who receives iron preparations should be taught the importance of reporting any gastric distress. The patient should be reassured that this complaint is

1. serious
2. evidence of a toxic reaction to the drug
3. used as a guide to establish effective dosage
4. an indication that the medication is producing the desired results

229. The patient who takes oral iron preparations is instructed to brush his teeth frequently. If he does not, the result will be

1. toothache
2. rapid decay
3. bleeding and hypertrophy of the gums
4. discoloring deposits on the teeth and gums

230. Even a small dose of ferrous sulfate will produce nausea and vomiting if it is given

1. on an empty stomach
2. well diluted
3. in enteric-coated form
4. during the meal

231. Ventriculin is a powder. To prepare it to give to a patient, the nurse is instructed

1. to dissolve it in water or orange juice
2. to place it in empty gelatin capsules
3. to mix it with food
4. to give it while it effervesces

232. The blood-building drugs are classi-fied as

1. analgesics   3. anticoagulants
2. hematinics   4. antacids

233. Nitrogen mustard is effective in con-trolling the progress of leukemia and Hodgkin's disease because it acts on cells

1. produced by the red bone marrow
2. that are rapidly and abnormally multiplying
3. that circulate in the blood stream
4. with deficient hemoglobin

234. The nurse who must prepare nitrogen mustard for I.V. use must know that it will not be effective unless it is prepared

1. under sterile technique
2. at the bedside
3. well in advance of its administration
4. immediately before it is to be used

235. The nurse must be extremely careful in her preparation of nitrogen mustard, for if any of the medication gets on the skin the result will be

1. a burn
2. dermatitis
3. ulceration
4. skin cancer

236. If the nurse should get any Mustargen on her skin during the process of preparation, the contaminated part must be

1. rinsed in 70% alcohol
2. placed under running water for 15 minutes
3. covered with sterile vaseline gauze
3. kept at rest for at least 24 hours

237. One big advantage of T.E.M. over nitrogen mustard is that it is effectively given

1. orally
2. by the nurse
3. parenterally
4. with meals

238. The prescribed time for giving T.E.M. is

1. at bedtime
2. between meals
3. a.c.
4. before breakfast

239. All the drugs classified as anticarcinogens are known to be toxic to

1. children
2. all the body cells
3. adults
4. malignant cells only

240. Amyl nitrite is classified as

1. a vasodilator
2. a vasoconstrictor
3. an antispasmodic
4. an anticoagulant

241. Amyl nitrite is one of the few drugs that are effective when given

1. so that the fumes can be inhaled
2. intravenously
3. intramuscularly
4. sublingually

242. If the blood vessels dilate too rapidly, the patient who has used amyl nitrite will complain of

1. severe headache
2. diarrhea
3. diaphoresis
4. diplopia

243. When the patient is first placed on digitalis, the order will provide for

1. large doses to be given until the desired concentration in the blood is reached
2. small doses to be given until the patient gets used to the medicine
3. blood pressure check before and after each dose
4. intravenous administration

244. Congestive heart failure improves when digitalis is given because it

1. slows up the pulse
2. increases the pulse rate
3. causes the auricles to contract more rapidly
4. allows the ventricles to contract with more force

245. Digitalis poisoning must be recognized early. The nurse will check for evidence of poisoning by

1. checking the blood pressure q.2.h.
2. checking the pulse before each dose is given
3. taking a rectal temperature B.I.D.
4. stopping the medicine when the respirations are below 12 per minute

246. When the nurse's observation indicates the beginning symptom of digitalis poisoning, it is her responsibility

1. to give the drug and report to the doctor
2. to omit the drug and report to the doctor
3. to omit one dose of the drug and then to start again
4. to cancel the order for the drug

247. Digitalis must not be given without the specific direction of the doctor whenever

    1. the systolic blood pressure is above 100
    2. the rectal temperature is subnormal
    3. the pulse is 60 or below
    4. the patient is flushed and perspiring

248. The diuretic action of digitalis is produced because of the ability of the drug

    1. to pull edematous fluid in from the tissues
    2. to make the patient thirsty and increase the fluid intake
    3. to relax the arteries in the kidney
    4. to improve the total circulation

249. Tincture (10% solution) of digitalis 1 c.c. is ordered. Using a minim measuring glass, the nurse will measure

    1. gtts. X   3. m. LX
    2. gtts. XV   4. m. XV

250. Digoxin 0.3 mg. (H) is ordered. The label on the vial reads 0.5 mg. in each c.c. To give the ordered 0.3 milligrams the nurse will need to measure

    1. m. IX   3. m. XV
    2. m. V   4. 0.5 c.c.

251. Dicumarol 300 mg. is ordered. The label on the bottle reads Dicumarol 0.3 Gm. per tablet. The nurse will need to give the patient

    1. 1 tablet   3. 3 tablets
    2. 2 tablets   4. 4 tablets

252. Heparin and Dicumarol are drugs classified as

    1. antihistamines   3. antiemetics
    2. anticoagulants   4. antispasmodics

253. Although heparin acts more rapidly than Dicumarol, Dicumarol will be the drug of choice after the patient goes home because it is

    1. safer to use without supervision
    2. taken orally
    3. faster in an emergency
    4. absorbed gradually

254. Dicumarol will be given for the purpose of

    1. speeding up the clotting time of the blood
    2. slowing up circulation of blood in the coronary arteries
    3. speeding up circulation of blood in the coronary arteries
    4. slowing up the clotting time of the blood

255. Symptoms of overdose of Dicumarol will be recognized when the patient

    1. is nauseated and vomits
    2. has a very rapid pulse
    3. bleeds from the gums, rectum, or other body cavity
    4. complains of sharp pains in the legs caused by the forming blood clots

256. Most of the vasodilator medications used in the treatment of hypertension will be ordered given

    1. q.d.   3. parenterally
    2. orally   4. topically

257. If the blood vessels dilate too rapidly when medications such as veratrum or Priscoline are given, the patient will

    1. faint   3. become edematous
    2. hemorrhage 4. feel fatigued

258. Rauwolfia preparations are helpful in many persons with hypertension because of the

    1. stimulating effects
    2. vasodilating effects
    3. tranquilizing effects
    4. ability to thin the blood

259. Priscoline is effective in the treatment of peripheral vascular diseases because of its action which

    1. dilates the walls of the blood vessels
    2. prevents blood clots
    3. dissolves blood clots
    4. stimulates vasospasm

260. When a medication tends to produce a severe <u>hypotension</u> following its administration, the patient should be instructed

    1. to remain active and ambulatory
    2. to stay in bed for an hour after receiving the medicine
    3. to take high caloric liquids
    4. to sit quietly until all symptoms disappear

261. The patient who is getting Priscoline must be protected from

    1. applications of heat
    2. decreased flow of blood in the extremities
    3. anything that will raise the blood pressure
    4. exposure to cold

262. Priscoline is used in the treatment of peripheral vascular diseases because it is valuable in the prevention of

    1. postoperative thrombosis
    2. embolism
    3. ulceration and gangrene
    4. vasodilatation of the capillaries

263. In the treatment of varicose ulcers, Varidase is used because of its action which

    1. prepares the area for healing by dissolving dead tissue
    2. stimulates the formation of pus
    3. increases circulation to the part
    4. protects the healthy cells in the part from further damage

264. Before Varidase has been dissolved, it can be kept in the medicine cupboard

    1. several weeks   3. indefinitely
    2. about 1 month   4. 1 week

265. Once the normal saline solution has been added to the bottle of Varidase, it must be

    a. used within 1 week
    b. kept in the refrigerator
    c. sterilized in the autoclave
    d. discarded when the precipitate appears

        1. all of the above
        2. a only
        3. a and b
        4. a, b, and d

266. When aspirin and sodium bicarbonate are given to relieve the symptoms of rheumatic fever, the medications are <u>more quickly absorbed</u> if

    1. the tablets are enteric-coated
    2. a large glass of water is taken with the medicine
    3. the medicine is mixed with the food at mealtime
    4. the medicine is in capsule form

267. The rheumatic fever child who is on large doses of aspirin over a long period should be watched for evidences of toxic symptoms such as

    1. ringing in the ears and dizziness
    2. headache and tympanitis
    3. edema
    4. blurred vision and spots before the eyes

268. It is never safe to leave a bottle of oil of wintergreen (methyl salicylate) at the bedside of a preschool child because

    1. self-administration will cause a skin reaction
    2. blisters are produced by the concentrated medicine
    3. the odor will upset the child's appetite
    4. it is fatal if taken internally

269. In severe cases of rheumatic fever, cortisone and ACTH have proven of value because of their ability

    1. to cut the disease process short
    2. to prolong the patient's life and permit the use of other treatment
    3. to clear up all infections
    4. to give the patient an interest in rehabilitation

270. Cortisone preparations, to be effective, must be kept at a required level in the blood. To do this, it will be necessary for the doctor

    1. to give the medicine in the vein
    2. to give the medicine I.M.
    3. to figure each dosage on the basis of kilogram weight of the patient
    4. to order a large initial dose and then smaller maintenance doses

271. Cortisone would be preferred to ACTH when the rheumatic fever child is being cared for at home because

    1. it is not so expensive
    2. the dose is not so large
    3. it is given orally
    4. it has no ill effects

272. It is currently believed that the blood level of penicillin should be kept constant for a long time in the child who has had rheumatic fever. This can be done by

    1. weekly injections of long-acting penicillin
    2. daily doses of oral penicillin
    3. steam inhalations of penicillin
    4. prophylactic doses before any surgery or dental care

273. If the dentist has been informed that his patient has had rheumatic fever, he can use prophylactic doses of

    1. Aspergum   3. ACTH
    2. cortisone   4. penicillin

274. If the blood level of penicillin is kept high in the child who has recovered from rheumatic fever, it should be possible for him

    1. to participate in limited recreational activities
    2. to avoid all upper respiratory infections
    3. to avoid recurring attacks of the disease
    4. to remain in a cold climate

275. Toxic symptoms have developed following the administration of one of the antituberculosis drugs. At this point, the nurse can expect that the doctor will

    1. stop all medications
    2. substitute another drug
    3. continue to give the drug in spite of symptoms
    4. stop the drug until all symptoms disappear

276. If the antituberculosis drugs are going to be effective in the treatment of this disease, they should be taken for a period of

    1. 6 to 8 weeks   3. 6 months to 1 year
    2. 3 to 6 months   4. 1 to 2 years

277. Streptomycin is a dry powder. Once it has been dissolved with sterile distilled water, the instructions caution the nurse

    1. to keep it in a locked medicine cupboard
    2. to keep it at room temperature indefinitely
    3. to refrigerate it if it is to be kept longer than 7 days
    4. to shake the bottle well to prevent a "settling out"

278. When streptomycin is effective in the treatment of tuberculosis, its action has

    1. coagulated the protein of the bacilli
    2. upset the reproductive ability of the tubercle bacilli
    3. upset the fluid balance of the bacilli
    4. dissolved the calcified areas in the lung

279. Streptomycin is being given in combination with other antituberculosis drugs. The streptomycin will be given

    1. daily   3. twice weekly
    2. B.I.D.   4. weekly

280. A toxic symptom of streptomycin that would make it dangerous to continue giving the medication is

    1. vomiting   3. dizziness
    2. diarrhea   4. deafness

281. The nurse must know how important it is to handle streptomycin carefully. If the drug comes in contact with the nurse, the result may be

    1. immunity to the drug
    2. infection with the tuberculosis
    3. a contact dermatitis
    4. distressing complications

282. The patient should be prepared to expect some <u>unpleasant</u> side reactions of streptomycin. One such symptom is

1. tenesmus   3. loss of memory
2. dizziness   4. diarrhea

283. If the patient is given streptomycin for any length of time, he will complain of

1. loss of appetite
2. nausea and vomiting
3. mental confusion and disorientation
4. tenderness at the site of injection

284. The side effects reported by the nurse have been responsible for discontinuing the administration of streptomycin. Side effects important enough to cancel this helpful medication are probably those of

1. nausea and vomiting
2. insomnia
3. lethargy and weakness
4. skin rash and fever

285. One side effect of dihydrostreptomycin that makes it a more dangerous drug than streptomycin is

1. irreversible deafness
2. continued dizziness
3. recurring skin rash
4. intractible jaundice

286. Streptomycin may have to be discontinued because of the toxic symptoms or because of the resistance of the bacilli. The drug usually substituted is

1. P.A.S.
2. isoniazid
3. dihydrostreptomycin
4. penicillin

287. P.A.S. is most effective in the treatment of

1. tuberculosis of the bone
2. pulmonary tuberculosis
3. miliary tuberculosis
4. tuberculosis meningitis

288. The antituberculosis quality of isoniazid or Nydrazid is responsible for

1. killing the tubercle bacilli and curing the patient
2. sterilizing the sputum
3. building up the general physical condition of the patient
4. weakening the tubercle bacillus so that the body can effectively fight the disease

289. Isoniazid may be the drug of choice for some patients instead of streptomycin. This is done because isoniazid

a. has no serious side effects
b. may be given either orally or I.M.
c. may be taken by the patient at home
d. is less expensive

1. a and c
2. b and d
3. a and b
4. all of the above

290. Isoniazid has proven very effective in the treatment of T.B. meningitis because of its ability

1. to decrease the activity of the bacilli
2. to concentrate in the brain and spinal cord
3. to limit the spread of infection to other parts of the body
4. to combine with other drugs

291. The patient treated with isoniazid may be a nursing problem because of the difficulty of

1. getting the patient to take his medication
2. keeping the weight within normal limits
3. constipation or diarrhea
4. keeping activity within the limits of the disease condition

292. P.A.S. will seldom be given alone. It is usually combined with

1. streptomycin and isoniazid
2. high protein foods
3. a vitamin supplement
4. streptomycin or isoniazid

293. The first combination of drugs used to treat the newly diagnosed T.B. patient will probably be

1. streptomycin and P.A.S.
2. streptomycin and isoniazid
3. streptomycin and dihydro-streptomycin
4. dihydrostreptomycin and P.A.S.

294. The patient who receives P.A.S. may be much safer for nontuberculous persons to be around. The presence of P.A.S. in the system often results in

1. reduction of the fever
2. disappearance of the bacilli from the sputum
3. calcification of the lung lesions
4. decreased irritability

295. A special effort should be made to give P.A.S. at mealtime. If it is not taken then, the nurse can expect the patient to complain of

1. constipation
2. dizziness
3. stomach discomfort
4. ringing in the ears

296. P.A.S. is frequently given to the patient receiving streptomycin. The purpose of the P.A.S. is

1. to prevent damage to the brain
2. to kill the tubercle bacilli
3. to slow up the development of resistance to the streptomycin
4. to speed up the healing effects of the streptomycin

297. P.A.S. has a side effect that often makes one aspect of the nursing care of the patient with tuberculosis easier. This side effect is helpful because it

1. increases the appetite
2. sedates the patient
3. lessens mental alertness
4. stimulates bowel elimination

298. The usual dose of P.A.S. is 12.0 grams or $\frac{...}{3}$ $\overline{iii}$. It is obvious that this medicine will be given

1. rectally
2. hypodermically
3. orally
4. intramuscularly

COMMUNICABLE DISEASES

(Answer sheet p. 323)

Knowledge of the vocabulary used to discuss communicable diseases is tested. The emphasis is on the nursing care of patients with the more common types of communicable disease.

1. DESQUAMATION means

   1. high temperature 3. peeling
   2. swelling   4. redness

2. ERYTHEMA means

   1. a rash   3. a weakening
   2. abnormal redness 4. a blood infection

3. ACTIVE IMMUNITY has been produced

   1. by some laboratory animal
   2. by some other human
   3. by the cells of the individual's body
   4. only by having the disease

4. ANTIBODY refers to

   1. an immune substance
   2. a substance given to start the process of immunity
   3. a weakened toxin
   4. the presence of bacteria in the blood

5. ATTENUATE is a verb that means

   1. to destroy bacteria
   2. to carry disease germs
   3. to touch a person or object with contaminated material
   4. to weaken the strength of a germ or a virus

6. CIRCUMORAL PALLOR describes

   1. the jaundiced sclera
   2. a white ring around the mouth
   3. blue fingertips
   4. a diagnostic sign

7. A CARRIER is

   1. one who passes on disease germs but does not have the disease himself
   2. an infected animal
   3. a fomite
   4. an animal that acts as a host to a parasite

8. An ANTIGEN refers to

   1. a substance that produces a high temperature
   2. freedom from bacteria
   3. a substance that can cause production of antibodies
   4. loss of appetite

9. FOMITES can be defined as

   1. all nonliving objects
   2. anything other than a sick person who can spread disease
   3. nonliving articles that contain disease germs
   4. any body secretion that carries disease producing organisms

10. COMMUNICABLE DISEASE means that the disease

   1. must be isolated
   2. is spread through the air
   3. is spread from one person to another by an infected animal or insect
   4. can be given by one person to another person

11. A CONTACT describes

   1. a person or animal who has been directly or indirectly exposed to disease producing material
   2. the act of touching anything contaminated
   3. an insect that picks up infected material on its feet and carries it to someone else
   4. anything that has been exposed to disease-producing organisms

12. The term CONTAGIOUS DISEASE describes

   1. all "catching" diseases
   2. a disease passed from one human to another by direct or indirect contact
   3. those diseases resulting from the bite of an animal or an insect
   4. all those diseases that must be placarded

13. CROSS INFECTION refers to

    1. any mixed infection
    2. an infection that becomes chronic
    3. a new infection added while another infection is present
    4. infection by a pus-producing organism

14. EXANTHEM refers to

    1. a rash   3. hyperemia
    2. scaling   4. pyrexia

15. The term MACULE describes

    1. a pimple
    2. an unraised spot on the skin or mucous membrane
    3. an urticaria
    4. a series of boils

16. The term PAROXYSM refers to

    1. convulsive movements
    2. a sudden return of symptoms followed by remission
    3. muscle rigidity
    4. muscle weakness alternating with spasticity

17. PAPULE describes

    1. an elevated eruption on the skin
    2. an elevated surface filled with pus
    3. an elevated surface filled with serum
    4. an elevated surface filled with blood

18. PANDEMIC is a term used to indicate

    1. a widespread disease in a community
    2. the occasional incidence of disease
    3. a disease is always present in the community
    4. widespread incidence of a disease

19. ORTHOTONOS describes a body position in which the

    1. rigid body is arched
    2. body is held rigid in a straight line
    3. weight of the body is carried on the heels and back of the head
    4. muscles are twitching

20. The INCUBATION PERIOD describes the

    1. length of the period of communicability
    2. onset of fever
    3. time between exposure and development of characteristic symptoms
    4. time between the onset of characteristic symptoms and the crisis

21. The term IMMUNITY means

    1. the inability to get a disease
    2. the ability of the body to resist and overcome a specific disease
    3. an inability to spread a disease
    4. those substances that protect from disease

22. The PORTAL OF ENTRY describes the

    1. site of the infection
    2. path by which disease germs leave the body
    3. prognosis of a disease
    4. body area where disease germs first enter

23. A VESICLE is

    1. a boil
    2. a rash that forms a scab
    3. an elevated skin lesion containing fluid
    4. an elevated skin lesion

24. PROPHYLAXIS means

    1. disease producing
    2. increased blood supply to a part
    3. an increase in the size of a part
    4. prevention

25. A PUSTULE is

    1. a rash
    2. a scaling rash
    3. an elevated skin lesion containing pus
    4. an elevated skin lesion containing serum

26. PATHOGENIC means

    1. preventive
    2. against fever
    3. disease producing
    4. freedom from germs

27. PRODROMAL refers to

   1. a characteristic set of symptoms
   2. a warning of a disease to follow
   3. the outcome of the illness
   4. the change in symptoms, for better or for worse

28. PASSIVE IMMUNITY is

   1. developed in response to the disease invasion
   2. immunity first built up by some other person or animal
   3. present at birth
   4. present only in some races

29. A WHEAL would be described as

   1. a white skin elevation surrounded by a red itching area
   2. a large inflamed area
   3. an area of jaundice
   4. an elevation of skin or mucous membrane filled with pus or serum

30. EPIDEMIC means

   1. scattered
   2. localized
   3. a large number with the disease in a local area
   4. the disease is widespread over the whole country

31. VIRULENT means

   1. widespread   3. very dangerous
   2. large numbers of   4. diluted

32. A group of students are having a ward class in the nurses station of a communicable-disease unit. Check the one behavior which indicates that the student does not understand and appreciate the principles of isolation technique.

   1. Nurse A opens both windows from the top and the bottom
   2. Nurse B places her purse on the floor
   3. Nurse C throws paper at the wastebasket, misses, then picks it up and places it in the basket
   4. Nurse D changes into a clean gown and mask before taking part in the class

33. ENDEMIC DISEASE is

   1. one in which there are many deaths
   2. one that is always present in a community
   3. a disease present only in certain seasons
   4. not reported

34. The natural immunity a baby has at birth is short-lasting. It is recommended that active immunization shots be started at the age of

   1. 3 months   3. 8 months
   2. 5 months   4. 10 months

35. The prodromal symptoms for many of the childhood communicable diseases are similar. These are most commonly listed as

   1. nausea and vomiting
   2. headache and diarrhea
   3. nausea and headaches
   4. symptoms of a common cold

36. Diseases that are transferred by way of the nose and throat discharges are often classified as "airborne." Such diseases require an isolation technique that includes

   a. care in a separate room
   b. use of mask by nursing personnel
   c. use of a gown by nursing personnel
   d. frequent, thorough handwashing

      1. a and b
      2. a, b, and d
      3. b and c
      4. all of the above

37. Several of the communicable diseases are characterized by a rash that desquamates. Those diseases that must be isolated until all peeling is completed include

   a. scarlet fever
   b. chicken pox
   c. smallpox
   d. typhoid fever

      1. all of the above
      2. b and c
      3. b only
      4. c and d

38. The most common and most serious complications of several of the childhood communicable diseases could be prevented if during the illness the child could be protected from

   1. people with upper respiratory infections
   2. drafts
   3. aspirating
   4. all stimulating and tiring activities

39. Two communicable diseases that are often fatal in children less than 1 year old can be prevented by active immunization. Immunizing shots early in the child's life should protect against

   a. measles
   b. mumps
   c. whooping cough
   d. diphtheria

      1. all of the above
      2. c and d
      3. a or b
      4. a and c

40. If the symptoms of a communicable disease are caused by toxins produced by the bacteria, active immunity would be stimulated by the antigen such as

   1. immune serum   3. antitoxin
   2. toxoid   4. vaccine

41. Communicable diseases that may be spread by carriers include

   a. scarlet fever
   b. typhoid fever
   c. diphtheria
   d. brucellosis

      1. all of the above
      2. all except d
      3. b and c
      4. a only

42. The diphtheria patient will find it easier to take fluids freely if the pain in the throat has been relieved by

   1. application of an ice collar
   2. penicillin troches given a.c.
   3. gentian violet throat swabs daily
   4. soda bicarbonate throat irrigations

43. Obstruction to respiration during diphtheria may be treated on an emergency basis by

   a. tracheotomy
   b. gavage
   c. intubation
   d. lavage

      1. any of the above, depending on the part affected
      2. a only
      3. c or d
      4. a or c

44. Diphtheria symptoms are serious and often dangerous to the life of the patient. As soon as this diagnosis is suspected, the patient should be given

   1. 3 doses of toxoid at 4 to 17 day intervals
   2. diphtheria antitoxin immediately
   3. large amounts of fluids to dilute the toxins
   4. mental preparation for a possible tracheotomy

45. Diphtheria is a serious disease and the most dangerous complications are

   1. difficult to diagnose
   2. the result of a virulent endotoxin
   3. the cause of the strict isolation routines
   4. heart failure and pneumonia

46. The most serious effects of mumps occur in those patients who are

   1. children 5 to 15
   2. adult males
   3. boys 4 to 12
   4. girls past puberty

47. Orchitis following mumps is most dreaded because

   1. the symptoms are so severe
   2. of the complicating mastitis
   3. the increased pulse and respiration are dangerous
   4. bilateral atrophy of the testicles will produce sterility

48. The common communicable disease responsible for the most childhood deaths is

1. measles
2. whooping cough
3. virus pneumonia
4. tetanus

49. When the infant or small child has whooping cough, the nursing-care plan must always include efforts

1. to provide good skin care and oral hygiene
2. to control the emotions
3. to stop the coughing paroxysms
4. to maintain adequate nutrition

50. Junior, age 5, was exposed to whooping cough two weeks ago while visiting his grandparents. Now that he is home, his family doctor has decided that the only effective protection can be obtained by

1. active immunization
2. racial immunity
3. passive immunization
4. convalescent immunity

51. Sally, age 7, lives next door to Junior. As soon as Junior's mother is advised of the whooping cough epidemic in grandmother's home town, Sally's mother consults her physician, who recommends Sally be protected by

1. active immunization
2. racial immunity
3. passive immunization
4. convalescent immunity

52. Sedative medications aimed at lessening the paroxysms of coughing in whooping cough are most effective when they are given

1. p.c. and h.s.
2. a.c. and h.s.
3. h.s.
4. q.i.d.

53. The symptom of chickenpox that requires the most nursing attention is

1. rash
2. anorexia
3. fever
4. headache

54. Nursing measures to keep the small child with chickenpox comfortable will be aimed at

1. preventing or relieving itching
2. protecting the eyes from glare
3. preventing nausea and vomiting
4. preventing convulsions

55. Measles, or rubeola, become serious and may lead to the death of the patient if complicated by

1. tetanus
2. a secondary infection
3. diphtheria
4. photophobia

56. Most measles patients should be placed in a room that allows adequate sunlight. In such a room the nurse should arrange for

1. the window shades to be closed tightly
2. dark glasses
3. hot, wet eye compresses
4. the bed to be turned away from the windows

57. Six months after the child has had measles he should have a thorough physical examination to determine the presence or absence of

1. sequelae and complications
2. mental retardation
3. pneumonia
4. a carrier condition

58. The infant has been exposed to measles. Protection that can prevent or modify an attack can be obtained from administration of

1. vaccine
2. toxoid
3. a Schick test
4. gamma globulin

59. One symptom considered essential to a positive diagnosis of German measles is

1. the characteristic rash
2. a sore throat
3. a temperature elevation to 104°F
4. swelling of the cervical glands

60. Koplik's spots appear as part of the prodromal symptoms of

    1. measles   3. measles, rubella
    2. measles, rubeola 4. scarlet fever

61. German, or three-day measles, is a disease with very mild symptoms and no ill effects except in

    1. little girls
    2. adult males
    3. pregnant women in the first trimester
    4. the very young, the very old, or those weakened by another disease

62. The nares and upper lip will need to be protected from excoriation during scarlet fever. The skin will be irritated by

    1. sordes that accompany the high fever
    2. nasal discharge
    3. localized infection
    4. sensitive, swollen tissues

63. A typhoid fever patient will have his activities limited and closely checked. Such a person can spread the disease as a result of

    1. carelessness about hand washing
    2. droplet infection
    3. contaminated nose wipes
    4. use of a common drinking cup

64. The typhoid fever patient complains of abdominal pain and thirst. The pulse rate has dropped; there is a marked pallor. The nurse would suspect the dreaded complication of

    1. cardiac failure
    2. internal hemorrhage or perforation
    3. bronchitis with impending pneumonia
    4. acute bowel obstruction

65. The nurse is responsible for caring for the typhoid fever patient in such a way that the community will be protected. One of the ways the nurse can do this is

    1. to stay away from movies or social meetings
    2. to order immunization shots for her family and neighbors
    3. to see that screens keep out flies and insects
    4. to notify the health officer

66. To care effectively for the typhoid fever patient and protect herself and the community, the nurse must recognize that

    a. the typhoid bacillus leaves the patient's body by way of the intestines
    b. nose and throat discharges are loaded with the virus
    c. complete isolation technique must be practiced
    d. the typhoid bacillus must enter a person's body through the G.I. tract

    1. all of the above
    2. b and c
    3. b only
    4. a and d

67. In the acute stage of typhoid fever the nurse should be suspicious if her check of cardinal symptoms seems to indicate

    1. an oral temperature of 104°F
    2. a respiratory rate between 20 and 26
    3. a pulse rate between 120 to 130
    4. any elevation of blood pressure

68. Smallpox is no longer a major public health problem in the United States. The incidence has been greatly reduced because of the widespread use of

    1. passive immunity acquired from horse serum
    2. dilute doses of gamma globulin
    3. antitoxin
    4. vaccine to produce active immunity

69. Symptoms that will appear in smallpox and will not be present in chickenpox include

    a. vesicles
    b. pustules
    c. odorous rash
    d. temperature elevation

    1. all of the above
    2. b only
    3. a, b, and c
    4. b and c

70. Rocky Mountain spotted fever is passed to humans by the bite of an infected

    1. animal   3. tick
    2. insect   4. flea

71. The patient who has tularemia most likely got the disease from one of the following sources:

   a. the bite of an infected mosquito
   b. eating poorly cooked, infected rabbit meat
   c. skinning diseased rabbits
   d. droplet infection from a neighbor with the disease

   1. a and b
   2. b and d
   3. b or c
   4. all of the above

72. The patient with tularemia often has open ulcers and draining, abscessed lymph nodes. Protective nursing technique requires the nurse

   1. to wear rubber gloves
   2. to insert an indwelling catheter
   3. to give only a shower bath
   4. to cover them with sterile dressings

73. Brucellosis may be tentatively diagnosed as tuberculosis based on the symptom of

   1. dyspnea
   2. hemoptysis
   3. temperature elevation every afternoon
   4. chest rales

74. The lengthy period of vague symptoms that characterize brucellosis and often interfere with arriving at an accurate diagnosis is responsible for the common mental attitude of

   1. depression   3. fatigue
   2. irritability   4. apprehension

75. During a malarial paroxysm diaphoresis is an important symptom. Electrolyte balance must be maintained by

   1. serving only sodium-free foods
   2. increased use of salt in the diet
   3. forcing fluids
   4. restricting fluids to control sweating

76. Liquids will be forced between chills in malaria. It is necessary to replace the fluid lost through

   1. diarrhea   3. tears
   2. hemorrhage   4. sweating

77. Because of the way malaria and tetanus infect humans, nursing technique will include

   1. full isolation procedure
   2. mask and gown
   3. careful disposal of respiratory discharges
   4. handwashing technique only

78. The child has already had immunizing shots to develop active immunity against tetanus. If, six months later, the child steps on a sharp, rusty nail, the doctor will restimulate the antibodies by giving

   1. horse serum   3. a booster shot
   2. the dead virus   4. an immune serum

79. Tetanus antitoxin is often given as an emergency measure following many types of accidental injuries. The nurse in the doctor's office or in the Emergency Room must keep in mind several facts about passive immunity substances:

   a. Foreign proteins may produce a fatal reaction
   b. Most antitoxins are produced in horse serum
   c. Sensitivity skin tests must always be done before any injection
   d. Sensitive persons may require several small doses rather than a single dose of antitoxin

   1. a and b
   2. a, c, and d
   3. a, b, and d
   4. all of the above

80. A nurse on private duty can feel justified in refusing a diagnosed case of rabies if she

   1. has not been immunized against the disease
   2. knows the disease is fatal
   3. has a dog at home
   4. has cuts or open wounds on her hands

81. The nursing care of the patient with rabies is concentrated on

   1. relief of respiratory paralysis
   2. prevention of cross contamination
   3. keeping the patient comfortable and quiet
   4. good oral and skin care with frequent baths and tepid sponges

REHABILITATION

(Answer sheet p. 325)

This section includes the general principles of rehabilitation, plus the application of these principles to those conditions that most commonly profit from rehabilitation techniques.

1. The basic principle underlying rehabilitation, regardless of the disease or the handicap, is to concentrate on

   1. the limitations
   2. necessary family adjustments
   3. acceptance of public attitude
   4. existing abilities

2. If the nurse is going to be of any value on the rehabilitation team, she must learn the importance of

   1. skills in hydrotherapy
   2. letting the patient help himself, even though it takes more time
   3. insisting on a postgraduate course before she works with the handicapped
   4. changing the attitudes of the family toward the handicap

3. The key to the successful or unsuccessful rehabilitation of any physically handicapped person is his

   1. motivation
   2. intelligence
   3. age
   4. personality development

4. Rehabilitation often progresses more rapidly in a special rehabilitation hospital or ward unit, because in such care units special effort is made

   1. to assign only skilled personnel
   2. to make assignments only on the case method
   3. to keep all personnel concerned informed of the therapy goals
   4. to provide all the needed equipment for rehabilitation activities

5. Until the physically handicapped person becomes able to care for his personal needs, rehabilitation activities must be presented with a recognition that the patient has exaggerated feelings of

   1. insecurity   3. self-pity
   2. hostility   4. dependency

6. When the person with a physical handicap must accept assistance from others, he may react by

   a. resentment of the fact that he needs help
   b. cooperating to the fullest with all requests
   c. expecting and depending on help
   d. insisting on special duty nurses

      1. all of the above
      2. a or c
      3. c or d
      4. a and d

7. Efforts to rehabilitate the adult with a physical handicap become increasingly difficult when the handicap has resulted in

   1. loss of status
   2. hospitalization
   3. institutionalization
   4. physical deformity

8. Once a physically handicapped person has been prepared for and placed in a position, it is equally important that rehabilitation workers occasionally check

   1. his physical state
   2. his efficiency
   3. to see that he is able to afford life's necessities
   4. to determine if both he and his employer are satisfied

9. Lack of acceptance of the physically handicapped on the job, in school, or socially is often based on nothing more than the fact that this person is

   1. pathetic
   2. dependent
   3. ugly in appearance
   4. different

10. If efforts to help the physically handicapped are based on emotion and sympathy, the outcome is most often

    1. lack of gratitude
    2. increased dependency
    3. insecurity
    4. emotional instability

11. Rehabilitation plans cannot progress satisfactorily until the handicapped person is ready to

    a. tolerate increased pain during therapy
    b. accept his limitations
    c. build on his assets
    d. learn new job skills

       1. all of the above
       2. a, c, and d
       3. b and c
       4. b only

12. The basic philosophy of rehabilitation that must guide nurses and all rehabilitation workers is

    1. to return the patient to economic independence
    2. to help the patient help himself
    3. to prevent overdependence
    4. to restore the patient to his former usefulness

13. The needs of any physically handicapped individual may include

    a. medical care and follow-up
    b. education
    c. vocational training
    d. social adjustment

       1. any of the above
       2. a or c
       3. b and d
       4. b and c

14. The nurse who really believes in the value of rehabilitation activities will be willing to allow her handicapped patient

    1. to be cared for only by the specialist
    2. to spend most of his day in hydrotherapy
    3. to practice self-care rather than do it for him
    4. to give in to the attentions of his family

15. The state and national governments share the cost of operating a State Board of Vocational Education and Rehabilitation. Any physically handicapped person can request, without cost if necessary, assistance in

    a. discovering work capacity and ability
    b. obtaining aids or prostheses to increase work ability
    c. obtaining extra preparation to do a job well
    d. finding and keeping a job

       1. all of the above
       2. any of the above
       3. b and c
       4. c only

16. Rehabilitation principles should be put into practice just as soon as the stroke patient regains consciousness. The reason for this is that

    1. muscles atrophy quickly with disease
    2. rehabilitation is needed to prevent contractures
    3. the patient is not given a chance to enjoy being an invalid
    4. only early rehabilitation methods will make it possible for the patient to take care of his personal needs

17. The paralyzed stroke patient will be given passive exercise for the purpose of

    1. preventing muscle contractures
    2. avoiding infections
    3. easing any pain
    4. forcing him to use the deformed part

18. The completely helpless stroke patient needs constant encouragement by his family and the nursing personnel. This is necessary to build up and maintain the patient's feeling

    1. that passive exercise is worth the effort
    2. of usefulness
    3. of hunger
    4. of faith in complete rehabilitation

19. Rehabilitation of the epileptic with grand mal seizures will be a discouraging job until

 1. newer medications will stop seizures
 2. the name of the disease is changed
 3. public attitude toward the disease changes
 4. all epileptics learn to accept the disease

20. The effective rehabilitation of a cardiac patient must consider

 a. the age of the patient
 b. the emotional reaction of the patient to the disease
 c. the degree of heart damage
 d. the patient's need to hold a job

  1. a, b and d
  2. c only
  3. a, b, and c
  4. all of the above

21. Rehabilitation of the cardiac child is made more difficult because of

 1. the attitude of the nurses
 2. the attitude of family and friends toward the diagnosis
 3. his inability to get enough education to earn a living later
 4. the lack of workshop facilities in most communities

22. Programs of the national and state Heart Associations that make it possible for many cardiac housewives to continue keeping house include

 1. housekeeping services
 2. paying for household help
 3. consultation service on the most efficient arrangement of the house
 4. building special housing units for cardiac families

23. Successful rehabilitation methods and the best job placement that provide employment security are essential for the cardiac adult

 1. to be happy in his job and increase his chance of longer life
 2. to accept the role of semi-invalid
 3. to pamper his heart condition
 4. to avoid the need for special privileges on the job

24. The older cardiac worker responds best to rehabilitation methods when it is possible

 1. to teach him a new skill requiring less physical and emotional energy
 2. to permit him to return to his old job with some restrictions
 3. to encourage him to move in with a son or a daughter
 4. to encourage retirement and life in an old peoples' home

25. If the cardiac worker can meet the physical demands of the job, it is possible for such a person

 1. to hold any job
 2. to return to his pre-illness activities
 3. to work as well on the job as noncardiacs
 4. to be employed in industry that hires the handicapped

26. Before the doctor can approve any job for the cardiac worker, he must

 1. get the employer to understand the need for restricted activity
 2. see what movements the job requires
 3. eliminate the emotional strains of the job
 4. balance the capacity of the cardiac with the physical demands of the job

27. Rehabilitation of the older man with heart trouble is more difficult because

 1. he does not like to learn a new job and find new friends
 2. his physical condition limits him
 3. his family does not understand why he must work for less pay
 4. he is afraid to get away from the protection of his family

28. The cardiac adult often insists that he feels well enough to do all the things his friends are doing. The nurse should recognize that such an attitude really means

 1. he is ready to do these things
 2. his medication is effective
 3. his emotional outlook is good
 4. he is not accepting the limitations of his diagnosis

29. The cardiac, child or adult, must understand his limitations and his capacity for play. To be effective, such instruction must also include

1. daily application of instructions
2. relatives and friends
3. group therapy classes
4. training in new recreation skills

30. Job placement of the cardiac is often difficult because

1. the patient does not want to go back to work
2. other people are afraid to work with him
3. the diagnosis makes the worker undependable
4. many employers are afraid to risk hiring him

31. Employers should be taught that it is safe to hire a known cardiac and place him in a safe position. The danger of employing a cardiac occurs when

1. the worker hides the fact that he is a cardiac
2. other employees object to working with the cardiac
3. the job requires overtime
4. the worker takes more time off than noncardiacs

32. The sheltered workshops sponsored by local Heart Associations are especially helpful to those cardiacs who

1. are ashamed of the disease
2. are afraid they are not well enough to safely work
3. need special supervision and treatment
4. must learn how to work

33. Any employer of a cardiac has a right to expect that employee to protect himself by

1. using all the safety measures
2. refusing to do any job that seems to be too strenuous
3. taking rest periods as he feels their need
4. following his doctor's recommendations

34. The one reaction to a diagnosis of heart disease that makes rehabilitation so difficult is

1. superstition   3. pride
2. fear   4. resentment

35. Successful physical and emotional rehabilitation of the amputee requires each nurse responsible for his care to insist that

1. he accept the fact that surgery has not changed him
2. he participate in ward games
3. he do as much as he can for himself
4. he take complete care of the stump

36. When a patient's muscles of speech are poorly coordinated, the nurse must appreciate that it is easier to understand him if

1. she can anticipate his thoughts
2. he talks to just one person
3. he is given time to express his thoughts
4. he is encouraged to speak rapidly

37. Preparation for rehabilitation of the patient with a laryngectomy should include conversation with him. The patient may have to respond by writing or forming words with his lips. This early activity is valuable because

1. the patient needs practice
2. emotionally, the patient needs extra attention
3. it paves the way for esophageal speech
4. it keeps the patient in the habit of communicating

38. The nurse may need to help the family adjust to the speech of the laryngectomized patient. The family must understand that esophageal speech becomes more difficult when their lack of understanding

1. causes the patient to withdraw
2. produces tension in the patient
3. increases the patient's respiratory rate
4. makes the patient afraid to practice

39. The blind person will suffer an initial shock when vision is lost. Later, the greatest resentment of the hospitalized blind person will result from

1. being cared for by strange persons
2. family indifference
3. the inability to move about freely
4. a feeling of hopelessness

40. The best way to help the blind person develop skill and self-confidence in feeding himself is

1. to place the same type of food in the same location on the plate
2. to insist that he feed himself from the beginning of his blindness
3. to provide only those foods that can be easily captured with a spoon
4. to provide many "finger foods"

41. The blind person should be encouraged to concentrate on sounds and develop an acute sense of hearing. This will be helpful to him in

1. identifying voices
2. getting around without a cane
3. determining direction or location
4. forgetting his lack of vision

42. Any teaching of a blind person must take into consideration that the lack of sight rules out much learning by

1. memorization
2. verbal direction
3. repetition
4. imitation

43. Achievement in minor activities will encourage the blind person to try other activities. It is most helpful if he can be taught very early

1. to concentrate on sounds
2. to put his belongings away where he can find them again
3. to care for his room and his clothes
4. to tell time

44. The blind person should be taught the importance of cleanliness and careful grooming. Carelessness in dress will be excused on the basis of blindness, but this is psychologically harmful because sighted persons tend

1. to take over his personal hygiene tasks
2. to pity the blind
3. to leave the blind person alone
4. to be cruelly critical

45. A good way to help the blind person feel useful is to ask him

1. to visit other handicapped patients
2. to show someone else how to master a skill
3. to care for all his personal needs
4. to wait on bed-fast patients

46. The blind person may be encouraged to have a window garden. The plants must be ones that

1. require little water
2. are brilliant in color
3. have distinctive leaves
4. have a fragrant odor

47. Effective rehabilitation of the blind will be limited until the person can be convinced that

1. personal and economic independence will be possible
2. there are still many things he can do
3. his life can go on just as before
4. use of a white cane will get him attention

48. The blind adult makes the best social adjustment when it becomes possible for him

1. to learn a job he can do at home
2. to use a cane without fear of the environment
3. to understand the cause of his handicap
4. to become economically independent

49. A mental mechanism frequently used by the blind and the deaf if they do not appreciate their limitations is that of

1. projection
2. compensation
3. identification
4. conversion

50. The sighted person should increase the blind individual's understanding of a new object by

1. combining explanation with examination
2. carefully planning a detailed description
3. stimulating the senses of smell and hearing
4. letting him touch it

51. The most effective rehabilitation of the blind will carefully consider the emotional reaction of the blind person to his handicap. The approach to the patient can best be planned if the nurse has been told whether

1. it will soon be possible for the patient to go home
2. there is any chance that the patient might be able to help himself
3. the blindness is the result of accident or disease
4. any treatment might restore the vision

52. Any plan for the rehabilitation of the blind would have to consider

a. the age of the patient
b. the previous educational level reached
c. any job experience
d. economic needs

1. b and c
2. a only
3. a and d
4. all except d

53. The sighted person can approach the blind more easily if blindness is not thought of as a handicap but rather as

1. an inconvenience
2. a temporary disability
3. a tragedy
4. chronic and progressive

54. You wish to set up a switchboard in your office and employ blind operators. To find out where equipment with Braille guides and directions on it can be obtained, you would expect to write to

1. The National Association for the Advancement of the Blind
2. The American Foundation for the Blind
3. The State Office of Blind Rehabilitation
4. the local Chamber of Commerce

55. A blind adult can keep up with current events and literature by means of

a. books in Braille
b. daily newspapers
c. radio
d. Talking Books

1. all of the above
2. a and b
3. all except b
4. d only

56. Participation in an occupational therapy program will help the blind person

1. to learn how to do things independently
2. to play
3. to socialize with other blind persons
4. to learn to follow directions

57. Rehabilitation of the blind requires repeated thorough instructions from the sighted. Occasionally, the only way the blind remembers important directions is to allow him

1. to get hurt
2. to get into difficulty under the supervision of the sighted
3. to remain in his room until he becomes more cooperative
4. to feel guilty whenever he forgets

58. Rehabilitation activities for the cleft lip or palate child will be ineffective in those instances in which parents overwork the mental mechanism of

1. rationalization
2. sublimation
3. substitution
4. overcompensation

59. Speech therapy following cleft-palate repair is frequently done in the form of games. The rules of the game will stress the importance of

1. matching words to pictures
2. putting ideas into action
3. socializing with less handicapped persons
4. careful listening and accurate reproduction of sounds

60. Rehabilitation techniques necessary to overcome the physical handicaps that accompany cleft palate include

a. speech therapy
b. supervision by the dental surgeon
c. lip reading
d. exercise games to strengthen palate muscles

    1. all of the above
    2. a only
    3. a, b, and d
    4. a and c

61. Members of the family, or friends, are more likely to become impatient with a deaf person than with a blind person because

1. it is harder to make the deaf understand
2. the deaf are more resentful of their handicap
3. the disability is not so obvious
4. personality deviations are more severe

62. The person who has a hearing loss, with or without a hearing aid, will benefit from a training program that includes his better use of

a. visual cues
b. observation
c. attention
d. speech skills

    1. d only
    2. a or c
    3. a, b, and c
    4. all of the above

63. The child who was born deaf may not be pleased with a hearing aid purchased for him just as he enrolls in school. The sounds he now hears may

1. be new sounds
2. be too stimulating
3. be confusing and frightening
4. interfere with his daydreams

64. One adjustment in speech that must be made by the nondeaf if the hard-of-hearing person is to lip read effectively is

1. to exaggerate all lip and tongue movements
2. to pause frequently
3. to use simple 4- or 5-letter words
4. to use only short sentences

65. When the nurse talks to a deaf person who understands by lip reading, the nurse must know that her words are recognized by

1. the facial expressions of the speaker
2. position and motion of the lips of the speaker
3. sound vibrations received
4. emphasis placed on each syllable

66. Instruction of a deaf person can best be done by a combination of

a. recorded directions
b. demonstrations
c. written instructions
d. diagrams

    1. all of the above
    2. c or d
    3. b only
    4. b, c, and d

67. Mr. X is being taught to operate a drill press. Mr. X is able to lip read. The supervisor will demonstrate the job step by step. To explain each step, the supervisor must

1. ask questions to see if the deaf person understands how and why
2. help the deaf person go through each step
3. stop the demonstration and face the deaf person during the explanation
4. depend upon information written on the blackboard

68. The nurse who works with the deaf or hard of hearing must gain and maintain his confidence. The nurse should not risk loss of this confidence by

    1. pretending to hear or understand when she does not
    2. shouting at the patient
    3. encouraging the patient to do all the talking
    4. talking instead of listening with interest

69. If a hard-of-hearing person is not able to lip read, the spoken words will reach him

    1. as a jumble of sounds without meaning
    2. but will not be correct
    3. after a brief delay
    4. only if vibrations are intensified

70. If the person has never heard, or has not heard well for a long time, rehabilitation activities must make it possible for the individual to learn to connect the sound with

    1. the written word
    2. what makes the sound
    3. the use of the object
    4. the area in which it is heard

71. One of the first requirements of learning the efficient use of a hearing aid is

    1. an understanding of its mechanics
    2. an appreciation of the expense of the equipment
    3. acceptance of the need for the prosthesis
    4. daily practice

72. Classes for the deaf or hard of hearing are often of psychological value because they

    1. point out the mental mechanisms used by the deaf
    2. stimulate competition among the members of the class
    3. demonstrate the value of lip reading
    4. teach job skills

73. A hard of hearing person should be taught that much can be understood of the general tone or feeling of a conversation by

    1. watching all the people taking part
    2. knowing the general subject under discussion
    3. adding his own comments to the discussion
    4. closely observing facial expressions

74. If the hard of hearing person pays close attention to the one who is speaking, he may not understand every word, but it should be possible for him

    1. to keep interested in the conversation
    2. to guess the mood by observing the gestures and facial expressions
    3. to get the general meaning of what is said
    4. to interrupt when the words are not clear

75. Mrs. X has been fitted with a hearing aid. This aid intensifies all sounds. If the aid is to be most effective, Mrs. X will now need to learn

    1. to instruct other people in the desirable way to speak to her
    2. to turn it off when people speak too loudly
    3. to carry on all conversation in a quiet room
    4. to ignore sounds that will distract her attention from the subject of interest

76. Johnny, age 8, is deaf. He is in the communicable disease section of the hospital with scarlet fever. The nurse can best communicate with this child by

    1. working through his mother
    2. play therapy
    3. writing her questions and directions
    4. standing with the light on her face

77. Rehabilitation efforts with deaf children must prepare them

    1. to be better than classmates without a defect
    2. to face reality
    3. to keep busy with solitary activities
    4. to strengthen all their other senses

78. The best way to encourage a deaf school child to master lip reading is

    1. set up a practice schedule
    2. allow him to play with only deaf children
    3. insist he repeat orally the things said to him
    4. talk to him often

79. The basic principle of rehabilitation is applied to the care of the burned patient when the nurse

    1. helps the patient help himself
    2. prevents all deformities
    3. has a positive emotional approach
    4. insists on regular physical therapy exercises

80. Rehabilitation techniques used on any orthopedic patient will concentrate on

    1. the patient's limitations
    2. the patient's existing abilities
    3. all the necessary family adjustments
    4. improving public attitudes

OBSTETRICS

(Answer sheets pp. 327–328)

This section includes the consideration of the anatomy and physiology of pregnancy and the development of the fetus as well as the prenatal care of the mother, care during labor and delivery and postnatal care. The immediate care of the newborn while it is still in the hospital is also covered.

1. The union of a sperm and an egg is called

    1. ovulation   3. menstruation
    2. fertilization   4. catamenia

2. The anatomical structure of the female allows an 8-pound baby to be born without excessive distress or danger because

    1. the contractions of the uterus force the birth
    2. the lining of the vagina normally lies in folds, permitting great distention
    3. the uterus is capable of stretching to 500 times its normal capacity
    4. of the short distance from the uterus to the perineum

3. The appearance of the menstrual flow is evidence that

    1. the female is not fertile
    2. the fertilized ovum has been planted on the lining of the uterus
    3. the ovum was not fertilized
    4. an examination for cancer of the uterus is urgent

4. The period each month when a mature egg is expelled from the ovary is called

    1. menopause   3. puberty
    2. menstruation   4. ovulation

5. After the egg is discharged from the ovary, unless it is fertilized, it remains alive a maximum of

    1. 3 days   3. 3 weeks
    2. 1 week   4. 4 days

6. Pregnancy is the result of

    1. cessation of the menstrual flow
    2. the deposit of sperm in the vagina
    3. 1 sperm entering 1 mature egg
    4. the egg attaching itself to the lining of the uterus

7. The only fertile period of the female is during the time

    1. of the menstrual flow
    2. the sperm is deposited
    3. the mature egg is alive
    4. the uterine lining is highly vascular

8. The fluid in the "water sac" or "bag of waters" is called the

    1. visceral fluid
    2. amniotic fluid
    3. pericardial fluid
    4. placenta

9. There is a physiological reason for the "bag of waters" breaking just a short time before the child is born. Its purpose at this time is

    1. to keep the baby from becoming dehydrated
    2. to wash out the vagina
    3. to get rid of the waste discharges of the infant
    4. to stretch the walls of the vagina

10. A day or two before ovulation, the uterus prepares for the entrance of the sperm into the uterus by

    1. pushing out the cervical mucus plug
    2. increasing the body temperature
    3. alkalizing the vaginal secretions
    4. dilating the cervix

11. Conception is defined as

    1. fertilization
    2. the union of a sperm with an ovum
    3. ovulation
    4. the passage of the ovum into the uterus

12. The amniotic fluid serves to protect the unborn baby by

    a. keeping its environment at constant temperature
    b. dilating the vagina
    c. absorbing shocks and vibrations
    d. diluting its waste products

        1. a and c   3. b, c, and d
        2. a only   4. all of the above

13. The health and nutrition of the pregnant woman during the first 3 months of pregnancy are so important because

    1. the complete development of the fetus takes place during this time
    2. immune substances are not yet available to the baby
    3. the chance of congenital deformity is greatest during this period
    4. the structural development of the baby has not yet started

14. The number of days in a lunar month is always

    1. 31   3. 24
    2. 28   4. 21

15. A baby is considered full term when it has been in the uterus

    1. 9-1/2 lunar months from the day of conception
    2. 10 calendar months from the first day of the last menstrual period
    3. 7 months
    4. 365 days

16. The mother supplies the baby with its needed food and oxygen supply in-directly through

    1. the amniotic sac
    2. the yolk sac
    3. the umbilical cord
    4. the embryo

17. The product of conception is no longer called an embryo at the end of the

    1. first month   3. third month
    2. second month   4. fourth month

18. The closer to full term it is before the baby is born, the greater its chances of living because of the increased development of

    1. its circulatory system
    2. its digestive system
    3. its nervous system
    4. its endocrine system

19. It takes longer for the fertilized egg to pass through the Fallopian tube than an unfertilized egg because

    1. the increasing size of the ovum slows up its progress
    2. the cilia of the tube resist its progress
    3. the uterus cannot receive it until it has reached a certain size
    4. the uterine lining must finish its preparations for pregnancy

20. All substances that reach the baby from the mother are filtered by the

    1. umbilical cord
    2. amniotic sac
    3. placenta
    4. uterine lining

21. The greasy vernix caseosa has a pro-tective function. If it did not cover the fetus,

    1. dehydration would occur
    2. the skin would get too soft
    3. the urine in the water sac would cause a rash
    4. the food supply from the mother would be affected

22. Some parts of the fetus do not function at all, or only occasionally, before birth. These parts are

    a. the lungs
    b. the stomach
    c. the kidneys
    d. the intestines

       1. all of the above
       2. a and b
       3. b and c
       4. c and d

23. The life of the fetus will be snuffed out if

    1. the nutritional intake of the mother is not adequate
    2. toxic substances are not screened by the placenta
    3. the flow of blood through the umbilical cord is stopped
    4. blood from the mother has a low hemoglobin count

24. The six- or seven-month fetus will be skinny and scrawny because

    1. all its nourishment has gone into completing the development of the nervous system
    2. its digestive system is not fully developed
    3. it is hyperactive up to this time
    4. it has not been in the uterus long enough to have fat pads deposited

25. The umbilical cord is essential to the life of the fetus because

    1. the blood from the mother to the baby is carried by this pathway
    2. the blood supply to and from the placenta is carried by this pathway
    3. the food supply needed by the infant is carried through the cord
    4. the waste products of the baby are eliminated through the cord

26. The doctor can hear and count the fetal heart tones when the fetus reaches the age of

    1. 2 months   3. 4 months
    2. 3 months   4. 5 months

27. The sex of the new baby is determined as soon as the

    1. sperm enter the vagina
    2. fertilized egg reaches the uterus
    3. sex chromosomes of the egg and sperm match up
    4. sex organs begin to develop

28. The most effective prenatal care can be possible only if the mother

    1. is accompanied by the father on most visits to the doctor
    2. visits the doctor before the end of the third month of pregnancy
    3. visits the doctor every 2 weeks during the early stages of pregnancy
    4. follows all the doctor's recommendations regularly

29. The symptom that often makes the prospective mother suspect she is pregnant is

    1. dysmenorrhea
    2. amenorrhea
    3. persistent headaches
    4. engorgement of breasts

30. On one of the expectant mother's early visits to the doctor it will be most important for him to determine

    1. her optimum weight
    2. the sex of the baby
    3. the presence of a uterine tumor
    4. her pelvic measurements

31. What laboratory test will be done on the expectant mother's first visit that will be aimed at preventing a deformity in her child?

    1. chest X-ray for tuberculosis
    2. blood examination for syphilis
    3. urinalysis for diabetes
    4. coagulation time to determine the ability of the blood to clot

32. The primipara may suspect pregnancy when the breasts

    1. ooze milk
    2. become painful
    3. deepen in color around the nipple
    4. atrophy

33. Each time the expectant mother visits her doctor he will check her

    1. E.K.G. and B.M.R.
    2. R.B.C. and hemoglobin
    3. B/P and urine
    4. differential blood count and bleeding time

34. Prospective parents benefit by attending Parents Classes because there they have an opportunity

    1. to meet other couples like themselves
    2. to get expert medical advice
    3. to share ideas and fears
    4. to get rid of all their superstitions

35. Routine urinalysis will determine

    1. the bacteria count
    2. the presence of albumin
    3. the presence of casts
    4. the acid level

36. The expectant mother will be advised by her dentist

    1. to drink 3 quarts of milk daily
    2. to take supplementary calcium tablets
    3. to brush her teeth after each meal, A.M. and H.S.
    4. have a dental examination every month for new cavities

37. The pregnant woman may avoid or lessen the discomforts of varicose veins if she is carefully instructed

   a. to rest frequently
   b. to avoid wearing round garters
   c. to rest with the feet elevated
   d. to take warm tub baths

      1. a only
      2. a and b
      3. b and c
      4. a, b, and c

38. The mother's total weight gain during pregnancy should not be more than

   1. 10 pounds   3. 35 pounds
   2. 20 to 25 pounds 4. 60 pounds

39. Some urinary symptoms will occur during pregnancy. These include

   a. oliguria
   b. dysuria during labor
   c. frequency during the last 4 to 6 weeks
   d. dysuria while the fetus is high in the abdomen

      1. all of the above at some time during the pregnancy
      2. d only
      3. a and d
      4. b and c

40. The most distressing symptom associated with glycosuria during pregnancy is

   1. extreme thirst
   2. frequency of urination
   3. boils
   4. pruritis

41. Edema of the feet and legs may occur in the later stages of pregnancy because

   1. the total volume of blood is greatly increased
   2. the fetus slows up the venous blood flow through the abdominal vessels
   3. shortness of breath interferes with flow of blood through the lungs
   4. the total work of the heart is greatly increased

42. Dyspnea in the later stages of pregnancy is greatest when the expectant mother

   1. is lying down
   2. assumes a squatting position
   3. reaches over her head
   4. sits in a deep, easy chair

43. Childbirth is made easier if the expectant mother has faithfully practiced strengthening her muscles by

   1. bending and squatting
   2. strenuous exercising
   3. holding the abdomen in with a boned corset
   4. panting "like a puppy dog"

44. The pregnant woman can best prepare for an easy delivery by

   1. psychotherapy and hypnosis
   2. working on the maternity floor of her local hospital
   3. observing an actual delivery
   4. exercises that strengthen the appropriate muscles and encourage relaxation

45. One of the best exercises advised for the pregnant woman throughout her pregnancy is

   1. golf
   2. walking outdoors
   3. bowling
   4. gardening that requires squatting

46. The effect of German measles on the unborn child will depend on

   1. the strength of the infecting virus
   2. stage of development of the embryo or fetus
   3. physical resistance of the mother
   4. health of the placenta

47. Superstitions concerning "marking" a baby do not make sense when the practical nurse understands

   1. that the placenta screens out most things damaging to the fetus
   2. this is seldom possible
   3. that emotions cannot be transferred to the fetus
   4. the nervous system of the fetus is not well enough developed to be affected

48. The only positive sign of pregnancy is

   1. the sound of fetal heart beats
   2. the absence of a menstrual period
   3. enlargement of the breasts
   4. a positive urine test

49. Symptoms of which the pregnant woman complains are most often caused by the increasing size of the uterus and its contents. Such symptoms include

    a. shortness of breath
    b. anuria
    c. backache
    d. constipation

        1. all of the above
        2. a or c
        3. b and d
        4. a, c, or d

50. The doctor will describe the condition as "quickening." The nurse can interpret this to the patient as meaning

    1. movement of the fetus
    2. settling of the fetus in the pelvis
    3. the start of labor pains
    4. the rupture of the bag of waters

51. Most of the nausea and vomiting of pregnancy will occur in

    1. the first trimester
    2. the second trimester
    3. the third trimester
    4. the first 3 weeks of pregnancy

52. If a well fitting, supportive brassiere keeps the expectant mother in good posture, it will help to prevent

    1. lordosis
    2. clumsiness
    3. a dragging feeling in the pelvis
    4. a backache

53. Shoes with low, broad heels, plus good posture, will do much to prevent prenatal complaints of

    1. vertigo   3. ataxia
    2. nausea   4. backache

54. Discomfort from several of the minor complications of pregnancy can be relieved by

    1. reducing the amount of exercise
    2. proper diet
    3. frequent rest periods with the legs elevated
    4. more frequent visits to the physician when the symptoms become too distressing

55. The nurse would encourage the prospective mother to report to her doctor immediately on the appearance of a danger sign such as

    1. a sick headache with nausea and vomiting
    2. vaginal bleeding
    3. painful breasts
    4. excessive appetite

56. Symptoms that the nurse must recognize as a warning of a severe complication of pregnancy include

    1. persistent headaches and dizziness
    2. nausea and vomiting
    3. mild cramping pains
    4. pains in the calf of the leg

57. Tub baths are usually not taken in the last 6 weeks of pregnancy chiefly because of the danger of

    1. stimulating contractions of the uterus
    2. breaking the bag of waters
    3. dilating the vagina
    4. slipping in the tub

58. A urinary symptom that occurs early in pregnancy and again in the last trimester as the result of pressure on the urinary organs is

    1. frequency   3. oliguria
    2. dysuria   4. hematuria

59. The expectant mother must be taught to recognize the difference in symptoms of "false labor" and of "true labor". True labor is present when

    1. the pains become regular and the time between pains gets shorter
    2. abdominal pains can be counted every ten minutes
    3. headache and dizziness are severe
    4. contractions are severe enough to cause pains in both legs

60. The "bloody show" is really

    1. the first indication of labor
    2. the first indication of a complication
    3. the mucus plug from the cervix
    4. the warning that the third stage of labor is about to begin

61. Symptoms of labor, singly or in combination, which indicate that the pregnant woman is ready to go to the hospital, will include

   a. bloody show
   b. bulging of the perineum
   c. contractions about every 10 minutes
   d. rupture of the amniotic sac

     1. a, b, and d
     2. a, b, and c
     3. a or d
     4. a, c, or d

62. Labor pains are most likely to <u>begin</u> in the

     1. perineum   3. vulva
     2. small of the back   4. cervical opening

63. To prevent the introduction of infectious material into the vaginal canal, the nurse must always shave pubic hair

     1. with a sterile razor
     2. after the area has been disinfected
     3. away from the vaginal opening
     4. after the patient has been draped with sterile sheets

64. The patient in the first stage of labor will be given an enema on admission to the O.B. service. The purpose of the enema at this time is

     1. to relieve pressure
     2. to clear the rectum for digital examination
     3. to dilate the cervix
     4. to relieve uterine cramps by applying heat

65. If the doctor wishes to do a rectal examination, the practical nurse must have available

   a. sterile gloves
   b. a flashlight
   c. clean gloves
   d. a lubricant

     1. a, b, and d
     2. c and d
     3. b, c, and d
     4. a and b

66. A rectal examination will provide information about

     1. fetal abnormalities present
     2. the degree of cervical dilatation
     3. the position of the baby
     4. the sex of the fetus

67. A rectal examination is done to determine the progress of labor. This examination is done while labor is in the

     1. first stage
     2. second stage
     3. third stage
     4. first 3-hour period

68. The procedure for timing uterine contractions begins by the nurse

     1. checking the pulse
     2. placing her fingertips over the fundus
     3. feeling the uterus through the rectum
     4. observing the movement of the abdominal wall

69. If the circular muscles of the cervix are to relax, the mother must be instructed

     1. to push at the height of each contraction
     2. to bear down at the end of each contraction
     3. to cooperate with each pain
     4. to keep from bearing down with the contractions

70. An enema will be given routinely if the pregnant woman is still in

     1. first stage of labor
     2. second stage of labor
     3. third stage of labor
     4. labor room

71. The nurse will recognize the "show" as

     1. the enlargement of the abdomen
     2. the appearance of the head at the vaginal opening
     3. a pinkish vaginal discharge
     4. the dilation of the cervix

72. The purpose of restricting solid food during the period of labor is to avoid

1. increased abdominal pressure
2. flatulence
3. increasing muscular peristalsis
4. possible aspiration later

73. It is important for the bladder to be emptied often during the first stage of labor, either by voiding or an indwelling catheter if necessary, in order

1. to relieve pressure
2. to protect the mother from infection
3. to avoid any obstruction to the baby's head as it moves downward in the pelvic cavity
4. to prevent puncturing the urethra during a contraction

74. The purpose of the uterine contractions during the first stage of labor is

1. to push the baby closer to the vaginal opening
2. rupture the bag of waters
3. push out the mucus plug
4. stretch the cervical opening

75. During the contractions of the first stage of labor, the nurse will encourage the mother

1. to refrain from bearing down with each contraction
2. to push downward with each contraction
3. to hold her breath to ease the pain
4. to take a whiff of gas

76. The student practical nurse is assigned to the Labor Room. If the patient complains of a headache, the student must recognize the importance of

1. an aspirin
2. morphine
3. cold compresses to the head
4. a blood pressure reading

77. The nurse will use all her skills to make the expectant mother comfortable before giving a pain-relieving medication because

1. the mother gets too comfortable
2. muscle contractions slow up
3. the medication may affect the fetus
4. cervical relaxation is speeded up

78. Any medications given to the mother during the first stage of labor would be classified as

1. narcotic   3. antiemetic
2. sedative   4. analgesic

79. It will be safe to leave the primipara in the Labor Room until

1. the bag of waters breaks
2. the head of the fetus can be seen at the vaginal opening
3. the contractions are 2 to 3 minutes apart
4. the doctor arrives and the delivery room is set up

80. A multipara in the second stage of labor would not be given

a. anything by mouth
b. an enema
c. an anesthetic
d. a bedpan

    1. b only
    2. a or b
    3. b or c
    4. all of the above

81. The multipara should be moved from the Labor Room to the Delivery Room as soon as

1. the cervix is completely dilated
2. "bloody show" is determined
3. she is admitted to the hospital
4. the head of the fetus can be seen

82. The stage of labor that will last the longest is

1. the first stage
2. the second stage
3. the third stage
4. the preliminary stage

83. The actual delivery of the baby from the vaginal canal of the mother occurs during

1. the first stage of labor
2. the second stage of labor
3. the third stage of labor
4. the fourth stage of labor

84. The contractions during the second stage of labor are important because they

1. push the baby along the vaginal canal
2. relax the muscles around the neck of the cervix
3. loosen the placenta from the wall of the uterus
4. turn the baby's head toward the mother's back

85. During the contractions of the second stage of labor the nurse will encourage the patient

1. to hold her breath
2. to bear down with each contraction
3. to breathe through her mouth
4. to relax completely

86. When the mother feels like bearing down, and the doctor does not wish her to do so, the nurse will instruct the mother

1. to squeeze the handle bars
2. to talk, to keep her mind off the pain
3. to count aloud during the contractions
4. to breathe through her mouth

87. When placenta previa has been diagnosed, a prolapsed cord should be expected because it is known that

1. uterine contractions will be more severe
2. the placental end of the cord is near the cervical outlet
3. the location of the placenta requires the cord to grow longer
4. the position of the baby will allow the cord to deliver first

88. A prolapsed cord can be expected whenever the presenting part of the fetus

1. is hydrocephalic
2. is in breech position
3. is in great distress from oxygen want
4. fails to press firmly into the cervical opening

89. If prolapse of the cord is not recognized promptly so that treatment can be started, the effect on the fetus will be

1. death due to anoxia
2. delay in delivery
3. development of cardiac complications
4. an increasingly difficult delivery

90. An emergency measure that attempts to keep the presenting part from pressing against the prolapse cord is

1. the relaxation of the mother
2. the elevation of the mother's hips
3. the clamping of the labia together
4. the positioning of the mother in the supine position

91. Once the cervix is dilated, the prolapsed cord is in danger of being pinched between

1. the presenting part and the pelvic bones
2. the presenting part and the vaginal walls
3. the placenta and the presenting part
4. the placenta and the anterior rectal wall

92. When the cervix is not fully dilated, pressure on the cord results from

1. the unruptured amniotic sac
2. interference of the "bloody show"
3. the forceful uterine contractions
4. its position between the cervix and the presenting part

93. The greatest pressure on a prolapsed cord comes when the presenting part is the

1. buttocks   3. head
2. foot   4. face

94. If the fetus is in distress and the cervix is not dilated, the nurse can expect that delivery will be by

1. high forceps
2. Cesarean section
3. low forceps
4. instruments stretching the cervix

95. The prolapsed cord and the distress of the fetus can be expected

1. to increase uterine contractions
2. to have no effect on the mother
3. to increase the severity of the pains
4. to add to the strain on the mother's heart

96. To save the life of the infant when the cord is prolapsed and the cervix is dilating slowly, delivery may be

1. forced
2. with instruments
3. delayed
4. by Cesarean section

97. The term "episiotomy" tells the student that

1. the delivery was with forceps
2. a Cesarean section was done
3. the presentation was breech
4. an incision was made in the perineum

98. The reason the doctor will do an episiotomy is

1. to repair tears that follow delivery
2. to deliver a large baby
3. to prevent stretching the hymen
4. to prevent tears during delivery

99. An episiotomy is an important aid to delivery when the condition of the baby makes it necessary

1. to deliver it rapidly
2. to turn the presenting part
3. to delay the expulsion of the head
4. to give it first aid

100. An episiotomy is done with very little loss of maternal blood. This is true because

1. only capillaries are cut
2. the presenting part acts as a pressure bandage
3. it will be sewed up at once
4. the blood supply to the perineum is minimal

101. The nurse can reassure the mother who has had her first episiotomy that this procedure

1. will not weaken uterine support
2. will not limit her movements
3. will not require stitches
4. prevented a more serious tear

102. The danger of incomplete removal of the placenta lies in

1. the continuing contraction of the uterine muscles
2. the failure to return to normal menstrual periods
3. the occurrence of postpartal hemorrhage
4. the prevention of further pregnancies

103. The final process of delivery is

1. the return of the mother to her room
2. the expulsion of the placenta
3. the cutting of the umbilical cord
4. the repair of any cervical tears

104. Cervical tears are common in all vaginal deliveries. Therefore, every new mother should be encouraged

1. to plan on at least 2 years between pregnancies
2. to prepare for delivery by hypnosis
3. to see her doctor for the 6-week postpartal check-up
4. to request delivery by Cesarean section

105. A deep cervical tear can be expected if delivery is

1. delayed over a period of several hours
2. done at home
3. complicated by sluggish uterine contractions
4. attempted before cervical dilatation is complete

106. During the first stage of labor the nurse can help to prevent cervical tears by frequently reminding the mother

1. to push with each pain
2. to keep her feet higher than her head
3. not to bear down with her pains
4. to keep the fundus massaged

107. Perineal tears occur as the result of

1. muscle weakness
2. the head suddenly popping through the vaginal opening
3. a difficult third stage of labor
4. birth that occurs before the mother can be properly prepared

108. Fecal incontinence would follow delivery that caused

1. a third degree cervical tear
2. a perineal laceration
3. a second-degree perineal tear
4. a third-degree perineal tear

109. The patient has excessive vaginal bleeding following delivery. The nurse should suspect a cervical tear if her examination of the patient reveals

1. a hard, contracted uterus
2. an elevation of blood pressure
3. acute pelvic pain
4. pieces of the placenta still attached to the uterine wall

110. The placental complication that places the fetus in the greatest danger occurs when the placenta is

1. separated from the uterus at the edges
2. attached low in the uterus
3. completely loosened from the uterus
4. hemorrhaging

111. The location of the placenta in the condition of placenta abruptio is

1. high in the uterus, at the normal point of attachment
2. over the opening of the Fallopian tube
3. near, or covering, the neck of the uterus
4. in the fundus

112. Placenta abruptio may be an unexpected complication of a normal delivery if the umbilical cord is

1. twisted   3. prolapsed
2. too short   4. pulsating

113. Placenta abruptio is dangerous to the mother in proportion to the extent of

1. trauma to the cervix
2. labor
3. anoxia
4. hemorrhage

114. All the observation and examination techniques the nurse has must be used to recognize the hemorrhage of placenta abruptio, since the bleeding may be

1. the only visible sign
2. latent
3. from the capillaries
4. internal and not visible

115. Uterine hemorrhage will force the blood between the muscle fibers of the uterus. This will result in

1. overactive muscle contraction
2. absorption of blood by the muscle cells
3. lethargic muscle contractions
4. rapid dilatation of the cervix

116. The most logical theory of the cause of placenta previa is the idea that there is some defect in

1. the preparation of the uterine lining at the normal level
2. the fertilized ovum
3. the hormones produced by the pituitary
4. the nutritional state of the mother before the time of conception

117. Delivery by Cesarean section will be necessary when the placenta is located

1. at the edge of the cervical os
2. below the presenting part
3. at the vaginal outlet
4. over the cervical os

118. The symptom of placenta previa that requires immediate medical attention is

1. painless vaginal bleeding
2. regularity of a bleeding cycle
3. the presence of meconium in the vagina
4. severe ovarian pains

119. An admission enema is contraindicated in a diagnosed condition of placenta previa. The enema is considered dangerous because

1. the emergency may not allow expulsion
2. the heat may dilate the cervix
3. intestinal contractions may increase uterine bleeding
4. the area must not be contaminated

120. An indication for delivery by Cesarean section would be previous surgery that had

1. scraped the lining of the uterus
2. removed uterine tumors
3. lowered the patient's pain threshold
4. amputated the cervix

121. A Cesarean section would be advised for the pregnant woman with heart trouble This would be done to protect her from the danger of

   1. fluid loss
   2. prolonged labor
   3. a prolapsed cord
   4. cervical or perineal tears

122. A complication of the Cesarean section which might be responsible for the death of the mother is

   1. placenta previa
   2. cervicitis
   3. pulmonary embolus
   4. uterine atony

123. The placenta has separated from the wall of the uterus before the cervix is fully dilated. A Cesarean section will be considered

   1. of little value
   2. the delivery of choice with mother's consent
   3. necessary to get the fetus delivered
   4. an emergency to save the baby

124. Following a Cesarean section, the major nursing care of the mother is determined by

   1. the abdominal incision
   2. the speed of the uterine contractions
   3. the number of lacerations received
   4. the amount of vaginal discharge

125. A second pregnancy would require a Cesarean section if the first delivery was by section because

   1. labor was long and difficult
   2. the bony outlet was too small
   3. the baby's life was in danger
   4. of malposition of the uterus

126. Most spontaneous abortions occur before the pregnancy has progressed to

   1. the third week   3. the fourth month
   2. the twelfth week   4. the fifth month

127. The doctor's use of the term "abortion" must often be interpreted to the lay person. The nurse recognizes this as a medical term meaning that

   1. the mother's condition made it necessary for the doctor to remove the fetus before term
   2. pregnancy was interrupted because of deformities evident in the fetus
   3. the loss of a fetus occurred before it was developed enough to live outside the uterus
   4. the cause was beyond the control of the mother or the doctor

128. Fetal malnutrition may be the cause of an abortion. Such malnutrition of the fetus occurs because

   1. of maternal malnutrition for one of many reasons
   2. constipation places undue pressure on the fetus
   3. stomach and intestinal peristalsis is increased
   4. a dietary deficiency decreases the clotting time

129. If the fertilized egg is not implanted in an area of the uterus that is well prepared to receive and nourish it, an abortion often results. Such a condition is present in

   1. placenta abruptio
   2. the presence of a systemic disease of the mother
   3. breech presentations
   4. placenta previa

130. The nurse may be able to reassure the mother following a "missed" abortion if she can help her to understand that the fetus

   1. was deformed
   2. was too young to live
   3. could have been saved if prenatal care had been adequate
   4. had been dead for several weeks

131. An abortion would be suspected if the patient complained of cramping pains, plus the passage of blood clots, followed by

   1. shock
   2. relief from pain
   3. massive vaginal hemorrhage
   4. uterine peristalsis

132. The classification of the abortion helps us to determine the status of the product of conception. The pregnant woman may go to full term and deliver a normal baby in spite of repeated symptoms of

1. threatened abortion
2. induced abortion
3. vaginal hemorrhage
4. severe uterine cramping

133. The patient has had an "incomplete" abortion. Vaginal bleeding will continue because

1. severe uterine contractions damage blood vessels
2. the uterus has been stripped of its lining membrane
3. some placental tissue remains in the uterus
4. the cervix remains dilated

134. When symptoms of abortion appear, the success of any treatment will depend on

1. the knowledge and skill of the physician
2. the ability of the mother to cooperate in the treatment plan
3. whether the fetus is dead or alive
4. the age of the fetus and the location of the placenta

135. Medically, the greatest danger of a criminal abortion is its effect on

1. future immoral behavior of the mother
2. community attitudes toward "free love"
3. the tax rate that must be increased to support illegitimate children
4. the life or the health of the mother

136. An ectopic pregnancy is defined as

1. a fertilization within the Fallopian tube
2. one that develops in the abdominal cavity
3. an embedding of the fertilized ovum outside the uterus
4. an ovarian pregnancy

137. The embryo will rupture into the abdominal cavity by the time it has reached the age of

1. 2 weeks   3. 2 months
2. 6 weeks   4. 3 months

138. A gonorrheal infection may narrow the Fallopian tube. Such a narrowing will allow

1. the unfertilized egg to pass out of the tube
2. the sperm to get into the tube but the fertilized egg cannot move out
3. the fertilized egg to attach to its lining wall
4. only the ovarian hormones to pass through it

139. One cause of a tubal pregnancy would be the blocking of the tubal opening into the uterus by

1. a fibroid tumor
2. a prolapsed fundus
3. the placenta
4. peristaltic contractions

140. The lumen of the Fallopian tube is only 1/16 of an inch in diameter. The embryo cannot grow to a very large size in such a small space and the pregnancy is usually terminated by

1. Cesarean section
2. being pushed out into the peritoneal cavity
3. death of the fetus
4. abortion

141. In the presence of abortion or tubal rupture the nurse knows that the product of conception will be

1. deformed   3. saved by surgery
2. dissolved   4. dead

142. The patient with a ruptured Fallopian tube will be in shock as the result of

a. emotional excitement
b. pain
c. abdominal distention
d. massive hemorrhage

1. all of the above
2. b only
3. a and c
4. b and d

143. Death of the patient with a tubal rupture can be prevented only by emergency measures that result in the removal of

1. the embryo
2. all the reproductive organs
3. the ruptured tube
4. both tubes and ovaries

144. The blood that escapes into the abdominal cavity following a tubal rupture will be responsible for the symptoms of

1. jaundice
2. edema
3. congestive heart failure
4. peritonitis

145. The nursing of a patient with tubal rupture will incorporate the principles of care of the patient

a. in shock
b. with hemorrhage
c. with a complicated laparotomy
d. who has lost her baby

   1. all of the above
   2. b and c only
   3. a, b, and c
   4. c and d

146. A pathologist's examination of a hydatidiform mole reveals that it is made up of

1. a deformed fetus
2. a cluster of blood clots
3. fetal cells organized as a tumor
4. placental tissue

147. Pregnancy has been diagnosed. If the doctor suspected that fetal development was not normal, he could correctly make a diagnosis of hydatidiform mole on the basis of

a. symptoms present
b. physical examination
c. special tests on the urine
d. X-ray

   1. none of the above
   2. all of the above
   3. a and d
   4. c only

148. When a hydatidiform mole is present, the fetus will die because of

1. changes in the placenta
2. hemorrhagic state
3. uterine cramping
4. cervical dilatation

149. The hydatidiform mole becomes a foreign substance within the uterus. This will explain the symptom of

1. hormone imbalance
2. severe uterine cramping
3. generalized muscle aching
4. abdominal distention

150. Whenever the nurse cares for the prenatal patient, whether in the hospital or at home, she must always remember the importance of

1. saving any expelled substance for laboratory examination
2. counting the fetal heart tones daily
3. insisting that the patient use the bedpan rather than the toilet
4. frequent urine examinations

151. The careful laboratory examination of the hydatidiform mole is for the purpose of determining

1. the presence of a fetus
2. the cause
3. any evidence of malignancy
4. any evidence of fetal deformity

152. If the Aschheim-Zondek urine pregnancy test remains positive after the mole has been expelled or removed, this is considered evidence of

1. continuing fetal growth
2. malignant metastasis
3. hormone imbalance
4. uterine infection

153. Of the several complications of pregnancy, toxemia ranks as

1. the most common complication
2. one of the most distressing to the mother
3. the greatest cause of deformity of the newborn
4. the most common serious complication

154. Following the removal of an hydatidiform mole, the mother may be afraid to consider future pregnancies unless she can be reassured that

1. this will only happen once to any individual
2. she has developed an immunity
3. another pregnancy right away will prevent a reoccurrence of such an abnormality
4. the incidence of such abnormalities is very low, less than 1% of all pregnancies

155. A condition of toxemia will be called eclampsia with the appearance of

1. albuminuria   3. edema
2. convulsions   4. hypertension

156. In every case of toxemia or eclampsia, regardless of the degree of severity, the nurse should expect to find evidence of

1. hypertension   3. hyperpnea
2. muscle twitching   4. mental confusion

157. A frequent predisposing cause of toxemia is a dietary deficiency of

1. vitamin A   3. protein
2. vitamin K   4. thiamine

158. It should be possible to prevent the progression of symptoms to the point of eclampsia by

1. an early visit to the obstetrician
2. prompt and continuous treatment of symptoms of toxemia
3. careful delivery techniques
4. bed rest and prompt hospitalization at the first symptom

159. Elevation of the blood pressure during the third trimester of pregnancy is a symptom of the dreaded complication of

1. hypertension   3. arteriosclerosis
2. toxemia   4. obesity

160. The urine is examined each time the pregnant woman visits the doctor. A serious complication of pregnancy is indicated by

1. albuminuria   3. crystalluria
2. glycosuria   4. polyuria

161. Toxemia will be suspected if the pregnant woman gains weight in excess of

1. 1/2 pound a week   3. 2 pounds a month
2. 2 pounds a week   4. 6 pounds a month

162. Toxemia is most likely to occur during the third trimester. For this reason the pregnant woman can expect her doctor to plan for

1. early hospitalization of the mother with heart disease
2. emergency admission to the hospital if symptoms appear
3. more frequent prenatal visits after the sixth month
4. a practical nurse to remain with the patient until delivery

163. Some prenatal examinations are done each time the pregnant woman visits the doctor. Those that are done for the purpose of recognizing the first symptoms of toxemia or pretoxemia include
a. weight
b. urinalysis
c. fetal heart tones
d. blood pressure

1. a, b, and d
2. d only
3. a and b
4. all of the above

164. If symptoms of toxemia are to be treated early enough to prevent eclampsia, then prenatal instruction must teach the pregnant woman that the doctor will need to know immediately if and whenever she experiences

1. albuminuria
2. a low backache
3. retention of fluid in the feet and ankles
4. severe, continuous headaches

165. The effects of toxemia on the fetus may be one or more of the following:
a. brain damage
b. premature delivery
c. intrauterine death
d. malpresentation

1. all of the above
2. b only
3. a and c
4. a, b, and c

166. When the patient with toxemia or eclampsis is admitted to the hospital, the nurse is responsible for frequent checking of signs and symptoms that may indicate progression of the condition. It is most important for the nurse to evaluate frequently

1. the environmental influences
2. the subjective symptoms
3. the dietary intake
4. the nurse's notes

167. The blood pressure reading is an important indication of the degree of seriousness of toxemia. The nurse will recognize the potential danger if the systolic blood pressure reading is

1. more than 150 millimeters of mercury
2. 10 millimeters or more above the usual B/P
3. higher than the diastolic pressure
4. 100 millimeters or higher

168. The nurse should appreciate that hyperemesis gravidarum can progress in seriousness to the point of

1. coma   3. death
2. convulsions 4. hyperpyrexia

169. The symptoms may be limited to nausea and vomiting. In this situation the nurse will not be concerned about ill effects on

1. the fetus
2. the nutritional state of the mother
3. the body metabolism
4. the electrolyte balance

170. The growing fetus can be the cause of hyperemesis gravidarum if

1. growth is too rapid
2. the mother is being deprived of essential nutrients
3. the child is not wanted
4. fetal toxins produce maternal toxemia

171. The most serious <u>systemic</u> symptoms that result from hyperemesis gravidarum are those of

1. nervous origin
2. dehydration
3. malnutrition
4. emotional imbalance

172. Emotions may be the basic cause of hyperemesis gravidarum. Such a functional cause would be suspected if

1. this were the first pregnancy
2. the mother were Para III
3. vomiting began soon after the first missed menstrual period
4. vomiting lasted longer than 1 month, and occurred after each meal

173. The loss of fluids through continuous vomiting will produce

a. oliguria
b. dry, inelastic skin
c. polydipsia
d. dry, cracked tongue

1. all of the above
2. a only
3. b and c
4. a, b, and d

174. The cause of hyperemesis gravidarum may be based on a need to obtain sympathy and attention from the husband or other members of the family. If this is the cause, the patient usually responds quickly to

1. complete isolation treatment
2. the hospital environment
3. I.M. injections
4. limited food intake

175. Sedatives may be given to help overcome the vomiting. Such sedation would be most effective if given

1. immediately after meals
2. by I.M.
3. 30 minutes a.c.
4. with plenty of fluid

176. When the nurse is caring for a patient with hyperemesis gravidarum, one <u>effective</u> approach is that of

1. censorship
2. disapproval
3. positive acceptance that the vomiting will soon stop
4. sympathetic understanding of the feelings of the patient

177. The patient vomits as soon as she finishes her tray. The usual procedure in such a situation is

    1. to delay cleaning the emesis basin or changing soiled linens
    2. to start I.V. fluids
    3. to ignore her call light when she signals the nurse
    4. to bring her a second tray immediately

178. Postpartal hemorrhage may be caused by

    a. failure of the uterine muscles to contract
    b. fatigue
    c. lack of adequate hemoglobin
    d. incomplete elimination of the placenta

        1. any of the above
        2. d only
        3. a or d
        4. b, c, and d

179. The danger of a postpartal infection in the vagina or cervix is the ease with which it can spread to

    1. the brain
    2. the peritoneum
    3. the circulatory system
    4. the fetus

180. Medication that is given after delivery to help prevent hemorrhage will

    1. increase the clotting time of the blood
    2. put the patient at complete rest
    3. contract uterine muscles
    4. increase the blood pressure

181. The lochia that appears immediately following delivery will be

    1. purulent   3. bloody
    2. serous   4. mucopurulent

182. The mother should be prepared to expect the discomforts of the postpartal period. One such discomfort is

    1. cramping
    2. muscle weakness
    3. a bloody discharge
    4. engorgement of the breasts

183. The nurse assigned to care for mothers after delivery is expected to observe and accurately describe the lochia. The importance of such observation is evident when

    1. a foul odor warns of the presence of an infection
    2. the doctor needs to determine the condition of the uterus
    3. release from the hospital depends on the nurse's reports
    4. the patient requests a vaginal douche

184. The nurse often finds it necessary to reassure the new mother that colostrum

    1. is a form of milk
    2. is probably valuable for its protective substances
    3. has all the nourishment of milk
    4. will change to milk if the mother's diet is adequate

185. After delivery, output of urine must be measured. The normal urine output would be

    1. concentrated   3. doubled
    2. decreased   4. increased

186. After delivery, the lochia may be collected on

    1. an absorbent pad
    2. a sterile sanitary napkin
    3. a tampon
    4. the clean sheet

187. A postpartal infection may be caused by

    1. poor resistance
    2. allowing the mother to be ambulatory
    3. contamination of the vulva with feces
    4. the high acidity of vaginal secretions

188. The nurse can contribute to the mother's need to move about in bed if she

    1. keeps telling the mother of its importance
    2. sets a routine time for practice
    3. lets the mother take her own bath
    4. always places desired articles just beyond easy reach

189. A postpartal complaint due to the stretching and relaxation of the abdominal muscles is

   1. constipation   3. after pains
   2. diaphoresis   4. urinary retention

190. The newly delivered patient is losing enough blood vaginally to be considered hemorrhaging. The student practical nurse could expect that her first step in the emergency care of this type of hemorrhage would be

   1. notification of the husband
   2. application of ice bags to the head
   3. massage of the fundus
   4. elevation of the bed on shock blocks

191. Once the baby has been delivered, the uterus will be massaged for the purpose of

   1. helping it to relax
   2. aiding its contraction
   3. giving the patient some attention
   4. quieting the patient

192. When milk fills the mother's breasts, this is known as a period of

   1. involution   3. engorgement
   2. puerperium   4. lactation

193. If the production of milk is to be stopped, it will be necessary

   a. to apply a tight binder
   b. to give saline cathartics
   c. to restrict fluid intake
   d. to pump the breasts T.I.D.

      1. all of the above
      2. a only
      3. a, c, and d
      4. b and c

194. The mother's breasts can be dried up, or congestion relieved, by the oral administration of

   1. adrenalin   3. stilbesterol
   2. testosterone   4. Cafergot

195. The 6-week physical examination of the mother is intended to allow the doctor to check
   a. the re-establishment of menstruation
   b. the position of the uterus
   c. the cervix for tears
   d. the breasts and the nipples

      1. a, b, and c
      2. b only
      3. b, c, and d
      4. all of the above

196. Check those conditions listed below in which it is no longer possible for pregnancy to occur:

   a. menstruation
   b. menopause
   c. a hysterectomy
   d. one sided salpingectomy

      1. all of the above
      2. b, c, or d
      3. b or c
      4. b only

197. The life of the newborn depends upon the ease with which it can be stimulated to cry. Such behavior is necessary because

   1. crying improves the circulation
   2. the alveoli must be filled with air
   3. it indicates a need for nourishment
   4. abnormal symptoms can be easily recognized

198. The black, tarry material expelled from the rectum of the newborn is called

   1. vernix caseosa   3. viable
   2. foramen ovale   4. meconium

199. The newborn has a "soft spot" on its head. The purpose of this spot is

   1. to allow for increased pressure of spinal fluid
   2. to protect the brain from intra-uterine pressures
   3. to protect the brain against pressures within the birth canal
   4. to permit easy adjustment to the pressure from the external environment

200. The breast-fed baby must be weighed

    a. after the bath
    b. before going to breast
    c. after feeding
    d. before visiting hours

        1. c only
        2. b and c
        3. a and d
        4. none of the above

201. The nurse learns that the newborn communicates its feelings and its needs through its

    1. kicking   3. movements
    2. smile   4. cry

202. The sensory end-organs that are best developed at birth are those that carry the messages of

    1. smell   3. touch
    2. taste   4. sight

203. The newborn is not fed immediately after it is born. This is because the baby needs time to allow it

    1. to get rid of collected mucus
    2. to build up an energy reserve
    3. to regulate its breathing
    4. to empty the bowel of fetal wastes

204. The newborn can be expected to lose some of its birth weight. This is due to the loss of

    a. mucus
    b. feces
    c. fluid through urination
    d. a warm environment

        1. all of the above
        2. c only
        3. a, b, and c
        4. a and c

205. A "cord paint" may be applied to the umbilical cord after it has been cut. This is done for the purpose of

    1. helping the cord to fall off
    2. stopping bleeding
    3. preventing infection
    4. keeping the cord from falling off too soon

206. Identification bracelets are placed on the newborn before it leaves the Delivery Room because

    1. it is easier while the baby is unwrapped
    2. the chart of the mother, with the correct spelling, is available
    3. the mother is present to answer any questions
    4. the chance of mixing babies is eliminated, since mother and baby have not been separated

207. The state law requires that silver nitrate or penicillin drops be placed in the eyes of the newborn. This is done in an effort to prevent

    1. blindness due to a gonorrheal infection
    2. the spread of diseases throughout the nursery
    3. infant deaths in the first few days after birth
    4. nipple infection in the mother

208. Any baby that weighs less than 2500 grams at birth should be cared for as a premature even if it has been in the uterus full term; 2500 grams is equal to

    1. 3 pounds   3. 5 pounds
    2. 4 pounds   4. 6 pounds

209. The normal stool of the newborn by the end of the fourth neonatal day will be described as

    1. yellow   3. greenish brown
    2. brown   4. black and tarry

210. Until the newborn takes its first breath, the lungs would be described as in a condition of

    1. anoxia   3. collapse
    2. atelectasis   4. hypertension

211. The nursing personnel will play an important part in the early personality development of a baby when it is necessary for it to be

    1. cared for in the nursery
    2. bottle fed
    3. in the hospital for weeks after birth
    4. isolated

212. The nurse can expect that the breast-fed baby will have more stools per day than the formula-fed baby. This is true because

1. the fat content is higher in breast milk
2. the CHO content is higher in a formula
3. the water content of breast milk is high
4. a formula is not so completely assimilated

213. The bottle-fed baby can get the needed T.L.C. (tender loving care) during its feeding if the adult responsible for the feeding will

1. sing or hum
2. relax
3. sit down in the rocking chair
4. hold and cuddle the baby

214. It is not true that the longer the baby remains in the uterus after term the fatter and more completely developed it will be. Instead it will lose weight because

1. the mother's tissues have given up providing nourishment
2. the umbilical cord does not continue to provide nourishment
3. the vernix caseosa is absorbed
4. it must depend on its own fat and protein for nourishment

215. The mother will need adequate reassurance and explanation if the new baby has some vaginal bleeding. The nurse understands that this has been caused by

1. premature stimulation of the ovarian hormones by the pituitary gland
2. the effect of female sex hormones, absorbed from the mother on the uterine lining of the baby
3. the increased total of circulating blood in the mother throughout the pregnancy
4. the hormone changes that normally are part of the birth process

216. The footprints of the newborn will be recorded

1. as soon as the cord is cut
2. in the Delivery Room
3. as soon as the baby is admitted to the Nursery
4. by the doctor who delivers the baby

217. A sterile bulb syringe should be placed in the corner of the incubator housing a newborn. Immediate use of this syringe would be necessary if the baby

1. became cyanotic
2. aspirated
3. had irregular respirations
4. became jaundiced

218. Spread of infection throughout the Nursery is avoided if each nurse who works on this unit will conscientiously

a. wash her hands before touching a baby
b. wipe out the scale with alcohol before weighing a baby
c. cover the scale with a disposable towel before weighing a baby
d. keep everything in the environment sterile

1. all of the above
2. a only
3. a, b, and c
4. b and c

219. The procedure for daily cleansing of the eyes of the newborn provides for

1. disinfecting drops
2. discarding the gauze sponge after it has passed over the eye once
3. irrigation with normal saline and a sterile bulb syringe
4. moving the gauze sponge from the outer canthus toward the inner canthus

220. After the baby has been returned to its crib, following feeding, it will usually be positioned on its

1. back
2. side
3. abdomen
4. left side

221. All babies must be closely observed for the first 12 hours after birth. The nurse will carefully check for any evidence of

1. bleeding from the cord
2. fecal impaction
3. internal malformations
4. club feet or harelip

222. The normal baby should still be seen by the doctor as often as

a. every month
b. every 2 months
c. every month for 3 months
d. every other month from age 4 to 12 months

1. a only
2. a and d
3. c and d
4. b and c

223. Behavior that can be expected of the baby at about 6 months of age includes the ability

1. to pull himself to an upright position
2. to walk without support
3. to sit alone for a short time
4. to feed himself

224. Most infants can be expected to begin to walk at about the age of

1. 1 year
2. 2 years
3. 18 months
4. 10 months

225. Circumcision can be described as the process of

1. enlarging the skin sac surrounding the penis
2. prophylaxis against cancer of the penis
3. cutting away the foreskin
4. exposing the glans penis

226. Cancer of the penis is prevented when the boy is circumcised at birth. Circumcision makes it impossible for

1. the penis to be irritated
2. elimination problems to occur
3. the penis to become infected
4. secretions to accumulate under the foreskin

227. The age of the baby at time of circumcision may depend on

a. religious customs
b. the physical condition of the baby
c. the convenience of the hospital personnel
d. the preference of the doctor

1. a and b
2. a, b, or d
3. c and d
4. all of the above

228. Circumcision is a surgical procedure. Legally, circumcision requires the hospital to obtain

1. certification of need from the doctor
2. written consent from the mother
3. witnessed signatures of both parents
4. the consent of the obstetric staff

229. The greatest postoperative danger to which the nursery personnel must be alert following a circumcision is

1. shock
2. hemorrhage
3. infection
4. cyanosis

230. The new mother asks the student why such stress is placed on circumcision so soon after birth. The student's knowledge of emotional growth and development will help her explain that

1. the poorly developed nervous and circulatory systems of the newborn make the procedure safe now
2. pain stimuli do not affect the baby in the neonatal period
3. psychological injury, common in the older child or adult, can be avoided if the surgery is done early
4. there is less danger of contamination and infection

231. If the penis bleeds freely following circumcision, vitamin K will be given for the purpose of

1. increasing the plasma proteins needed for coagulation
2. preventing blood clots
3. providing material to produce prothrombin and increase coagulation
4. speeding up absorption of substances needed for blood coagulation

232. To prevent infection in the penis following a circumcision, the operated area is covered with a sterile petrolatum gauze and

1. changed each time the diaper is soiled during the first 24 hours
2. wiped off frequently with an alcohol sponge
3. penicillin is given I.M., B.I.D.
4. the dressing is not removed during the first 24 hours P.O.

233. Icterus Neonatorum will be evident

1. immediately after birth
2. after the second week of life
3. around the third neonatal day
4. within the first 36 hours

234. Physiological jaundice is normal in many newborn. The yellow color occurs when the rapid destruction of the red blood cells

1. stimulates replacement with immature cells
2. goes on faster than cells are replaced
3. lowers the hemoglobin level
4. makes it possible for bilirubin to circulate in the bloodstream

235. If the jaundice is diagnosed as icterus neonatorum, the nurse can reassure the mother that

a. the baby's health will not be affected
b. surgery will produce a permanent cure
c. the symptoms will disappear before she takes the baby home
d. the jaundice will fade by the end of 2 weeks

    1. all of the above
    2. d only
    3. b and c
    4. a and d

236. The nurse can be sure nothing is wrong with the production and flow of bile in the baby with icterus neonatorum because

1. the stools will be a normal color
2. urine will be concentrated
3. the appetite will be good
4. sleep is normal

237. If the baby is born with red blood cells that are fragile, the number breaking will depend on changes on the osmotic pressure. In such a case jaundice would be present

1. at birth
2. intermittently
3. continuously
4. only when the baby is awake

238. The typical stool of the baby with an obstruction of the bile ducts would be described as

1. greasy   3. clay-colored
2. diarrheal   4. green

239. When the pigments are eliminated in the saliva, nursing care must include frequent

1. collections of specimens to go to the laboratory
2. oral hygiene
3. change of clothing and linens
4. rinsing with mouthwash to change the taste

240. Hemorrhage is a constant danger for the child with obstruction of the bile ducts. This is true because

1. vitamin K is not assimilated when bile is lacking in the small intestine
2. prothrombin, essential to clotting, is lost in excessive amounts
3. elements essential to clotting are eliminated in the feces
4. the red blood cells rupture so readily

241. The symptom that will be most distressing to the jaundiced baby is

1. loose stools
2. inability to digest fats
3. urine that irritates
4. itching

242. Jaundice due to obstruction of the bile ducts occasionally appears in the first few days of life. This is serious because the diagnosis is likely to be confused with

1. the Rh factor
2. syphilitic jaundice
3. icterus neonatorum
4. hepatitis

243. The Nursery nurse can check on the normality or abnormality of the baby's feet. An easy test is

1. to check the Babinski reflex
2. to study the footprints
3. to place the feet in a position opposite of normal
4. to stand the baby upright and note the direction the heel turns

244. A very noticeable sign of bilateral dislocation that can readily be observed in the newborn is

1. the increased sensitivity of the muscles of the legs
2. the cry of pain as the baby is picked up
3. the unequal length of the two legs
4. the broadening and flattening of the buttocks

245. When conjunctivitis is the result of the silver nitrate drops placed in the baby's eyes, the cause is classified as

1. bacterial
2. virus
3. poor technique in the Delivery Room
4. chemical irritation

246. The baby may develop a gonorrheal conjunctivitis after prophylactic drops have been placed in its eyes. The source of such infection is usually

1. the mother's contaminated hands
2. medication of a strength too weak to be effective
3. poor nursery techniques
4. another infant

247. A baby born at home without the assistance of doctor or nurse would not have the advantage of prophylactic eye drops. If such a baby develops a gonorrheal conjunctivitis, we would suspect that it had been exposed to the germs

1. after the delivery
2. as it came through the birth canal
3. in the use of contaminated nursing equipment
4. while being fed

248. Conjunctivitis, regardless of the cause, will have an accompanying swelling of the eyelids. Such swelling is caused by

1. bacterial invasion
2. the collection of white blood cells
3. infiltration of tissues with exudate from the blood stream
4. increased blood supply to the part, brought about by the elevated temperature

249. When the baby is not treated for a gonorrheal conjunctivitis, the final damage will be

1. destruction of the cornea
2. visual disturbances
3. generalized gonorrheal infection
4. sterility

250. Nursing care will be done to prevent spread of gonorrheal conjunctivitis from the infected eye to the unaffected eye. All treatments will be given with the baby positioned

1. on its back
2. in the dorsal recumbent position
3. on the nurse's lap
4. on the affected side

251. Smears are taken of the material that accumulates in the baby's eyes for the purpose of determining

1. the medications to be ordered
2. the nursing care needed
3. the causative organism
4. the extent of injury to the eye

252. The nurse who cares for the baby with gonorrheal conjunctivitis must constantly remember than the gonococcus organism is

1. rapidly fatal
2. readily transferred to the eyes of the nurse
3. dangerous because it is a venereal disease
4. one of the hardest organisms to kill

253. If the conjunctivitis is due to the silver nitrate drops, the nurse can expect the symptoms to appear

1. before the baby goes home
2. no sooner than 72 hours after birth
3. in the 24 hours after birth
4. sometime within the first week of life

254. A symptom that is present in gonorrheal conjunctivitis and is seldom, if ever, a problem in other types of conjunctivitis is

1. blindness
2. photophobia
3. infected mucous membrane
4. swollen eyelids

255. Impetigo in the newborn is especially undesirable because of

1. the reaction of the parents to the disfiguring appearance of the baby
2. the ease with which an epidemic can occur
3. the danger of infection in the lesions
4. serious systemic symptoms

256. Spread of impetigo will be decreased if the nurse is aware that the causative organism can survive

1. in dust
2. for hours in a moist environment
3. without oxygen
4. scrubbing with soap and water

257. The lesions of impetigo are most likely to be noticed first

1. on the soles of the feet
2. in the groin
3. on the face
4. on hairy parts of the body

258. The characteristic lesion of impetigo is

1. the papule   3. the pustule
2. the vesicle   4. the golden crust

259. The yellow crust so typical of impetigo is the result of

1. the vesicle rupturing and the serum drying on the surface
2. pus formation
3. the vesicles running together to form large crusts
4. injury to the surrounding tissue

260. Crusts of impetigo are usually removed by the doctor or the nurse. This is done for the purpose of

1. stimulating healing
2. applying the medication more effectively
3. preventing the spread of the disease
4. building up the skin resistance

261. The crusts of impetigo are loosened effectively with

1. antibiotic ointments
2. soda-bicarbonate soaks
3. warm compresses of magnesium sulfate
4. continuous hot, wet dressings

262. Impetigo is prevented or its spread controlled when all Nursery personnel conscientiously follow the stated routine of

1. a daily bath
2. handwashing between caring for each baby
3. cap, mask, and gown technique
4. limiting visitors

263. The fungus causing thrush is most likely to be found in

1. hospital-prepared formula
2. the respiratory secretions of nursery personnel
3. the feces of one of the infants
4. the vaginal secretions of one of the mothers

264. The lesions of thrush will be found

1. on the tongue
2. in the cheek
3. over the tonsil area
4. scattered all over the mouth

265. Unless the Nursery nurse has been taught to look for and recognize the lesions of thrush, they may be mistaken for

1. milk curds   3. fever blisters
2. Koplick's spots 4. papillae

266. A characteristic of lesions of thrush that will help in positive identification of the disease is their tendency

1. to rinse off easily
2. to leave a raw, bleeding area when scraped off
3. to disappear when the mouth is swabbed with boric acid
4. to affect the baby's appetite

267. The only symptom of thrush that may be distressing to the baby is that of

1. a feeling of roughness to the lesions
2. pain
3. soreness in the mouth during nursing
4. a bad taste from the medicine

268. The rapid spread of thrush throughout the Nursery is most likely to be caused by

1. an infected nurse
2. unclean bottles and nipples
3. poor technique on the part of the examining doctor
4. unsterilized water

269. It is not recommended that an attempt be made to prevent thrush in the newborn by

1. setting standards of formula preparation
2. cautioning the mother to keep her breasts and hands clean
3. rigid handwashing techniques
4. frequent, daily oral swabbing

270. A predisposing factor to an epidemic of infectious diarrhea in a newborn Nursery is

1. poor bath technique
2. inadequacy of the diet
3. overcrowding
4. poor isolation techniques

271. A frequent cause of an epidemic of bacterial infectious diarrhea in the newborn Nursery is

1. a healthy employee who is a carrier
2. poor feeding techniques
3. flies in the Nursery
4. the drinking water

272. Infectious diarrhea cannot be considered under control in an obstetric department so long as

1. babies are still being delivered
2. no change has been made in nursing personnel
3. some babies have diarrhea
4. visiting hours are not restricted

273. The nurse should suspect the onset of infectious diarrhea in any baby that has

1. blood in the stool
2. mucus in the stool
3. a clay-colored, liquid stool
4. more than 2 watery stools in 24 hours

274. Prodromal symptoms of infectious diarrhea include

1. sore mouth
2. anorexia and fretfulness
3. unexplained coma
4. constipation and irritability

275. A typical stool passed by a baby with infectious diarrhea would be described as

1. full of blood and mucus
2. green, foul-smelling, and passed explosively
3. yellow-brown and watery
4. mostly mucous, tinged with fecal material

276. The systemic symptoms that put the baby in greatest danger are those that result from

1. loss of weight
2. exhaustion due to frequent stools
3. intercurrent infection
4. dehydration

277. The sulfa preparation that is effectively used in treating both contacts and infected infants with infectious diarrhea is

1. Aureomycin
2. bacitracin
3. Gantrisin
4. sulfathiazole

278. A hospital policy that is aimed at preventing an outbreak of infectious diarrhea in the newborn Nursery requires all Nursery personnel to have

1. Staphylococcus immunity
2. vaccinations
3. throat cultures
4. weekly physical examinations

279. The mortality rate of infectious diarrhea in a newborn Nursery varies from 50 to 100%. As a result, when this disease is present in a nursery, health authorities will

1. inspect the O.B. department more often
2. establish rigid health standards for all hospital personnel
3. close the infected nursery to new admissions
4. require an admission physical examination

The IBM answer sheets which follow have been perforated for easy removal from the book. It is suggested that the user detach the appropriate answer sheet, study an individual test question and fill in the selected answer on the IBM form. In this way the review will simulate the actual process of taking the licensing examination.

The Key of correct answers is available in a separate booklet. When the answer you have selected does not agree with the key, try to decide which of the test techniques mentioned in the Introduction has been violated

PERSONAL HYGIENE
(pp. 1-8)

SCORES

1	5
2	6
3	7
4	8

NAME _____ DATE _____
LAST   FIRST   MIDDLE

SCHOOL _____ CITY _____

DATE OF BIRTH _____ AGE _____ SEX _____ M OR F

GRADE OR CLASS _____ INSTRUCTOR _____

NAME OF TEST _____ PART _____

SAMPLE:

1—1 a country
1—2 a mountain
1—3 an island
1—4 a city
1—5 a state

1. Chicago is

DIRECTIONS: Read each question and its numbered answers. When you have decided which answer is correct, blacken the corresponding space on this sheet with the special pencil. Make your mark as long as the pair of lines, and move the pencil point up and down firmly to make a heavy black line. If you change your mind, erase your first mark completely. Make no stray marks; they may count against you.

BE SURE YOUR MARKS ARE HEAVY AND BLACK.
ERASE COMPLETELY ANY ANSWER YOU WISH TO CHANGE.

Answer grid, columns numbered 1 2 3 4 5 for each question:

Questions 1–30, 31–60, 61–90, 91–120, 121–150

Printed by the International Business Machines Corporation, Dayton, N. J., U.S.A.

IBM FORM I.T.S. 1000 B 108

297

VOCATIONAL ADJUSTMENTS
(pp. 9–15)

SCORES

1	5
2	6
3	7
4	8

NAME _____
LAST   FIRST   MIDDLE

SCHOOL _____
CITY

DATE _____

DATE OF BIRTH _____   AGE _____   SEX _____ M OR F

GRADE OR CLASS _____   INSTRUCTOR _____

NAME OF TEST _____   PART _____

DIRECTIONS: Read each question and its numbered answers. When you have decided which answer is correct, blacken the corresponding space on this sheet with the special pencil. Make your mark as long as the pair of lines, and move the pencil point up and down firmly to make a heavy black line. If you change your mind, erase your first mark completely. Make no stray marks; they may count against you.

SAMPLE:

1—1 a country
1—2 a mountain
1—3 an island
1—4 a city
1—5 a state

1. Chicago is

BE SURE YOUR MARKS ARE HEAVY AND BLACK.
ERASE COMPLETELY ANY ANSWER YOU WISH TO CHANGE.

Printed by the International Business Machines Corporation, Dayton, N. J., U. S. A.   IBM FORM I.T.S. 1000 B 108

GROWTH AND DEVELOPMENT
(pp. 17-36)

NAME _____
LAST   FIRST   MIDDLE

SCHOOL _____
CITY

DATE _____

DATE OF BIRTH _____

GRADE OR CLASS _____ INSTRUCTOR _____

NAME OF TEST _____

AGE _____ SEX _____ M OR F

PART _____

SCORES

1 _____ 5 _____
2 _____ 6 _____
3 _____ 7 _____
4 _____ 8 _____

DIRECTIONS: Read each question and its numbered answers. When you have decided which answer is correct, blacken the corresponding space on this sheet with the special pencil. Make your mark as long as the pair of lines, and move the pencil point up and down firmly to make a heavy black line. If you change your mind, erase your first mark completely. Make no stray marks; they may count against you.

SAMPLE:

1. Chicago is
   1—1 a country
   1—2 a mountain
   1—3 an island
   1—4 a city
   1—5 a state

Printed by the International Business Machines Corporation, Dayton, N. J., U.S.A.   IBM FORM I.T.S. 1000 B 108

SCORES

5
6
7
8

1
2
3
4

1 2 3 4 5	1 2 3 4 5	1 2 3 4 5	1 2 3 4 5	1 2 3 4 5
151	181	211	241	271
152	182	212	242	272
153	183	213	243	273
154	184	214	244	274
155	185	215	245	275
156	186	216	246	276
157	187	217	247	277
158	188	218	248	278
159	189	219	249	279
160	190	220	250	280
161	191	221	251	281
162	192	222	252	282
163	193	223	253	283
164	194	224	254	284
165	195	225	255	285

BE SURE YOUR MARKS ARE HEAVY AND BLACK.
ERASE COMPLETELY ANY ANSWER YOU WISH TO CHANGE.

1 2 3 4 5	1 2 3 4 5	1 2 3 4 5	1 2 3 4 5	1 2 3 4 5
166	196	226	256	286
167	197	227	257	287
168	198	228	258	288
169	199	229	259	289
170	200	230	260	290
171	201	231	261	291
172	202	232	262	292
173	203	233	263	293
174	204	234	264	294
175	205	235	265	295
176	206	236	266	296
177	207	237	267	297
178	208	238	268	298
179	209	239	269	299
180	210	240	270	300

MIDDLE

FIRST

LAST

NAME

IBM FORM I.T.S. 1100 B 107-2

NUTRITION AND DIET THERAPY
PART I
(pp. 37–54)

NAME _____ LAST _____ FIRST _____ MIDDLE _____ DATE _____ DATE OF BIRTH _____ AGE _____ SEX M OR F

SCHOOL _____ CITY _____ GRADE OR CLASS _____ INSTRUCTOR _____

NAME OF TEST _____ PART _____

SCORES

1	5
2	6
3	7
4	8

DIRECTIONS: Read each question and its numbered answers. When you have decided which answer is correct, blacken the corresponding space on this sheet with the special pencil. Make your mark as long as the pair of lines, and move the pencil point up and down firmly to make a heavy black line. If you change your mind, erase your first mark completely. Make no stray marks; they may count against you.

SAMPLE:
1—1 a country
1—2 a mountain
1—3 an island
1—4 a city
1—5 a state

1. Chicago is

BE SURE YOUR MARKS ARE HEAVY AND BLACK.
ERASE COMPLETELY ANY ANSWER YOU WISH TO CHANGE.

(Answer grid, questions 1–150, each with response options 1 2 3 4 5)

(OVER)

SCORES

5
6
7
8

1
2
3
4

MIDDLE

FIRST

LAST

NAME

	1	2	3	4	5		1	2	3	4	5		1	2	3	4	5		1	2	3	4	5		1	2	3	4	5
151						181						211						241						271					
152						182						212						242						272					
153						183						213						243						273					
154						184						214						244						274					
155						185						215						245						275					
156						186						216						246						276					
157						187						217						247						277					
158						188						218						248						278					
159						189						219						249						279					
160						190						220						250						280					
161						191						221						251						281					
162						192						222						252						282					
163						193						223						253						283					
164						194						224						254						284					
165						195						225						255						285					

BE SURE YOUR MARKS ARE HEAVY AND BLACK.
ERASE COMPLETELY ANY ANSWER YOU WISH TO CHANGE.

	1	2	3	4	5		1	2	3	4	5		1	2	3	4	5		1	2	3	4	5		1	2	3	4	5
166						196						226						256						286					
167						197						227						257						287					
168						198						228						258						288					
169						199						229						259						289					
170						200						230						260						290					
171						201						231						261						291					
172						202						232						262						292					
173						203						233						263						293					
174						204						234						264						294					
175						205						235						265						295					
176						206						236						266						296					
177						207						237						267						297					
178						208						238						268						298					
179						209						239						269						299					
180						210						240						270						300					

304

IBM FORM I.T.S. 1100 B 107-2

NUTRITION AND DIET THERAPY
PART II
(pp. 55-73)

NAME _____
LAST   FIRST   MIDDLE

SCHOOL _____
CITY

DATE OF BIRTH _____ AGE _____ SEX _____ M OR F

GRADE OR CLASS _____ INSTRUCTOR _____

NAME OF TEST _____ PART _____

SCORES

1	5
2	6
3	7
4	8

DIRECTIONS: Read each question and its numbered answers. When you have decided which answer is correct, blacken the corresponding space on this sheet with the special pencil. Make your mark as long as the pair of lines, and move the pencil point up and down firmly to make a heavy black line. If you change your mind, erase your first mark completely. Make no stray marks; they may count against you.

SAMPLE:
1. Chicago is

1—1 a country
1—2 a mountain
1—3 an island
1—4 a city
1—5 a state

BE SURE YOUR MARKS ARE HEAVY AND BLACK.
ERASE COMPLETELY ANY ANSWER YOU WISH TO CHANGE.

Printed by the International Business Machines Corporation, Dayton, N. J., U. S. A.   IBM FORM I.T.S. 1000 B 108

(OVER)

	1 2 3 4 5		1 2 3 4 5		1 2 3 4 5		1 2 3 4 5		1 2 3 4 5
151		181		211		241		271	
152		182		212		242		272	
153		183		213		243		273	
154		184		214		244		274	
155		185		215		245		275	
156		186		216		246		276	
157		187		217		247		277	
158		188		218		248		278	
159		189		219		249		279	
160		190		220		250		280	
161		191		221		251		281	
162		192		222		252		282	
163		193		223		253		283	
164		194		224		254		284	
165		195		225		255		285	

BE SURE YOUR MARKS ARE HEAVY AND BLACK.
ERASE COMPLETELY ANY ANSWER YOU WISH TO CHANGE.

	1 2 3 4 5		1 2 3 4 5		1 2 3 4 5		1 2 3 4 5		1 2 3 4 5
166		196		226		256		286	
167		197		227		257		287	
168		198		228		258		288	
169		199		229		259		289	
170		200		230		260		290	
171		201		231		261		291	
172		202		232		262		292	
173		203		233		263		293	
174		204		234		264		294	
175		205		235		265		295	
176		206		236		266		296	
177		207		237		267		297	
178		208		238		268		298	
179		209		239		269		299	
180		210		240		270		300	

306

IBM FORM I.T.S. 1100 B 107-2

NURSING ARTS
PART I
(pp. 74-101)

NAME _____ LAST _____ FIRST _____ MIDDLE

SCHOOL _____ CITY _____

DATE OF BIRTH _____ **DATE** _____

GRADE OR CLASS _____ **INSTRUCTOR** _____

AGE _____ **SEX** M OR F

NAME OF TEST _____ **PART** _____

SCORES

1	5
2	6
3	7
4	8

SAMPLE:

1—1 a country
1—2 a mountain
1—3 an island
1—4 a city
1—5 a state

1. Chicago is

DIRECTIONS: Read each question and its numbered answers. When you have decided which answer is correct, blacken the corresponding space on this sheet with the special pencil. Make your mark as long as the pair of lines, and move the pencil point up and down firmly to make a heavy black line. If you change your mind, erase your first mark completely. Make no stray marks; they may count against you.

BE SURE YOUR MARKS ARE HEAVY AND BLACK.
ERASE COMPLETELY ANY ANSWER YOU WISH TO CHANGE.

SCORES

5
6
7
8

1
2
3
4

MIDDLE

FIRST

LAST

NAME

	1 2 3 4 5		1 2 3 4 5		1 2 3 4 5		1 2 3 4 5		1 2 3 4 5
151		181		211		241		271	
152		182		212		242		272	
153		183		213		243		273	
154		184		214		244		274	
155		185		215		245		275	
156		186		216		246		276	
157		187		217		247		277	
158		188		218		248		278	
159		189		219		249		279	
160		190		220		250		280	
161		191		221		251		281	
162		192		222		252		282	
163		193		223		253		283	
164		194		224		254		284	
165		195		225		255		285	

BE SURE YOUR MARKS ARE HEAVY AND BLACK.
ERASE COMPLETELY ANY ANSWER YOU WISH TO CHANGE.

	1 2 3 4 5		1 2 3 4 5		1 2 3 4 5		1 2 3 4 5		1 2 3 4 5
166		196		226		256		286	
167		197		227		257		287	
168		198		228		258		288	
169		199		229		259		289	
170		200		230		260		290	
171		201		231		261		291	
172		202		232		262		292	
173		203		233		263		293	
174		204		234		264		294	
175		205		235		265		295	
176		206		236		266		296	
177		207		237		267		297	
178		208		238		268		298	
179		209		239		269		299	
180		210		240		270		300	

IBM FORM I.T.S. 1100 B 107-2

NURSING ARTS
PART II
(pp. 102–115)

NAME _____ LAST _____ FIRST _____ MIDDLE _____ DATE _____

SCHOOL _____ CITY _____

DATE OF BIRTH _____ AGE _____ SEX _____ M OR F

GRADE OR CLASS _____ INSTRUCTOR _____

NAME OF TEST _____ PART _____

SCORES

1	5
2	6
3	7
4	8

DIRECTIONS: Read each question and its numbered answers. When you have decided which answer is correct, blacken the corresponding space on this sheet with the special pencil. Make your mark as long as the pair of lines, and move the pencil point up and down firmly to make a heavy black line. If you change your mind, erase your first mark completely. Make no stray marks; they may count against you.

SAMPLE:

1–1 a country
1–2 a mountain
1–3 an island
1–4 a city
1–5 a state

1. Chicago is

BE SURE YOUR MARKS ARE HEAVY AND BLACK.
ERASE COMPLETELY ANY ANSWER YOU WISH TO CHANGE.

Printed by the International Business Machines Corporation, Dayton, N. J., U.S.A.   IBM FORM I. T. S. 1000 B 108

NURSING ARTS
PART III
INTEGRATED EXAMINATION
(pp. 116-126)

(OVER)

SCORES

5 6 7 8

1 2 3 4

NAME   LAST   FIRST   MIDDLE

BE SURE YOUR MARKS ARE HEAVY AND BLACK.
ERASE COMPLETELY ANY ANSWER YOU WISH TO CHANGE.

151 152 153 154 155 156 157 158 159 160 161 162 163 164 165 166 167 168 169 170 171 172 173 174 175 176 177 178 179 180

181 182 183 184 185 186 187 188 189 190 191 192 193 194 195 196 197 198 199 200 201 202 203 204 205 206 207 208 209 210

211 212 213 214 215 216 217 218 219 220 221 222 223 224 225 226 227 228 229 230 231 232 233 234 235 236 237 238 239 240

241 242 243 244 245 246 247 248 249 250 251 252 253 254 255 256 257 258 259 260 261 262 263 264 265 266 267 268 269 270

271 272 273 274 275 276 277 278 279 280 281 282 283 284 285 286 287 288 289 290 291 292 293 294 295 296 297 298 299 300

310

IBM FORM I.T.S. 1100 B 107-2

SCORES

1	5
2	6
3	7
4	8

NAME _____ LAST ___ FIRST ___ MIDDLE ___ DATE ___

SCHOOL _____ CITY ___

DATE OF BIRTH ___ AGE ___ SEX M or F ___

GRADE OR CLASS ___ INSTRUCTOR ___

NAME OF TEST ___ PART ___

SAMPLE:

1. Chicago is

1—1 a country
1—2 a mountain
1—3 an island
1—4 a city
1—5 a state

DIRECTIONS: Read each question and its numbered answers. When you have decided which answer is correct, blacken the corresponding space on this sheet with the special pencil. Make your mark as long as the pair of lines, and move the pencil point up and down firmly to make a heavy black line. If you change your mind, erase your first mark completely. Make no stray marks; they may count against you.

BE SURE YOUR MARKS ARE HEAVY AND BLACK.
ERASE COMPLETELY ANY ANSWER YOU WISH TO CHANGE.

(Answer grid, items 1–150, each with columns 1 2 3 4 5)

SCORES

5
6
7
8

1
2
3
4

	1 2 3 4 5		1 2 3 4 5		1 2 3 4 5		1 2 3 4 5		1 2 3 4 5
151		181		211		241		271	
152		182		212		242		272	
153		183		213		243		273	
154		184		214		244		274	
155		185		215		245		275	
156		186		216		246		276	
157		187		217		247		277	
158		188		218		248		278	
159		189		219		249		279	
160		190		220		250		280	
161		191		221		251		281	
162		192		222		252		282	
163		193		223		253		283	
164		194		224		254		284	
165		195		225		255		285	

BE SURE YOUR MARKS ARE HEAVY AND BLACK.
ERASE COMPLETELY ANY ANSWER YOU WISH TO CHANGE.

	1 2 3 4 5		1 2 3 4 5		1 2 3 4 5		1 2 3 4 5		1 2 3 4 5
166		196		226		256		286	
167		197		227		257		287	
168		198		228		258		288	
169		199		229		259		289	
170		200		230		260		290	
171		201		231		261		291	
172		202		232		262		292	
173		203		233		263		293	
174		204		234		264		294	
175		205		235		265		295	
176		206		236		266		296	
177		207		237		267		297	
178		208		238		268		298	
179		209		239		269		299	
180		210		240		270		300	

NAME   LAST   FIRST   MIDDLE

IBM FORM I.T.S. 1100 B 107-2

ANATOMY AND PHYSIOLOGY
PART II
APPLIED ANATOMY AND PHYSIOLOGY
(pp. 145–164)

SCORES

1   5

2   6

3   7

4   8

NAME _____
LAST   FIRST   MIDDLE

SCHOOL _____ CITY _____

DATE _____

DATE OF BIRTH _____

GRADE OR CLASS _____ INSTRUCTOR _____

NAME OF TEST _____

AGE _____ SEX _____ M or F

PART _____

SAMPLE:

1—1 a country
1—2 a mountain
1—3 an island
1—4 a city
1—5 a state

1. Chicago is

DIRECTIONS: Read each question and its numbered answers. When you have decided which answer is correct, blacken the corresponding space on this sheet with the special pencil. Make your mark as long as the pair of lines, and move the pencil point up and down firmly to make a heavy black line. If you change your mind, erase your first mark completely. Make no stray marks; they may count against you.

BE SURE YOUR MARKS ARE HEAVY AND BLACK.
ERASE COMPLETELY ANY ANSWER YOU WISH TO CHANGE.

(Answer grid: items 1–150, each with response columns 1 2 3 4 5)

1 … 31 … 61 … 91 … 121 …
2 … 32 … 62 … 92 … 122 …
3 … 33 … 63 … 93 … 123 …
4 … 34 … 64 … 94 … 124 …
5 … 35 … 65 … 95 … 125 …
6 … 36 … 66 … 96 … 126 …
7 … 37 … 67 … 97 … 127 …
8 … 38 … 68 … 98 … 128 …
9 … 39 … 69 … 99 … 129 …
10 … 40 … 70 … 100 … 130 …
11 … 41 … 71 … 101 … 131 …
12 … 42 … 72 … 102 … 132 …
13 … 43 … 73 … 103 … 133 …
14 … 44 … 74 … 104 … 134 …
15 … 45 … 75 … 105 … 135 …
16 … 46 … 76 … 106 … 136 …
17 … 47 … 77 … 107 … 137 …
18 … 48 … 78 … 108 … 138 …
19 … 49 … 79 … 109 … 139 …
20 … 50 … 80 … 110 … 140 …
21 … 51 … 81 … 111 … 141 …
22 … 52 … 82 … 112 … 142 …
23 … 53 … 83 … 113 … 143 …
24 … 54 … 84 … 114 … 144 …
25 … 55 … 85 … 115 … 145 …
26 … 56 … 86 … 116 … 146 …
27 … 57 … 87 … 117 … 147 …
28 … 58 … 88 … 118 … 148 …
29 … 59 … 89 … 119 … 149 …
30 … 60 … 90 … 120 … 150 …

Printed by the International Business Machines Corporation, Dayton, N. J., U.S.A.   IBM FORM I.T.S. 1000 B 108

SCORES

5 6 7 8

1 2 3 4

	1 2 3 4 5		1 2 3 4 5		1 2 3 4 5		1 2 3 4 5		1 2 3 4 5
151		181		211		241		271	
152		182		212		242		272	
153		183		213		243		273	
154		184		214		244		274	
155		185		215		245		275	
156		186		216		246		276	
157		187		217		247		277	
158		188		218		248		278	
159		189		219		249		279	
160		190		220		250		280	
161		191		221		251		281	
162		192		222		252		282	
163		193		223		253		283	
164		194		224		254		284	
165		195		225		255		285	

BE SURE YOUR MARKS ARE HEAVY AND BLACK.
ERASE COMPLETELY ANY ANSWER YOU WISH TO CHANGE.

	1 2 3 4 5		1 2 3 4 5		1 2 3 4 5		1 2 3 4 5		1 2 3 4 5
166		196		226		256		286	
167		197		227		257		287	
168		198		228		258		288	
169		199		229		259		289	
170		200		230		260		290	
171		201		231		261		291	
172		202		232		262		292	
173		203		233		263		293	
174		204		234		264		294	
175		205		235		265		295	
176		206		236		266		296	
177		207		237		267		297	
178		208		238		268		298	
179		209		239		269		299	
180		210		240		270		300	

MIDDLE

FIRST

LAST

NAME

314

IBM FORM I.T.S. 1100 B 107-2

CONDITIONS OF ILLNESS
(pp. 165-178)

SCORES

1 —— 5
2 —— 6
3 —— 7
4 —— 8

1 ——
2 ——

NAME ———— LAST ———— FIRST ———— MIDDLE ———— DATE OF BIRTH ———— DATE ———— AGE ———— SEX M OR F

SCHOOL ———— CITY ———— GRADE OR CLASS ———— INSTRUCTOR ———— PART ————

NAME OF TEST ————

DIRECTIONS: Read each question and its numbered answers. When you have decided which answer is correct, blacken the corresponding space on this sheet with the special pencil. Make your mark as long as the pair of lines, and move the pencil point up and down firmly to make a heavy black line. If you change your mind, erase your first mark completely. Make no stray marks; they may count against you.

SAMPLE:

1—1 a country
1—2 a mountain
1—3 an island
1—4 a city
1—5 a state

1. Chicago is

BE SURE YOUR MARKS ARE HEAVY AND BLACK.
ERASE COMPLETELY ANY ANSWER YOU WISH TO CHANGE.

(columns of answer bubbles numbered 1–150, each with choices 1 2 3 4 5)

Printed by the International Business Machines Corporation, Dayton, N. J., U.S.A.

IBM FORM I.T.S. 1000 B 108

315

SCORES

5
6
7
8

1
2
3
4

	1 2 3 4 5		1 2 3 4 5		1 2 3 4 5		1 2 3 4 5		1 2 3 4 5
151		181		211		241		271	
152		182		212		242		272	
153		183		213		243		273	
154		184		214		244		274	
155		185		215		245		275	
156		186		216		246		276	
157		187		217		247		277	
158		188		218		248		278	
159		189		219		249		279	
160		190		220		250		280	
161		191		221		251		281	
162		192		222		252		282	
163		193		223		253		283	
164		194		224		254		284	
165		195		225		255		285	

BE SURE YOUR MARKS ARE HEAVY AND BLACK.
ERASE COMPLETELY ANY ANSWER YOU WISH TO CHANGE.

	1 2 3 4 5		1 2 3 4 5		1 2 3 4 5		1 2 3 4 5		1 2 3 4 5
166		196		226		256		286	
167		197		227		257		287	
168		198		228		258		288	
169		199		229		259		289	
170		200		230		260		290	
171		201		231		261		291	
172		202		232		262		292	
173		203		233		263		293	
174		204		234		264		294	
175		205		235		265		295	
176		206		236		266		296	
177		207		237		267		297	
178		208		238		268		298	
179		209		239		269		299	
180		210		240		270		300	

MIDDLE

FIRST

LAST

NAME

316

SCORES

NAME _____ DATE _____
LAST   FIRST   MIDDLE

SCHOOL _____
CITY

DATE OF BIRTH _____   AGE _____   SEX _____
M OR F

GRADE OR CLASS _____   INSTRUCTOR _____

NAME OF TEST _____   PART _____

SAMPLE:
1—1 a country
1—2 a mountain
1—3 an island
1—4 a city
1—5 a state

1. Chicago is

DIRECTIONS: Read each question and its numbered answers. When you have decided which answer is correct, blacken the corresponding space on this sheet with the special pencil. Make your mark as long as the pair of lines, and move the pencil point up and down firmly to make a heavy black line. If you change your mind, erase your first mark completely. Make no stray marks; they may count against you.

BE SURE YOUR MARKS ARE HEAVY AND BLACK.
ERASE COMPLETELY ANY ANSWER YOU WISH TO CHANGE.

SCORES

5
6
7
8

1
2
3
4

	1 2 3 4 5		1 2 3 4 5		1 2 3 4 5		1 2 3 4 5		1 2 3 4 5
151		181		211		241		271	
152		182		212		242		272	
153		183		213		243		273	
154		184		214		244		274	
155		185		215		245		275	
156		186		216		246		276	
157		187		217		247		277	
158		188		218		248		278	
159		189		219		249		279	
160		190		220		250		280	
161		191		221		251		281	
162		192		222		252		282	
163		193		223		253		283	
164		194		224		254		284	
165		195		225		255		285	

BE SURE YOUR MARKS ARE HEAVY AND BLACK.
ERASE COMPLETELY ANY ANSWER YOU WISH TO CHANGE.

	1 2 3 4 5		1 2 3 4 5		1 2 3 4 5		1 2 3 4 5		1 2 3 4 5
166		196		226		256		286	
167		197		227		257		287	
168		198		228		258		288	
169		199		229		259		289	
170		200		230		260		290	
171		201		231		261		291	
172		202		232		262		292	
173		203		233		263		293	
174		204		234		264		294	
175		205		235		265		295	
176		206		236		266		296	
177		207		237		267		297	
178		208		238		268		298	
179		209		239		269		299	
180		210		240		270		300	

MIDDLE

FIRST

LAST

NAME

318

IBM FORM I.T.S. 1100 B 107-2

MEDICAL AND SURGICAL DISEASES AND NURSING
PART II
(pp. 206–226)

SCORES

1	5
2	6
3	7
4	8

NAME _____
LAST   FIRST   MIDDLE

DATE _____ DATE OF BIRTH _____ AGE _____ SEX _____ N OR F

SCHOOL _____ CITY _____ GRADE OR CLASS _____ INSTRUCTOR _____ PART _____

NAME OF TEST _____

SAMPLE:

1—1 a country
1—2 a mountain
1—3 an island
1—4 a city
1—5 a state

1. Chicago is

DIRECTIONS: Read each question and its numbered answers. When you have decided which answer is correct, blacken the corresponding space on this sheet with the special pencil. Make your mark as long as the pair of lines, and move the pencil point up and down firmly to make a heavy black line. If you change your mind, erase your first mark completely. Make no stray marks; they may count against you.

BE SURE YOUR MARKS ARE HEAVY AND BLACK.
ERASE COMPLETELY ANY ANSWER YOU WISH TO CHANGE.

(Answer grid items 1–150, each with columns 1 2 3 4 5)

Printed by the International Business Machines Corporation, Dayton, N. J., U.S.A.   IBM FORM I.T.S. 1000 B 108

(OVER)

SCORES

5
6
7
8

1
2
3
4

MIDDLE
FIRST
LAST
NAME

151	181	211	241	271
152	182	212	242	272
153	183	213	243	273
154	184	214	244	274
155	185	215	245	275
156	186	216	246	276
157	187	217	247	277
158	188	218	248	278
159	189	219	249	279
160	190	220	250	280
161	191	221	251	281
162	192	222	252	282
163	193	223	253	283
164	194	224	254	284
165	195	225	255	285

BE SURE YOUR MARKS ARE HEAVY AND BLACK.
ERASE COMPLETELY ANY ANSWER YOU WISH TO CHANGE.

166	196	226	256	286
167	197	227	257	287
168	198	228	258	288
169	199	229	259	289
170	200	230	260	290
171	201	231	261	291
172	202	232	262	292
173	203	233	263	293
174	204	234	264	294
175	205	235	265	295
176	206	236	266	296
177	207	237	267	297
178	208	238	268	298
179	209	239	269	299
180	210	240	270	300

320

IBM FORM I.T.S. 1100 B 107-2

PHARMACOLOGY AND DRUGS AND SOLUTIONS
(pp. 227-252)

NAME _____
LAST   FIRST   MIDDLE

SCHOOL _____
CITY _____

SCORES

1 _____	5 _____
2 _____	6 _____
3 _____	7 _____
4 _____	8 _____

DATE _____

DATE OF BIRTH _____

GRADE OR CLASS _____ INSTRUCTOR _____

NAME OF TEST _____

AGE _____ SEX _____ M OR F

PART _____

DIRECTIONS: Read each question and its numbered answers. When you have decided which answer is correct, blacken the corresponding space on this sheet with the special pencil. Make your mark as long as the pair of lines, and move the pencil point up and down firmly to make a heavy black line. If you change your mind, erase your first mark completely. Make no stray marks; they may count against you.

SAMPLE:

1—1 a country
1—2 a mountain
1—3 an island
1—4 a city
1—5 a state

1. Chicago is

BE SURE YOUR MARKS ARE HEAVY AND BLACK.
ERASE COMPLETELY ANY ANSWER YOU WISH TO CHANGE.

(Answer grid: items 1–150, each with numbered answer spaces 1 2 3 4 5, arranged in columns 1–30, 31–60, 61–90, 91–120, 121–150)

(OVER)

SCORES

5 6 7 8

1 2 3 4

NAME   LAST   FIRST   MIDDLE

	1 2 3 4 5		1 2 3 4 5		1 2 3 4 5		1 2 3 4 5		1 2 3 4 5
151		181		211		241		271	
152		182		212		242		272	
153		183		213		243		273	
154		184		214		244		274	
155		185		215		245		275	
156		186		216		246		276	
157		187		217		247		277	
158		188		218		248		278	
159		189		219		249		279	
160		190		220		250		280	
161		191		221		251		281	
162		192		222		252		282	
163		193		223		253		283	
164		194		224		254		284	
165		195		225		255		285	

BE SURE YOUR MARKS ARE HEAVY AND BLACK.
ERASE COMPLETELY ANY ANSWER YOU WISH TO CHANGE.

	1 2 3 4 5		1 2 3 4 5		1 2 3 4 5		1 2 3 4 5		1 2 3 4 5
166		196		226		256		286	
167		197		227		257		287	
168		198		228		258		288	
169		199		229		259		289	
170		200		230		260		290	
171		201		231		261		291	
172		202		232		262		292	
173		203		233		263		293	
174		204		234		264		294	
175		205		235		265		295	
176		206		236		266		296	
177		207		237		267		297	
178		208		238		268		298	
179		209		239		269		299	
180		210		240		270		300	

IBM FORM I.T.S. 1100 B 107-2

COMMUNICABLE DISEASES
(pp. 253–259)

BE SURE YOUR MARKS ARE HEAVY AND BLACK.
ERASE COMPLETELY ANY ANSWER YOU WISH TO CHANGE.

323

REHABILITATION
(pp. 261-269)

NAME _____
LAST   FIRST   MIDDLE   DATE _____

SCHOOL _____ CITY _____

DATE OF BIRTH _____ AGE _____ SEX M OR F

GRADE OR CLASS _____ INSTRUCTOR _____

NAME OF TEST _____ PART _____

SCORES

1	5
2	6
3	7
4	8

DIRECTIONS: Read each question and its numbered answers. When you have decided which answer is correct, blacken the corresponding space on this sheet with the special pencil. Make your mark as long as the pair of lines, and move the pencil point up and down firmly to make a heavy black line. If you change your mind, erase your first mark completely. Make no stray marks; they may count against you.

SAMPLE:
1—1 a country
1—2 a mountain
1—3 an island
1—4 a city
1—5 a state

1. Chicago is

BE SURE YOUR MARKS ARE HEAVY AND BLACK.
ERASE COMPLETELY ANY ANSWER YOU WISH TO CHANGE.

(Answer grid, items 1–150, columns 1–5)

Printed by the International Business Machines Corporation, Dayton, N. J., U. S. A.

IBM FORM I.T.S. 1000 B 108

OBSTETRICS
(pp. 271-294)

SCORES

NAME _____ LAST _____ FIRST _____ MIDDLE _____ DATE _____ DATE OF BIRTH _____ AGE _____ SEX M or F

SCHOOL _____ CITY _____ GRADE OR CLASS _____ INSTRUCTOR _____

NAME OF TEST _____ PART _____

1 _____ 5 _____
2 _____ 6 _____
3 _____ 7 _____
4 _____ 8 _____

DIRECTIONS: Read each question and its numbered answers. When you have decided which answer is correct, blacken the corresponding space on this sheet with the special pencil. Make your mark as long as the pair of lines, and move the pencil point up and down firmly to make a heavy black line. If you change your mind, erase your first mark completely. Make no stray marks; they may count against you.

SAMPLE:

1—1 a country
1—2 a mountain
1—3 an island
1—4 a city
1—5 a state

1. Chicago is

BE SURE YOUR MARKS ARE HEAVY AND BLACK.
ERASE COMPLETELY ANY ANSWER YOU WISH TO CHANGE.

(Answer grid: items 1–150, each with response columns 1 2 3 4 5, arranged in columns 1–30, 31–60, 61–90, 91–120, 121–150)

Printed by the International Business Machines Corporation, Dayton, N. J., U.S.A.   IBM FORM I.T.S. 1000 B 108

SCORES

5 | 6 | 7 | 8

1 | 2 | 3 | 4

MIDDLE

FIRST

LAST

NAME

	1 2 3 4 5		1 2 3 4 5		1 2 3 4 5		1 2 3 4 5		1 2 3 4 5
151		181		211		241		271	
152		182		212		242		272	
153		183		213		243		273	
154		184		214		244		274	
155		185		215		245		275	
156		186		216		246		276	
157		187		217		247		277	
158		188		218		248		278	
159		189		219		249		279	
160		190		220		250		280	
161		191		221		251		281	
162		192		222		252		282	
163		193		223		253		283	
164		194		224		254		284	
165		195		225		255		285	

BE SURE YOUR MARKS ARE HEAVY AND BLACK.
ERASE COMPLETELY ANY ANSWER YOU WISH TO CHANGE.

	1 2 3 4 5		1 2 3 4 5		1 2 3 4 5		1 2 3 4 5		1 2 3 4 5
166		196		226		256		286	
167		197		227		257		287	
168		198		228		258		288	
169		199		229		259		289	
170		200		230		260		290	
171		201		231		261		291	
172		202		232		262		292	
173		203		233		263		293	
174		204		234		264		294	
175		205		235		265		295	
176		206		236		266		296	
177		207		237		267		297	
178		208		238		268		298	
179		209		239		269		299	
180		210		240		270		300	

IBM FORM I.T.S. 1100 B 107-2